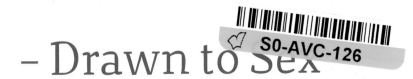

– Drawn to Sex

The Basics

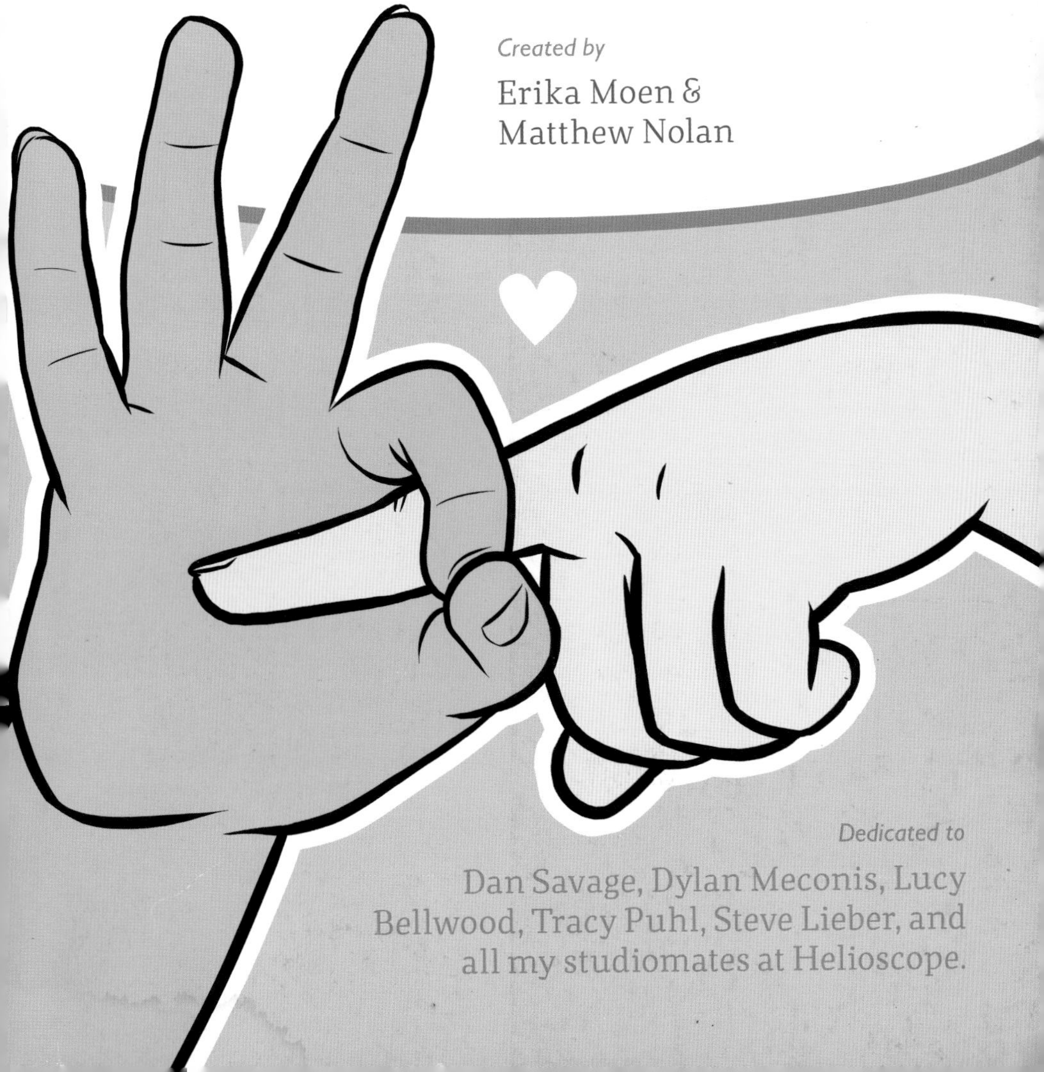

Created by

Erika Moen &
Matthew Nolan

Dedicated to

Dan Savage, Dylan Meconis, Lucy Bellwood, Tracy Puhl, Steve Lieber, and all my studiomates at Helioscope.

Published by Erika Moen Comics & Illustration, LLC
Helioscope Studio
333 SW 5th Ave, Suite 500
Portland, OR 97204
Matthew Nolan, creator
Erika Moen, creator

Published by Limerence Press
Limerence Press is an imprint of Oni Press, Inc.
Joe Nozemack, founder & chief financial officer
James Lucas Jones, publisher
Charlie Chu, v.p. of creative & business development
Brad Rooks, director of operations
Melissa Meszaros, director of publicity
Margot Wood, director of sales
Sandy Tanaka, marketing design manager
Amber O'Neill, special projects manager
Troy Look, director of design & production
Hilary Thompson, senior graphic designer
Kate Z. Stone, graphic designer
Sonja Synak, junior graphic designer
Angie Knowles, digital prepress lead
Ari Yarwood, executive editor
Sarah Gaydos, editorial director of licensed publishing
Robin Herrera, senior editor
Desiree Wilson, associate editor
Alissa Sallah, administrative assistant
Jung Lee, logistics associate
Scott Sharkey, warehouse assistant

Editorial Assists by: Ari Yarwood
Design by: Matthew Nolan, Erika Moen

OhJoySexToy.com
twitter.com/ErikaMoen
facebook.com/ErikaMoenComics
erikamoen.com

LimerencePress.com
twitter.com/limerencepress
limerencepress.tumblr.com

First edition: November 2018

Retail Market ISBN: 978-1-62010-544-3

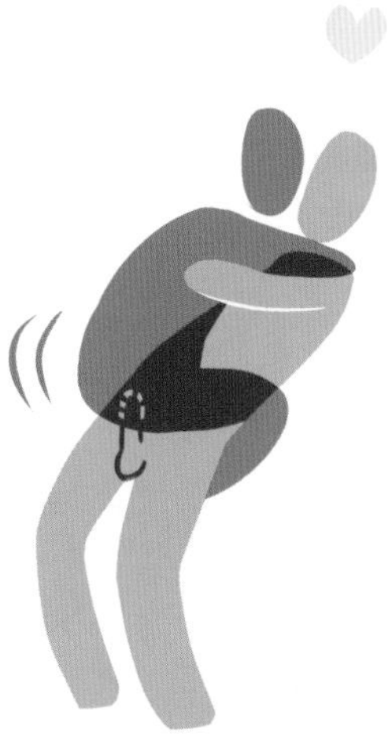

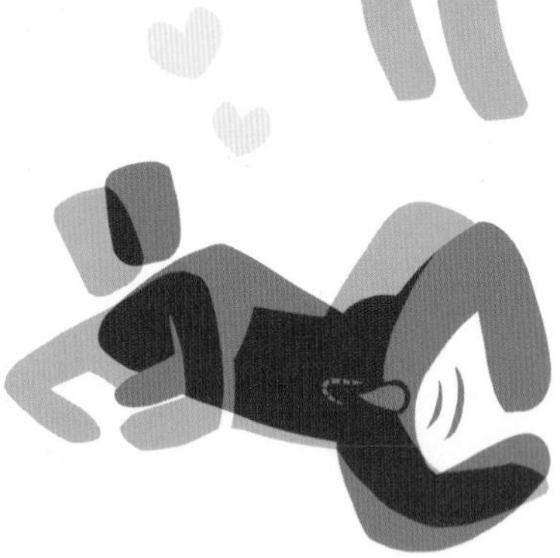

PRINTED IN HONG KONG.

Library of Congress Control Number: 2018940820
1 2 3 4 5 6 7 8 9 10

Index

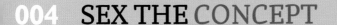

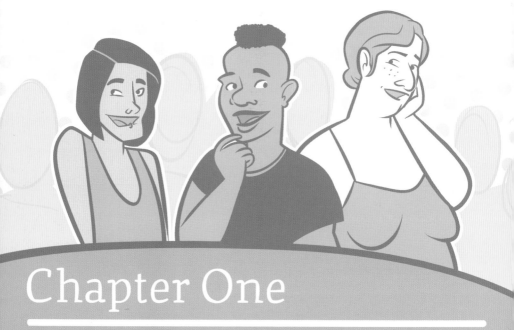

Chapter One

Sex the Concept

Hello, my Dearest Perverts! Welcome to our book! Grab a tea, find yourself a quiet spot, and come adventure with us as we explore sex education! I'm Erika and, together with my partner Matt, we've been making all sorts of silly sex positive comics for yeaaars now. What you hold in your hands is a collection of *just* our educational strips! We're hoping it'll cover some of the more basic questions about sex, give you some good fundamentals about the theories and practices of this subject, and hopefully make you laugh while you're learning something new (or maybe brushing up on familiar material!).

Think of this book as a tasty appetizer before the meal that will be your knowledge of sex education. Our comics serve as a quick introduction to subjects that have much more depth to them than we have the space to include here. If a topic catches your eye, we encourage you to do more research on it at Planned Parenthood and Scarleteen's websites, which are excellent resources!

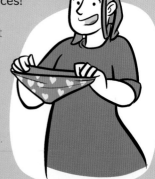

In this chapter we're talking about S-E-X. Like, what does it even MEAN? What COUNTS? When are you ready for it, and how does stuff like consent and sex positivity even work? That all sounds simple at first, right? But when you look closer and dive in, you'll find it's a super deep and interesting world with more going on than you would have guessed.

Take a breath, relax, and dive on in as we explore SEX.

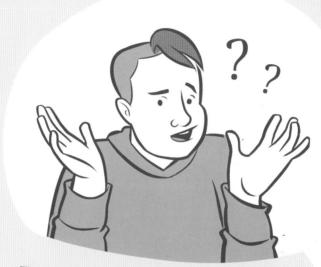

Am I Ready For Sex?

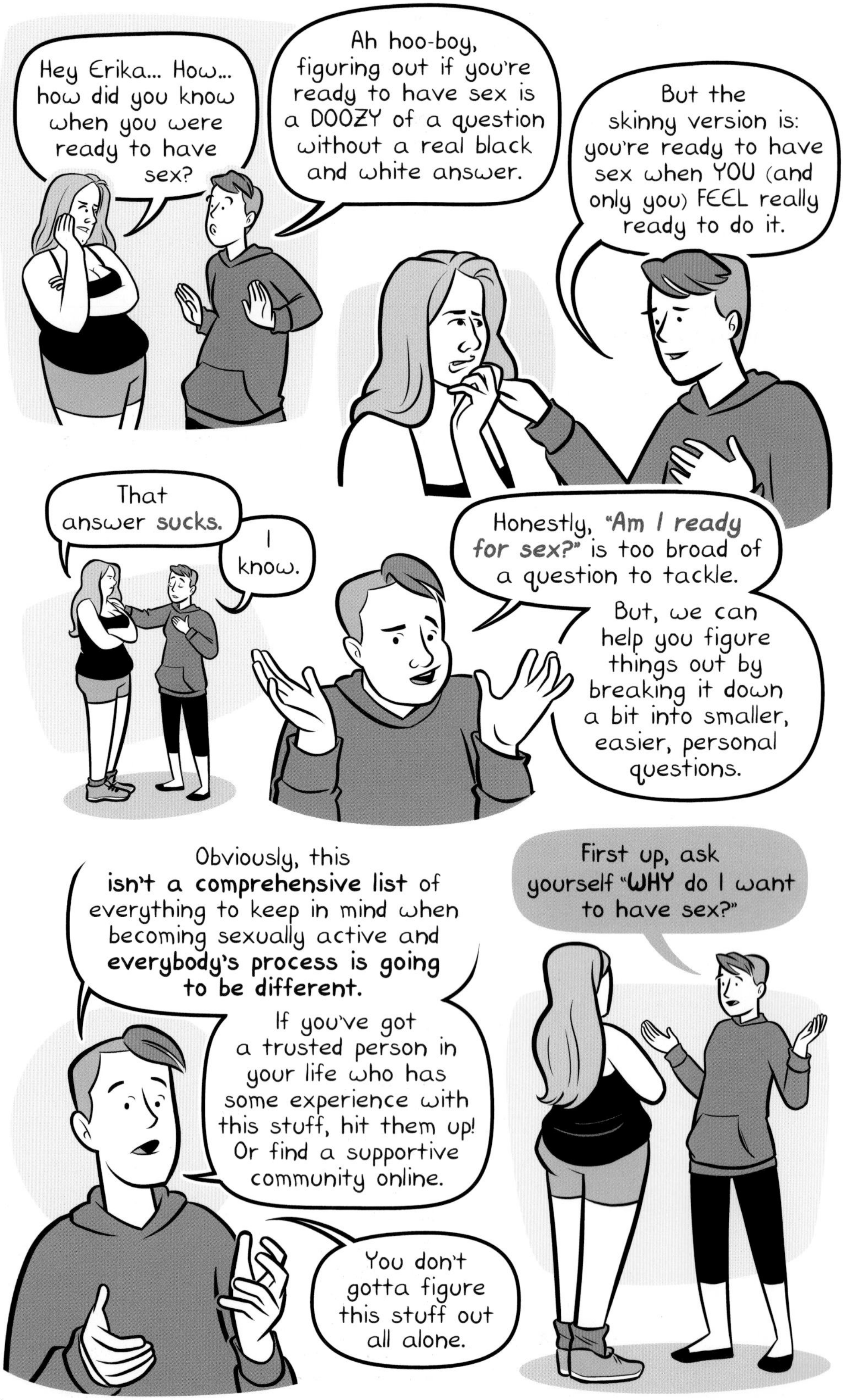
Hey Erika... How... how did you know when you were ready to have sex?
Ah hoo-boy, figuring out if you're ready to have sex is a DOOZY of a question without a real black and white answer.
But the skinny version is: you're ready to have sex when YOU (and only you) FEEL really ready to do it.
That answer **sucks.**
I know.
Honestly, ***"Am I ready for sex?"*** is too broad of a question to tackle.
But, we can help you figure things out by breaking it down a bit into smaller, easier, personal questions.
Obviously, this **isn't a comprehensive list** of everything to keep in mind when becoming sexually active and **everybody's process is going to be different.**
If you've got a trusted person in your life who has some experience with this stuff, hit them up! Or find a supportive community online.
You don't gotta figure this stuff out all alone.
First up, ask yourself "**WHY** do I want to have sex?"

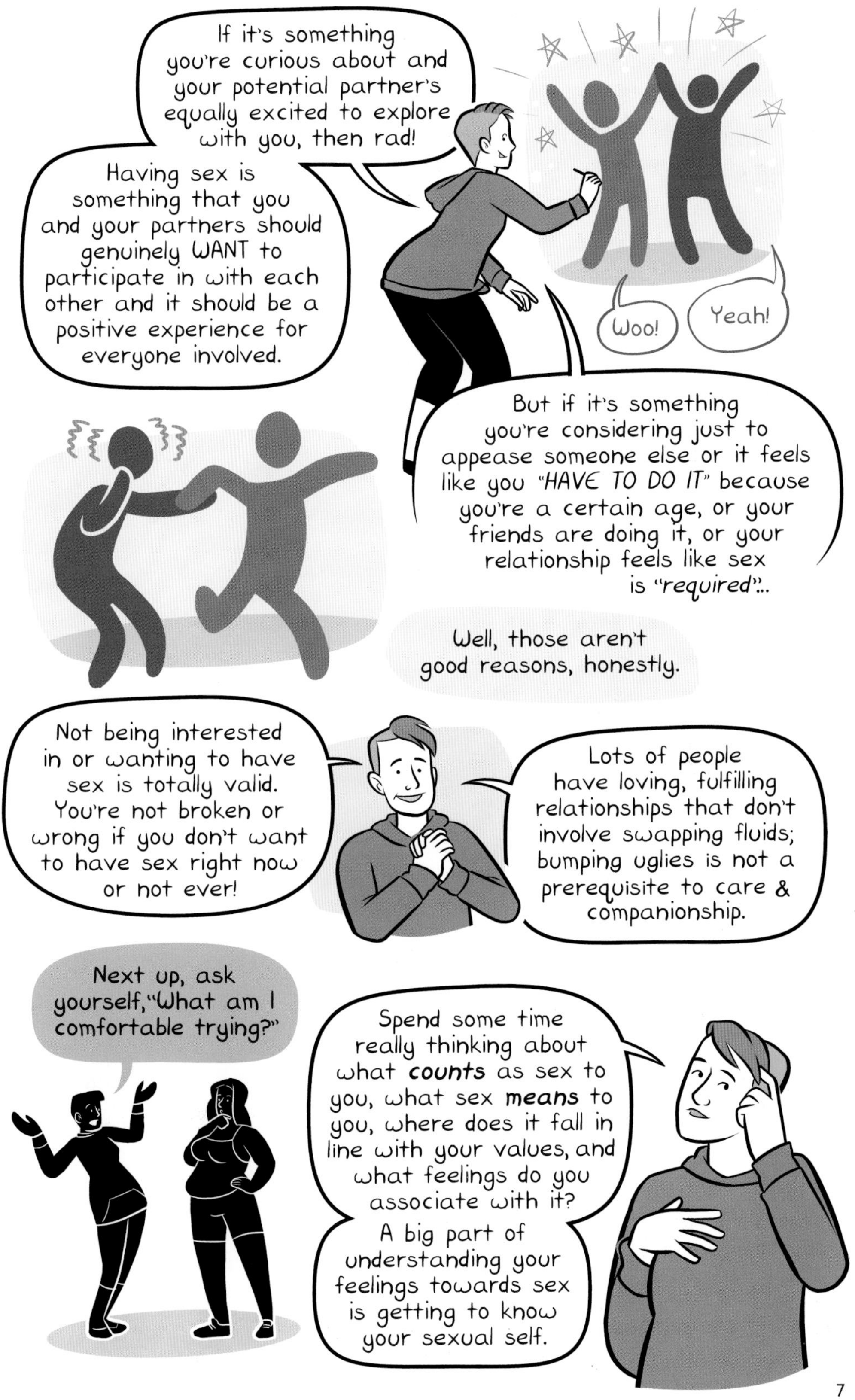
Having sex is something that you and your partners should genuinely WANT to participate in with each other and it should be a positive experience for everyone involved.
If it's something you're curious about and your potential partner's equally excited to explore with you, then rad!
Woo!
Yeah!
But if it's something you're considering just to appease someone else or it feels like you "HAVE TO DO IT" because you're a certain age, or your friends are doing it, or your relationship feels like sex is "required"...
Well, those aren't good reasons, honestly.
Not being interested in or wanting to have sex is totally valid. You're not broken or wrong if you don't want to have sex right now or not ever!
Lots of people have loving, fulfilling relationships that don't involve swapping fluids; bumping uglies is not a prerequisite to care & companionship.
Next up, ask yourself, "What am I comfortable trying?"
Spend some time really thinking about what **counts** as sex to you, what sex **means** to you, where does it fall in line with your values, and what feelings do you associate with it?
A big part of understanding your feelings towards sex is getting to know your sexual self.

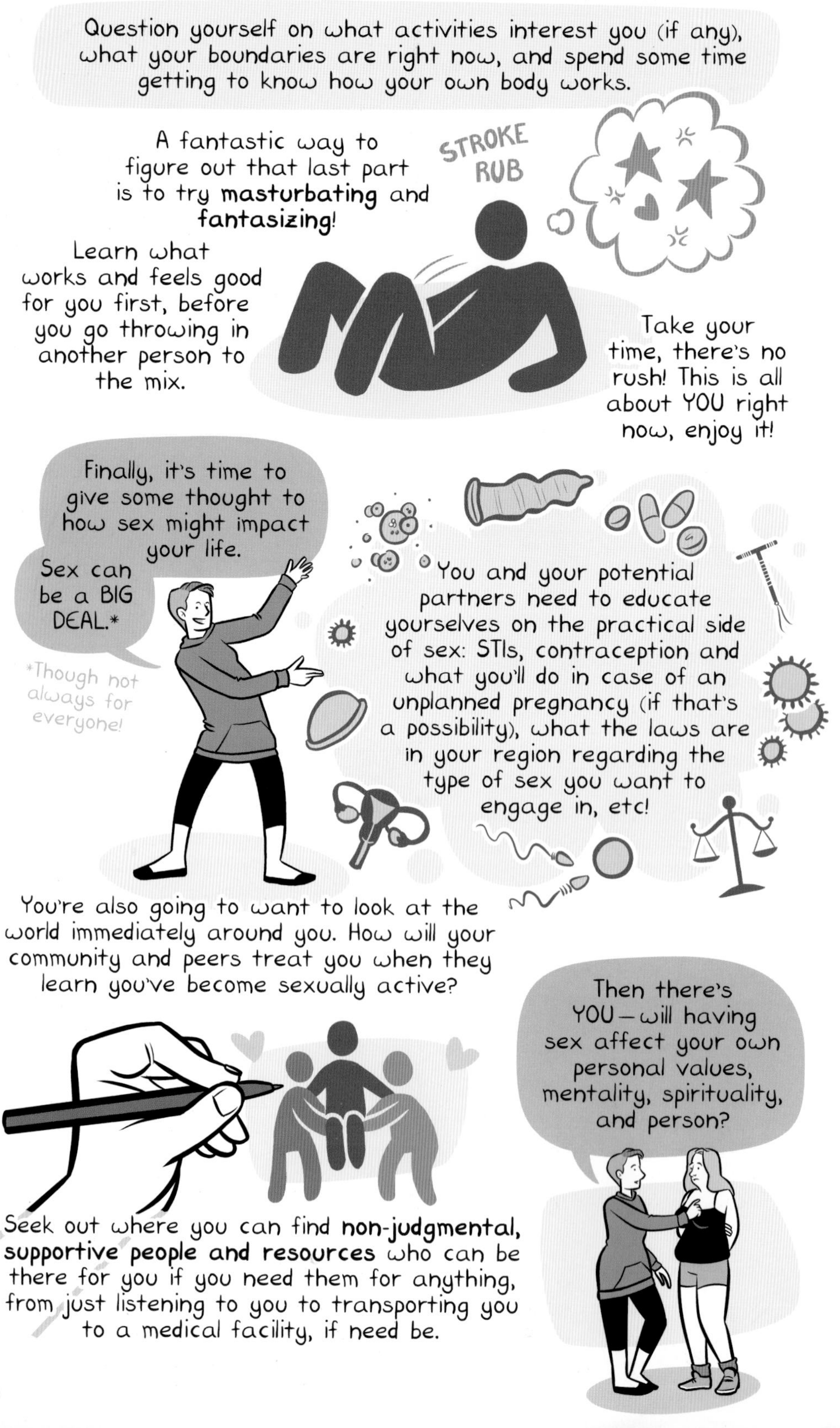

Question yourself on what activities interest you (if any), what your boundaries are right now, and spend some time getting to know how your own body works.
A fantastic way to figure out that last part is to try **masturbating** and **fantasizing**!
STROKE
RUB
Learn what works and feels good for you first, before you go throwing in another person to the mix.
Take your time, there's no rush! This is all about YOU right now, enjoy it!
Finally, it's time to give some thought to how sex might impact your life.
Sex can be a BIG DEAL.*
*Though not always for everyone!
You and your potential partners need to educate yourselves on the practical side of sex: STIs, contraception and what you'll do in case of an unplanned pregnancy (if that's a possibility), what the laws are in your region regarding the type of sex you want to engage in, etc!
You're also going to want to look at the world immediately around you. How will your community and peers treat you when they learn you've become sexually active?
Then there's YOU—will having sex affect your own personal values, mentality, spirituality, and person?
Seek out where you can find **non-judgmental, supportive people and resources** who can be there for you if you need them for anything, from just listening to you to transporting you to a medical facility, if need be.

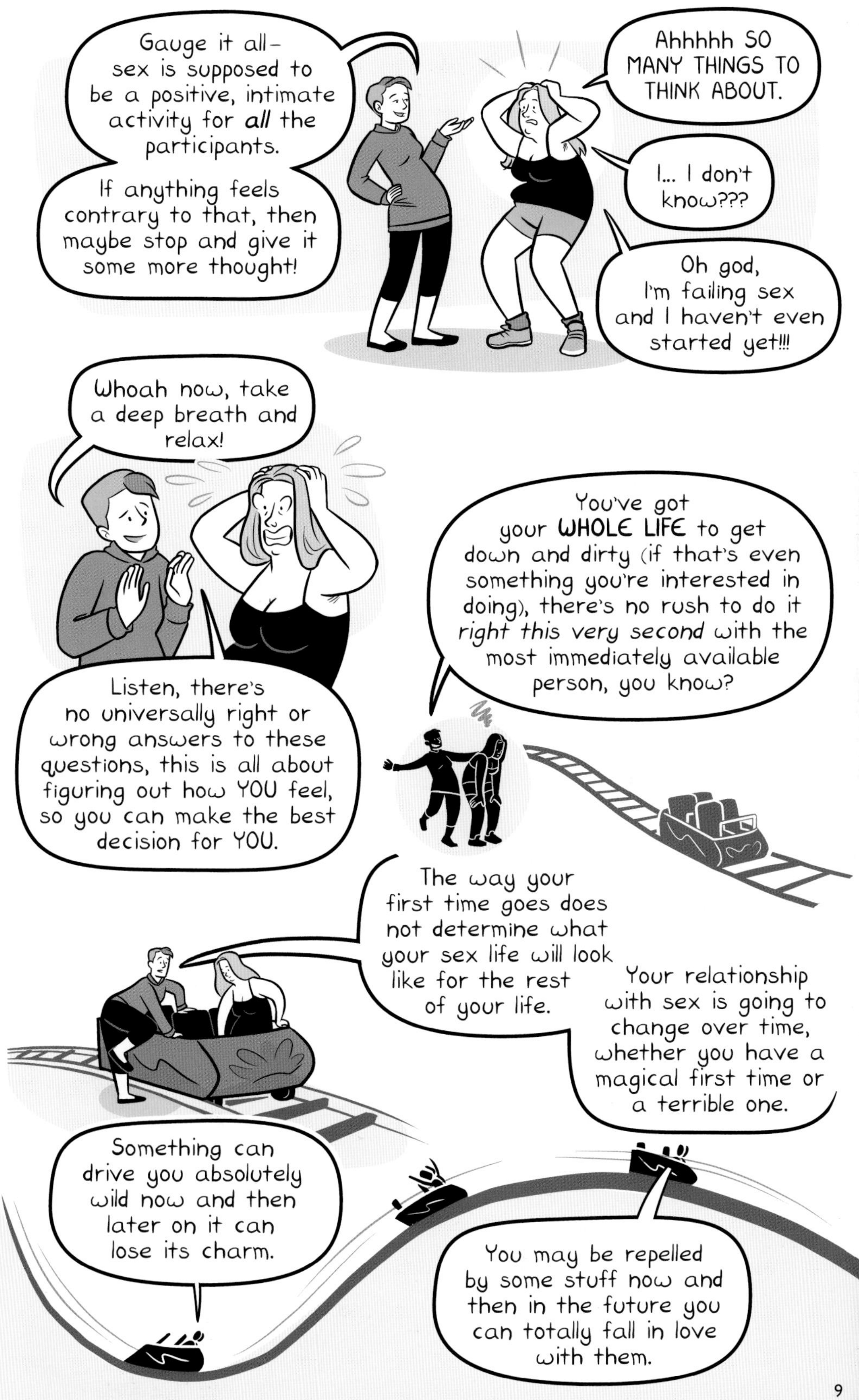
Gauge it all– sex is supposed to be a positive, intimate activity for *all* the participants.
If anything feels contrary to that, then maybe stop and give it some more thought!
Ahhhhh SO MANY THINGS TO THINK ABOUT.
I... I don't know???
Oh god, I'm failing sex and I haven't even started yet!!!
Whoah now, take a deep breath and relax!
Listen, there's no universally right or wrong answers to these questions, this is all about figuring out how YOU feel, so you can make the best decision for YOU.
You've got your **WHOLE LIFE** to get down and dirty (if that's even something you're interested in doing), there's no rush to do it *right this very second* with the most immediately available person, you know?
The way your first time goes does not determine what your sex life will look like for the rest of your life.
Your relationship with sex is going to change over time, whether you have a magical first time or a terrible one.
Something can drive you absolutely wild now and then later on it can lose its charm.
You may be repelled by some stuff now and then in the future you can totally fall in love with them.

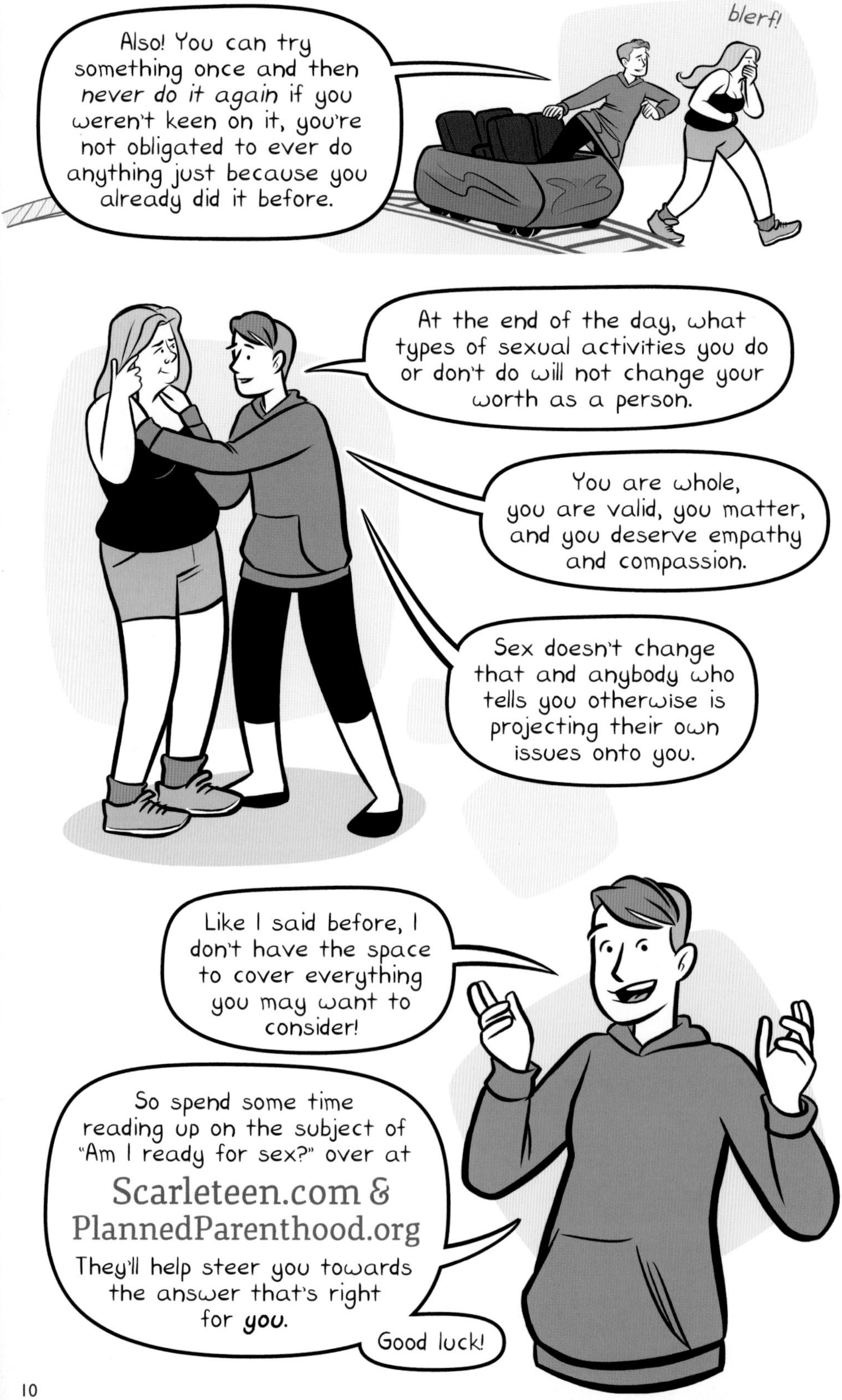

Also! You can try something once and then *never do it again* if you weren't keen on it, you're not obligated to ever do anything just because you already did it before.
blerf!
At the end of the day, what types of sexual activities you do or don't do will not change your worth as a person.
You are whole, you are valid, you matter, and you deserve empathy and compassion.
Sex doesn't change that and anybody who tells you otherwise is projecting their own issues onto you.
Like I said before, I don't have the space to cover everything you may want to consider!
So spend some time reading up on the subject of "Am I ready for sex?" over at Scarleteen.com & PlannedParenthood.org They'll help steer you towards the answer that's right for **you**.
Good luck!

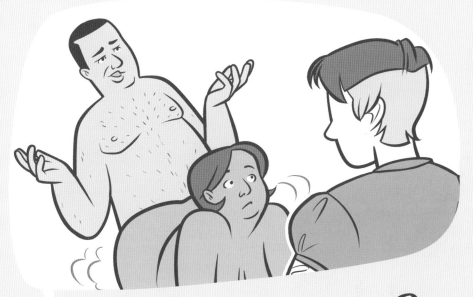

What IS Sex?

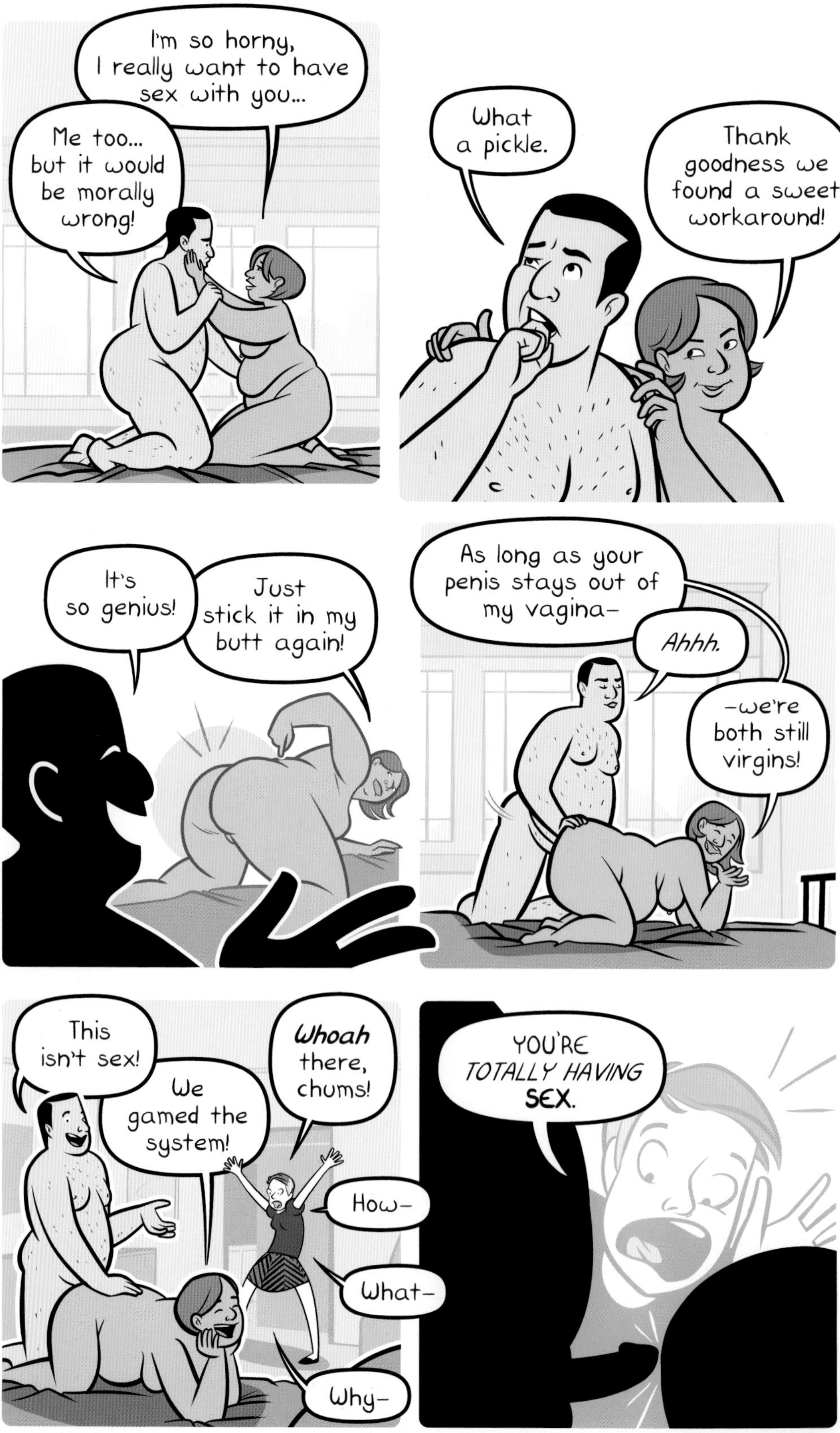
I'm so horny, I really want to have sex with you...
Me too... but it would be morally wrong!
What a pickle.
Thank goodness we found a sweet workaround!
It's so genius!
Just stick it in my butt again!
As long as your penis stays out of my vagina–
Ahhh.
–we're both still virgins!
This isn't sex!
We gamed the system!
Whoah there, chums!
How–
What–
Why–
YOU'RE TOTALLY HAVING SEX.

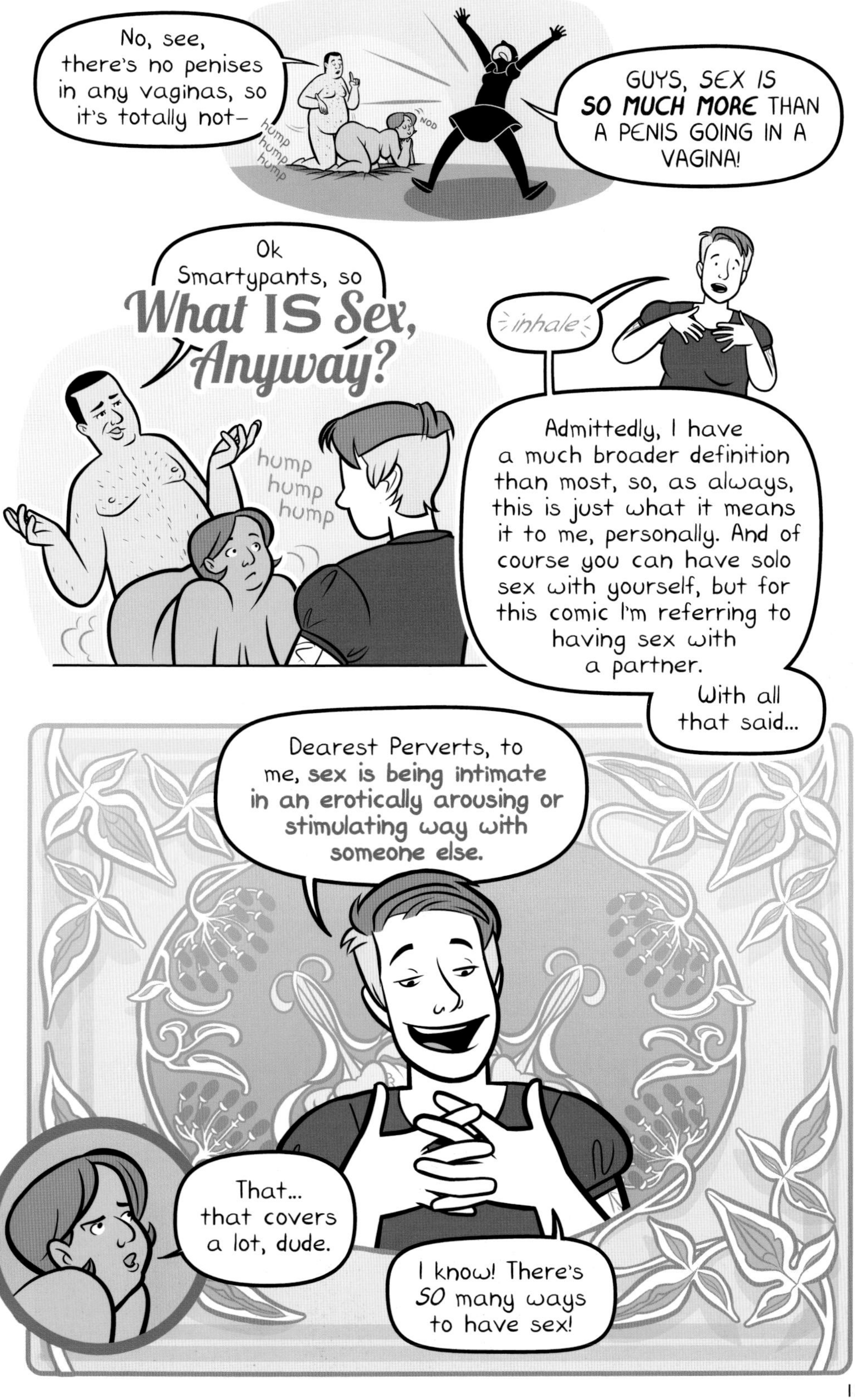
No, see, there's no penises in any vaginas, so it's totally not–
hump hump hump
NOD
GUYS, SEX IS **SO MUCH MORE** THAN A PENIS GOING IN A VAGINA!
Ok Smartypants, so
What IS Sex, Anyway?
hump hump hump
inhale
Admittedly, I have a much broader definition than most, so, as always, this is just what it means it to me, personally. And of course you can have solo sex with yourself, but for this comic I'm referring to having sex with a partner.
With all that said...
Dearest Perverts, to me, **sex is being intimate in an erotically arousing or stimulating way with someone else.**
That... that covers a lot, dude.
I know! There's *SO* many ways to have sex!

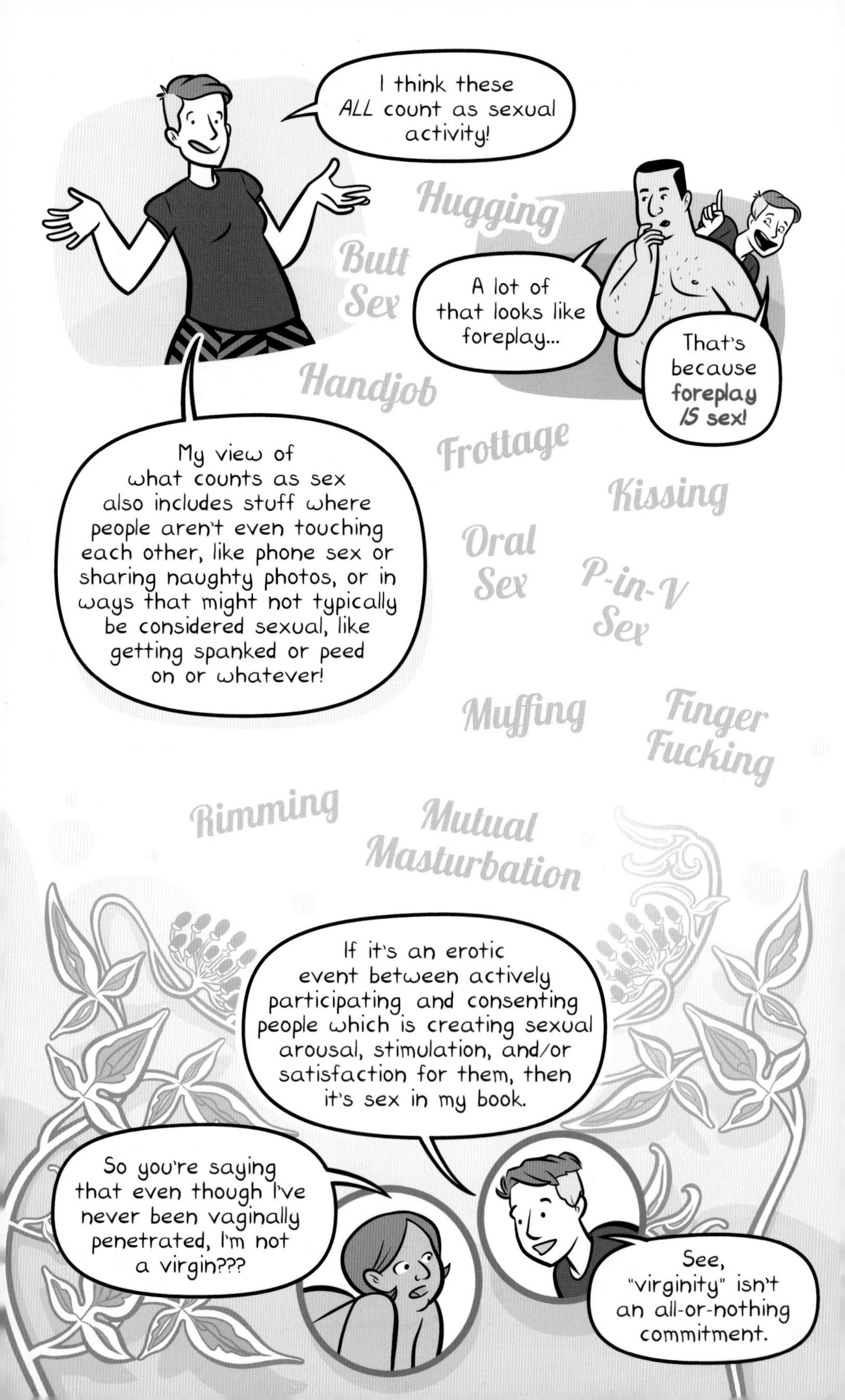

I think these ALL count as sexual activity!
Hugging
Butt Sex
A lot of that looks like foreplay...
That's because foreplay IS sex!
Handjob
Frottage
Kissing
My view of what counts as sex also includes stuff where people aren't even touching each other, like phone sex or sharing naughty photos, or in ways that might not typically be considered sexual, like getting spanked or peed on or whatever!
Oral Sex
P-in-V Sex
Muffing
Finger Fucking
Rimming
Mutual Masturbation
If it's an erotic event between actively participating and consenting people which is creating sexual arousal, stimulation, and/or satisfaction for them, then it's sex in my book.
So you're saying that even though I've never been vaginally penetrated, I'm not a virgin???
See, "virginity" isn't an all-or-nothing commitment.

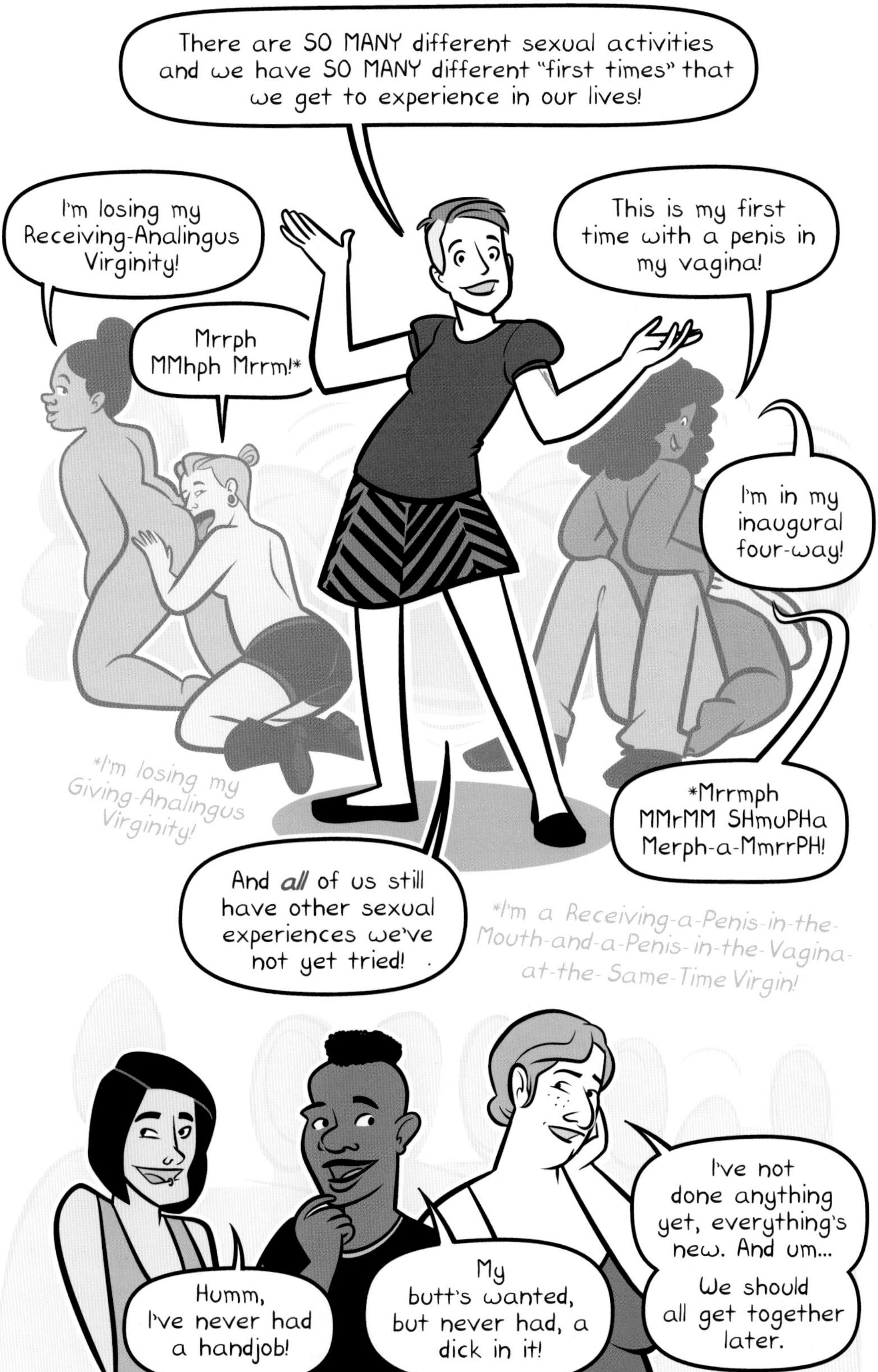

There are SO MANY different sexual activities and we have SO MANY different "first times" that we get to experience in our lives!
I'm losing my Receiving-Analingus Virginity!
Mrrph MMhph Mrrm!*
*I'm losing my Giving-Analingus Virginity!
This is my first time with a penis in my vagina!
I'm in my inaugural four-way!
*Mrrmph MMrMM SHmuPHa Merph-a-MmrrPH!
*I'm a Receiving-a-Penis-in-the-Mouth-and-a-Penis-in-the-Vagina-at-the-Same-Time Virgin!
And *all* of us still have other sexual experiences we've not yet tried!
Humm, I've never had a handjob!
My butt's wanted, but never had, a dick in it!
I've not done anything yet, everything's new. And um...
We should all get together later.

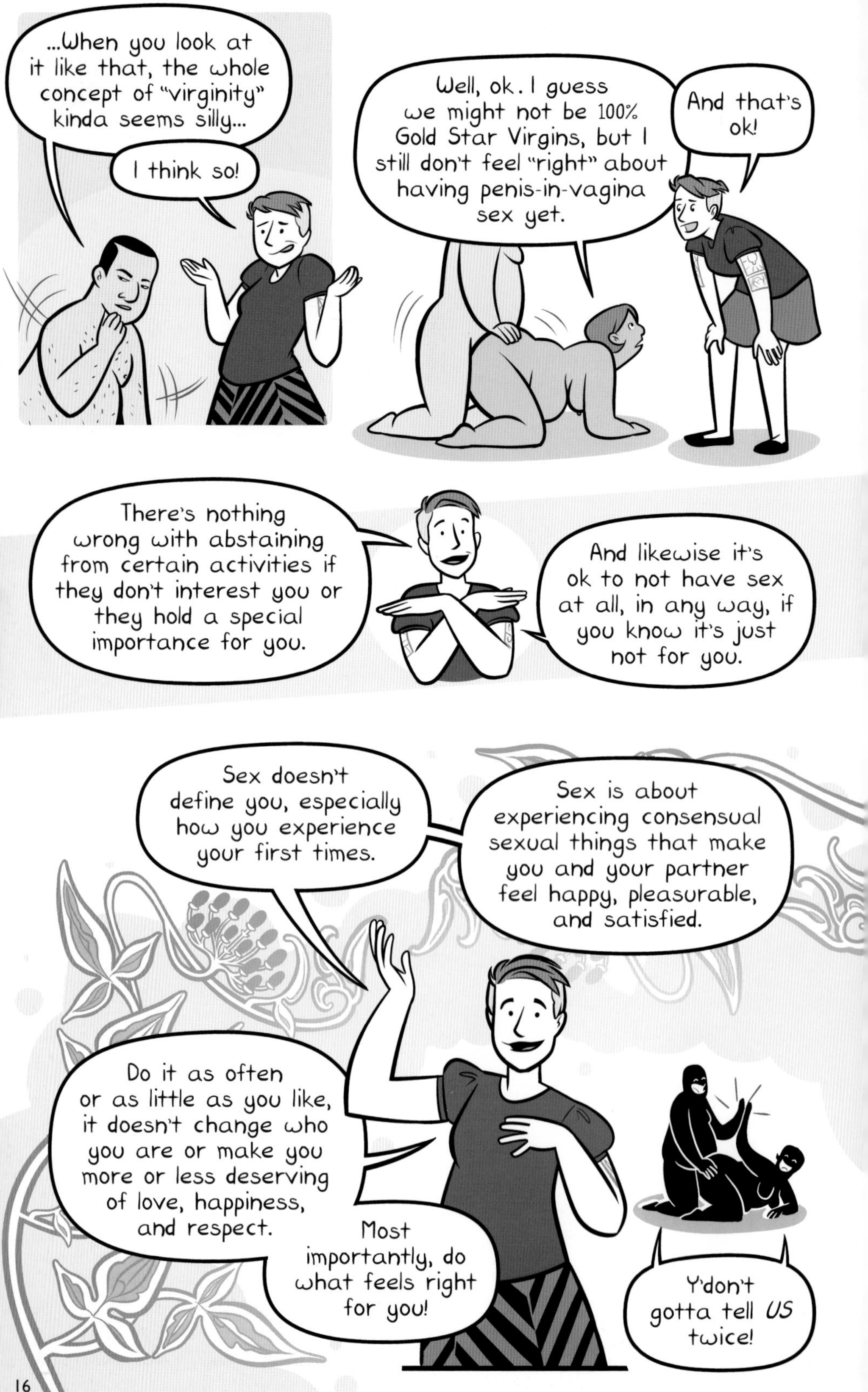
...When you look at it like that, the whole concept of "virginity" kinda seems silly...
I think so!
Well, ok. I guess we might not be 100% Gold Star Virgins, but I still don't feel "right" about having penis-in-vagina sex yet.
And that's ok!
There's nothing wrong with abstaining from certain activities if they don't interest you or they hold a special importance for you.
And likewise it's ok to not have sex at all, in any way, if you know it's just not for you.
Sex doesn't define you, especially how you experience your first times.
Sex is about experiencing consensual sexual things that make you and your partner feel happy, pleasurable, and satisfied.
Do it as often or as little as you like, it doesn't change who you are or make you more or less deserving of love, happiness, and respect.
Most importantly, do what feels right for you!
Y'don't gotta tell *US* twice!

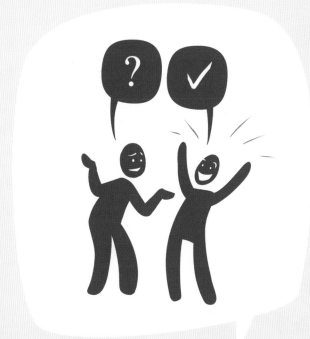

Consent

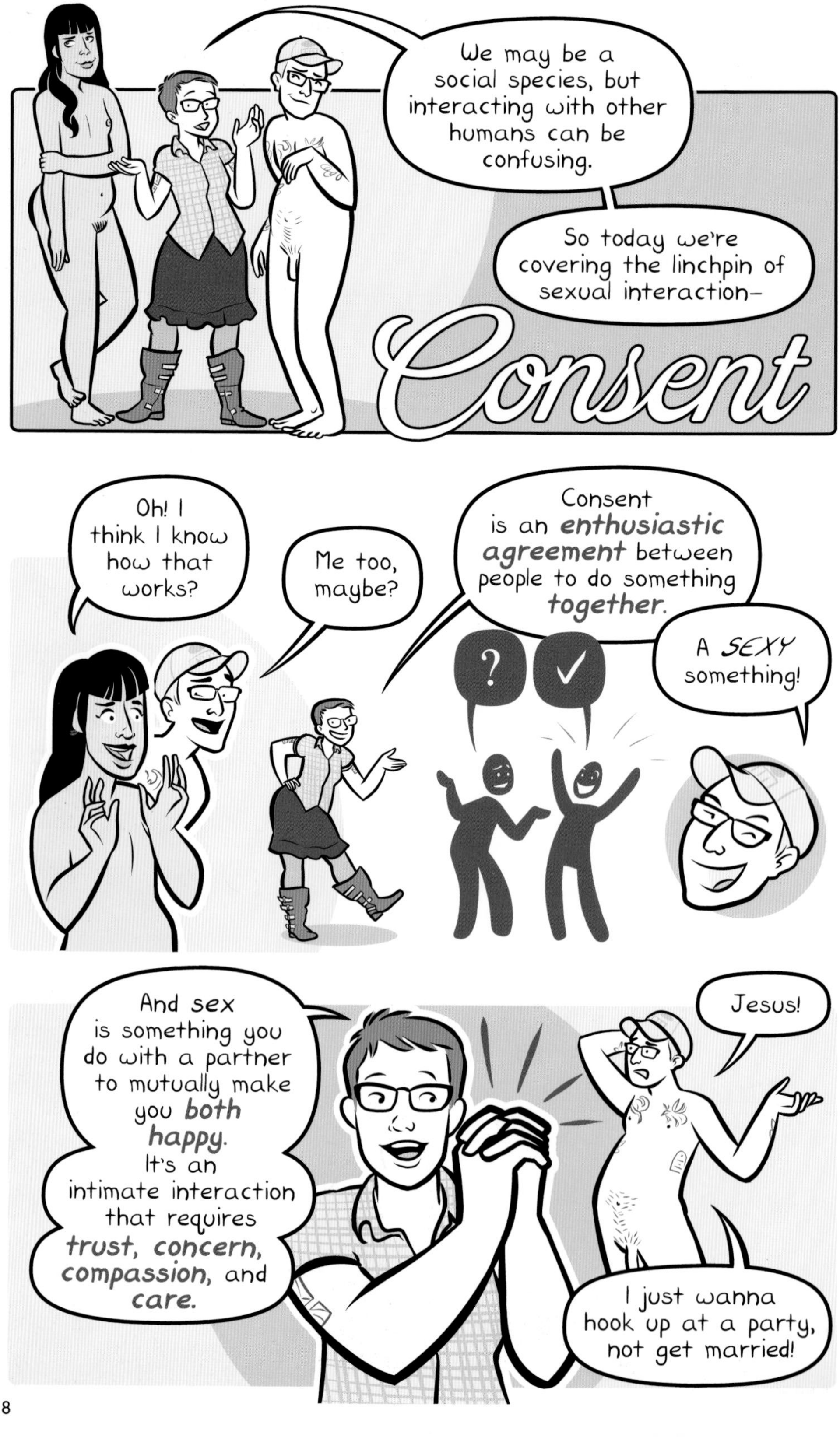
We may be a social species, but interacting with other humans can be confusing.
So today we're covering the linchpin of sexual interaction–
Consent
Oh! I think I know how that works?
Me too, maybe?
Consent is an **enthusiastic agreement** between people to do something **together**.
?
✓
A *SEXY* something!
And sex is something you do with a partner to mutually make you **both happy**. It's an intimate interaction that requires **trust, concern, compassion,** and **care.**
Jesus!
I just wanna hook up at a party, not get married!

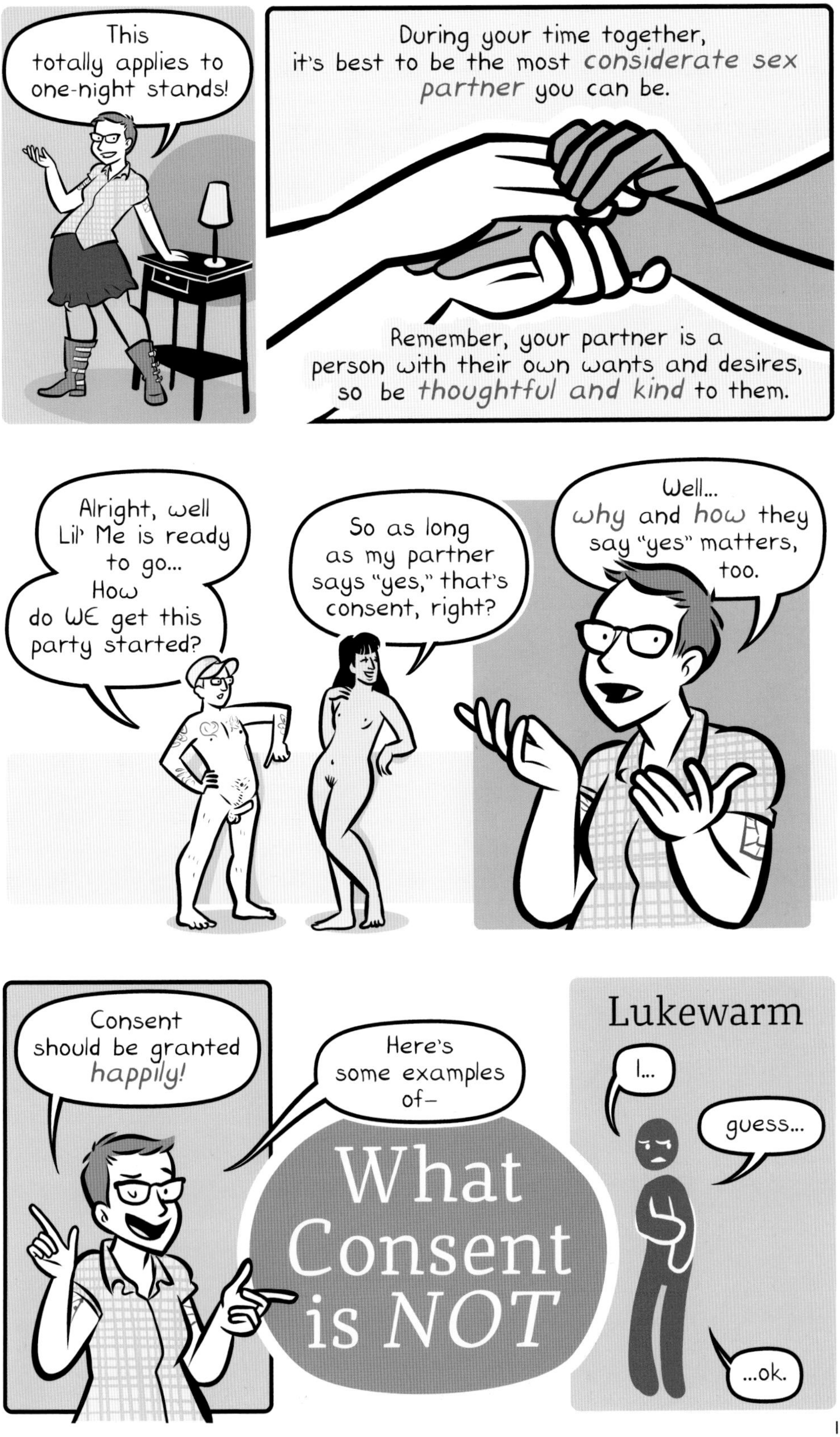
This totally applies to one-night stands!
During your time together, it's best to be the most considerate sex partner you can be.
Remember, your partner is a person with their own wants and desires, so be thoughtful and kind to them.
Alright, well Lil' Me is ready to go... How do WE get this party started?
So as long as my partner says "yes," that's consent, right?
Well... why and how they say "yes" matters, too.
Consent should be granted happily!
Here's some examples of–
What Consent is NOT
Lukewarm
I...
guess...
...ok.

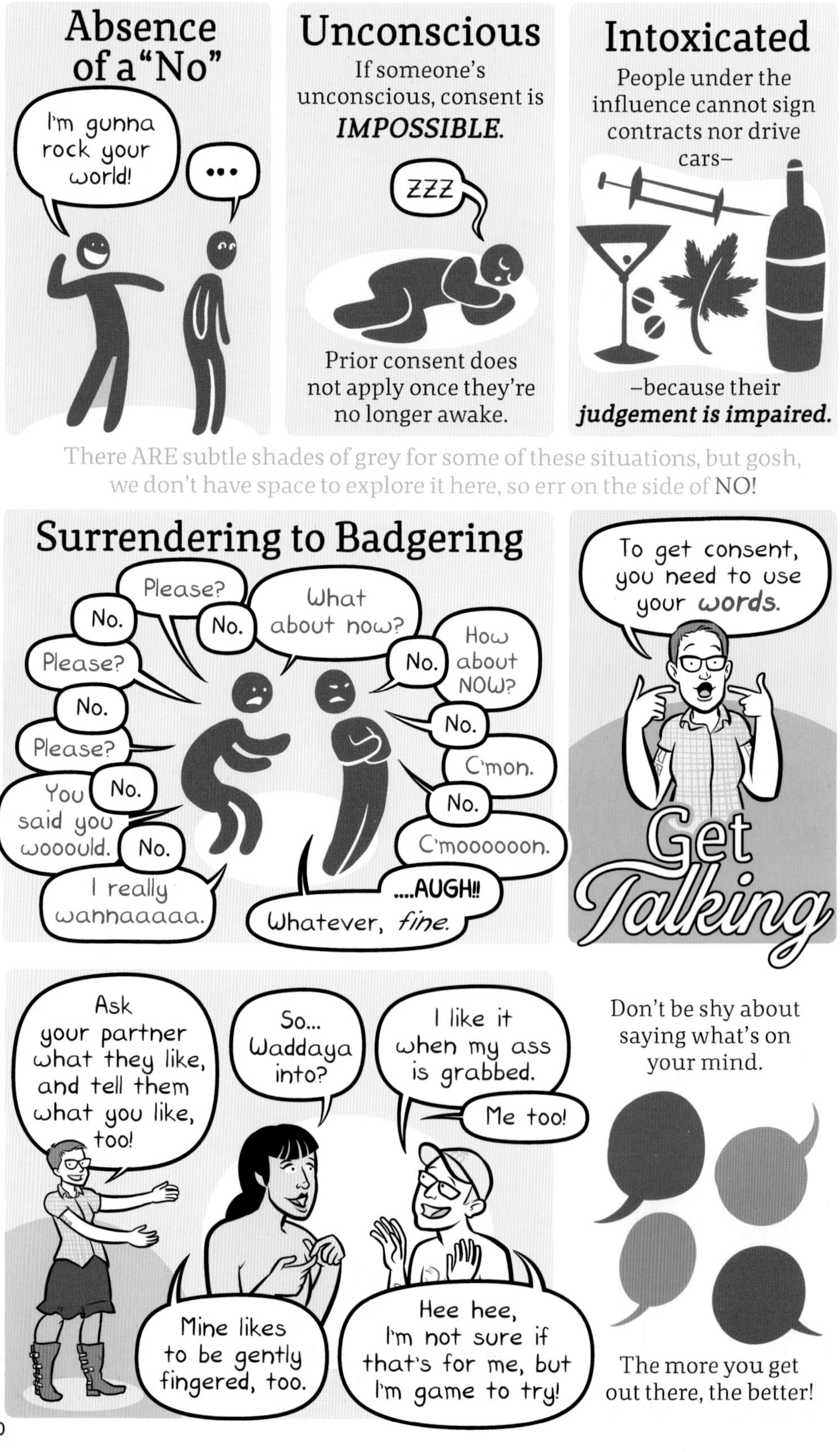

Absence of a "No"
I'm gunna rock your world!
...
Unconscious
If someone's unconscious, consent is IMPOSSIBLE.
ZZZ
Prior consent does not apply once they're no longer awake.
Intoxicated
People under the influence cannot sign contracts nor drive cars–
–because their judgement is impaired.
There ARE subtle shades of grey for some of these situations, but gosh, we don't have space to explore it here, so err on the side of NO!
Surrendering to Badgering
Please?
No.
No.
What about now?
Please?
No.
How about NOW?
No.
Please?
No.
You said you wooould.
No.
C'mon.
No.
No.
C'mooooooon.
I really wannaaaaa.
....AUGH!!
Whatever, fine.
To get consent, you need to use your words.
Get Talking
Ask your partner what they like, and tell them what you like, too!
So... Waddaya into?
I like it when my ass is grabbed.
Me too!
Mine likes to be gently fingered, too.
Hee hee, I'm not sure if that's for me, but I'm game to try!
Don't be shy about saying what's on your mind.
The more you get out there, the better!

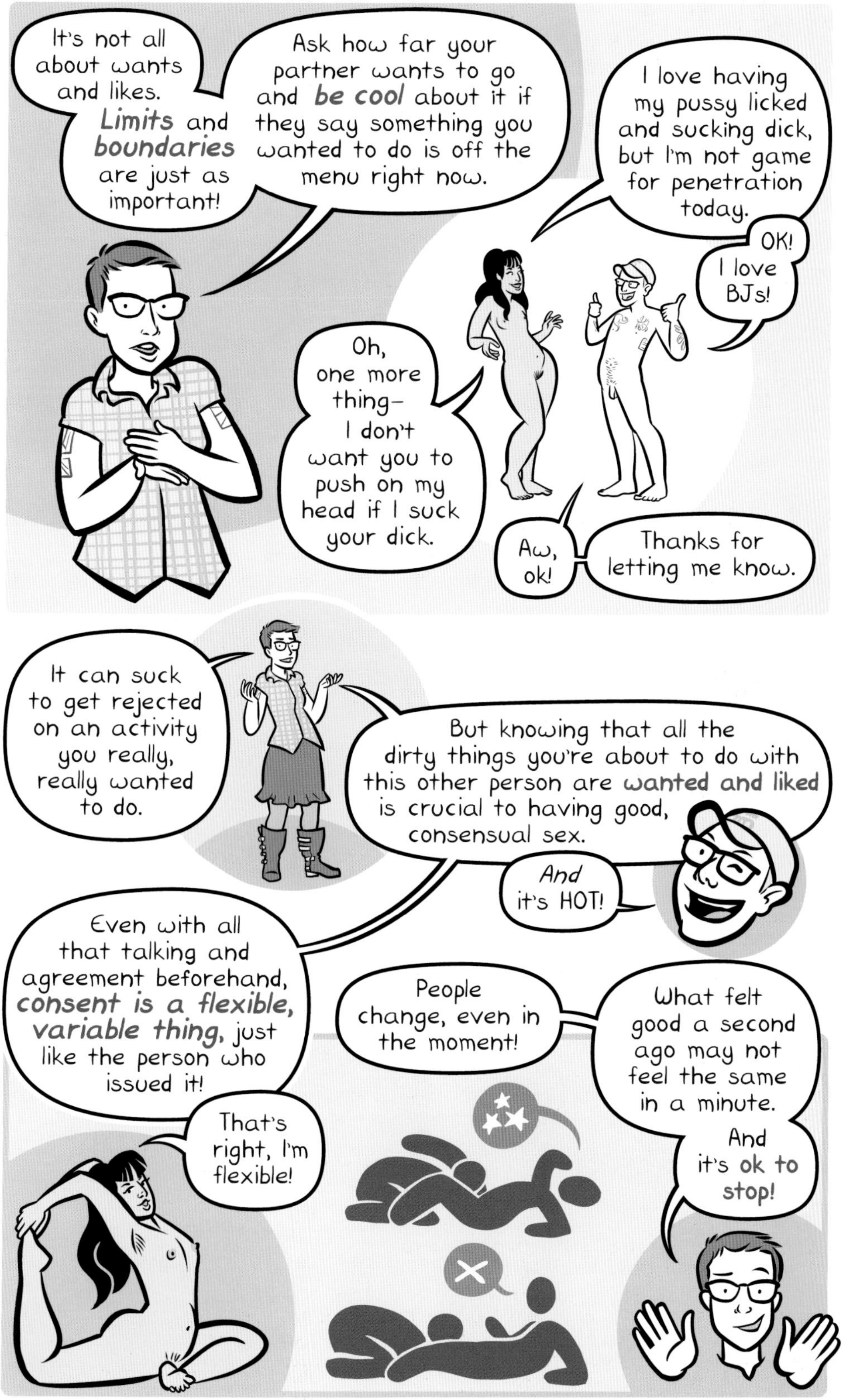
It's not all about wants and likes. Limits and boundaries are just as important!
Ask how far your partner wants to go and be cool about it if they say something you wanted to do is off the menu right now.
I love having my pussy licked and sucking dick, but I'm not game for penetration today.
OK! I love BJs!
Oh, one more thing– I don't want you to push on my head if I suck your dick.
Aw, ok!
Thanks for letting me know.
It can suck to get rejected on an activity you really, really wanted to do.
But knowing that all the dirty things you're about to do with this other person are wanted and liked is crucial to having good, consensual sex.
And it's HOT!
Even with all that talking and agreement beforehand, consent is a flexible, variable thing, just like the person who issued it!
That's right, I'm flexible!
People change, even in the moment!
What felt good a second ago may not feel the same in a minute.
And it's ok to stop!

Revoking Consent

Keep checking in with your partner.
Speak up when something doesn't feel right.

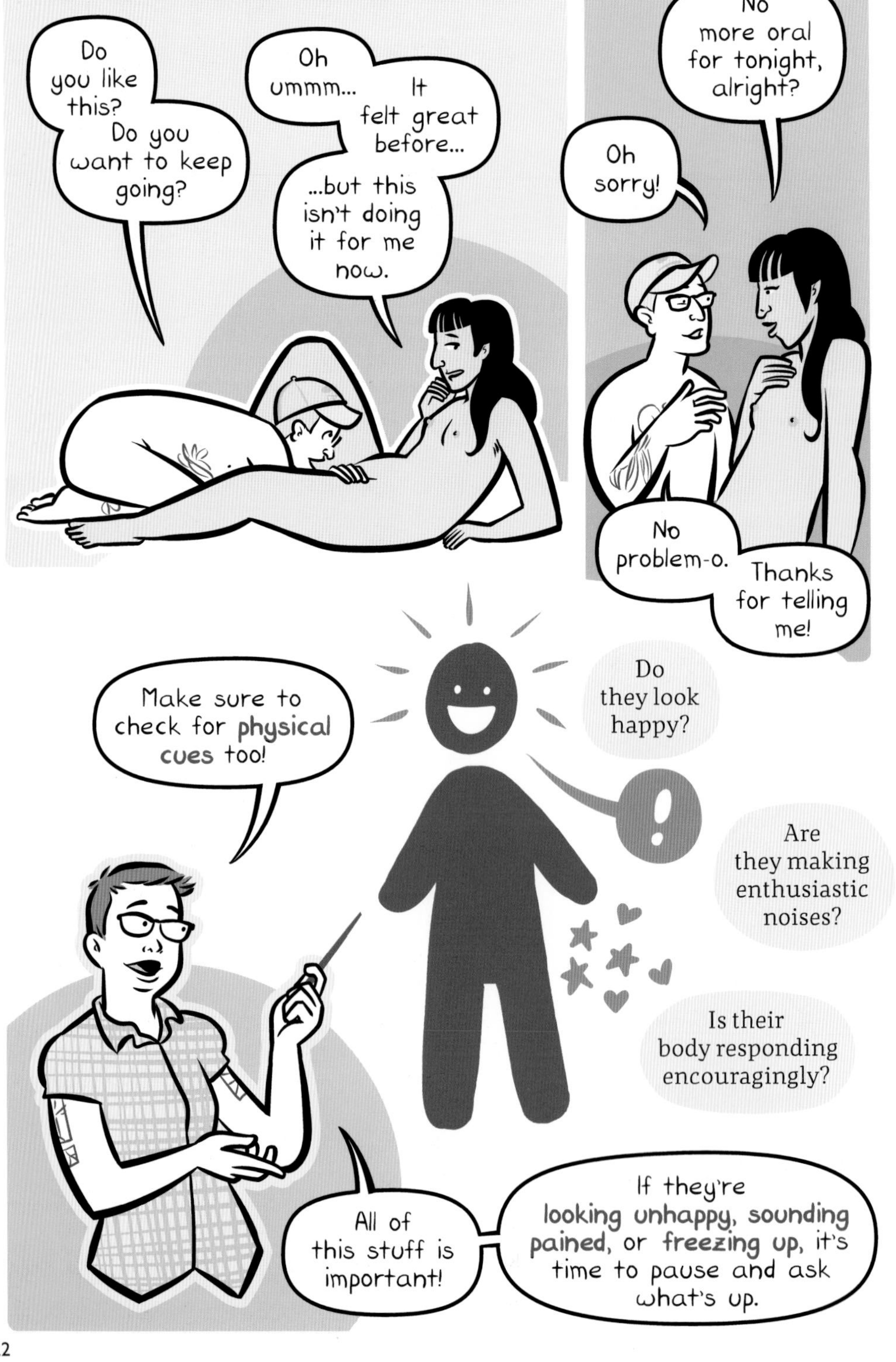
Do you like this? Do you want to keep going?
Oh ummm... It felt great before...
...but this isn't doing it for me now.
No more oral for tonight, alright?
Oh sorry!
No problem-o.
Thanks for telling me!
Make sure to check for physical cues too!
Do they look happy?
Are they making enthusiastic noises?
Is their body responding encouragingly?
All of this stuff is important!
If they're looking unhappy, sounding pained, or freezing up, it's time to pause and ask what's up.

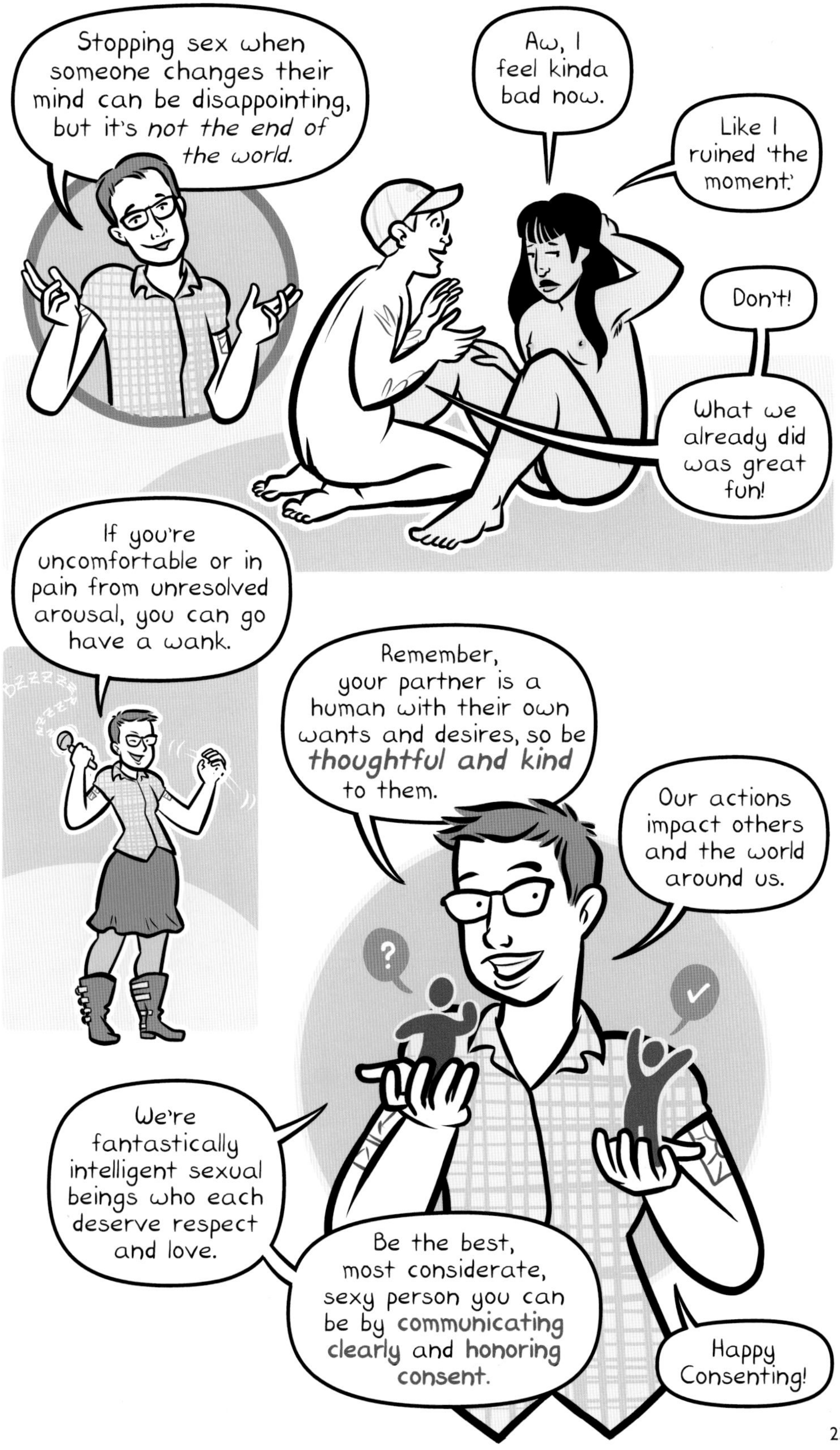
Stopping sex when someone changes their mind can be disappointing, but it's *not the end of the world.*
Aw, I feel kinda bad now.
Like I ruined 'the moment.'
Don't!
What we already did was great fun!
If you're uncomfortable or in pain from unresolved arousal, you can go have a wank.
BZZZZ
Remember, your partner is a human with their own wants and desires, so be **thoughtful and kind** to them.
Our actions impact others and the world around us.
?
We're fantastically intelligent sexual beings who each deserve respect and love.
Be the best, most considerate, sexy person you can be by **communicating clearly** and **honoring consent.**
Happy Consenting!

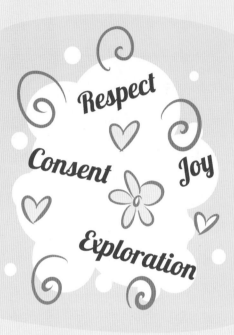

Respect

Consent

Joy

Exploration

Sex Positivity

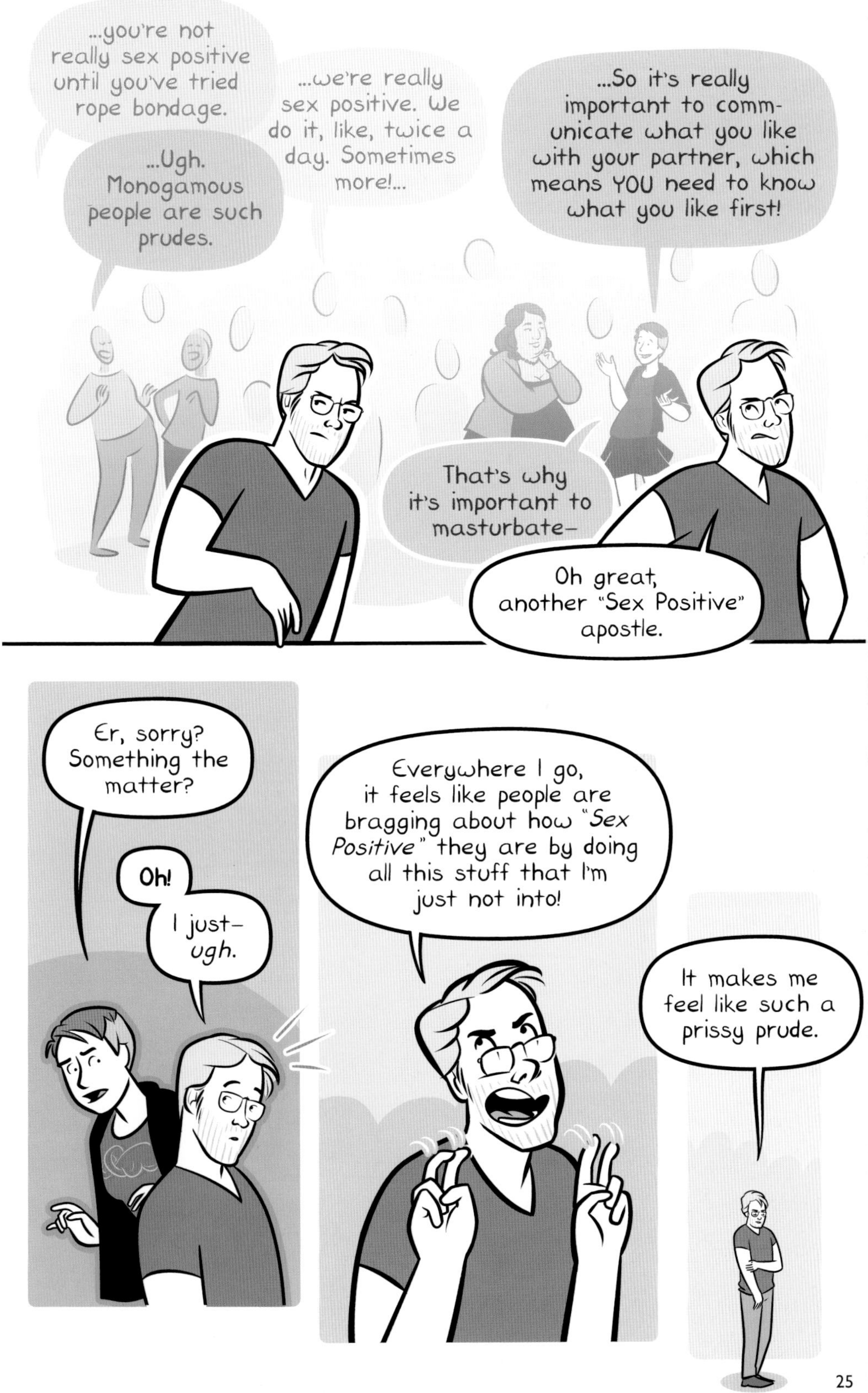
...you're not really sex positive until you've tried rope bondage.
...Ugh. Monogamous people are such prudes.
...we're really sex positive. We do it, like, twice a day. Sometimes more!...
...So it's really important to communicate what you like with your partner, which means YOU need to know what you like first!
That's why it's important to masturbate–
Oh great, another "Sex Positive" apostle.
Er, sorry? Something the matter?
Oh!
I just– *ugh.*
Everywhere I go, it feels like people are bragging about how "*Sex Positive*" they are by doing all this stuff that I'm just not into!
It makes me feel like such a prissy prude.

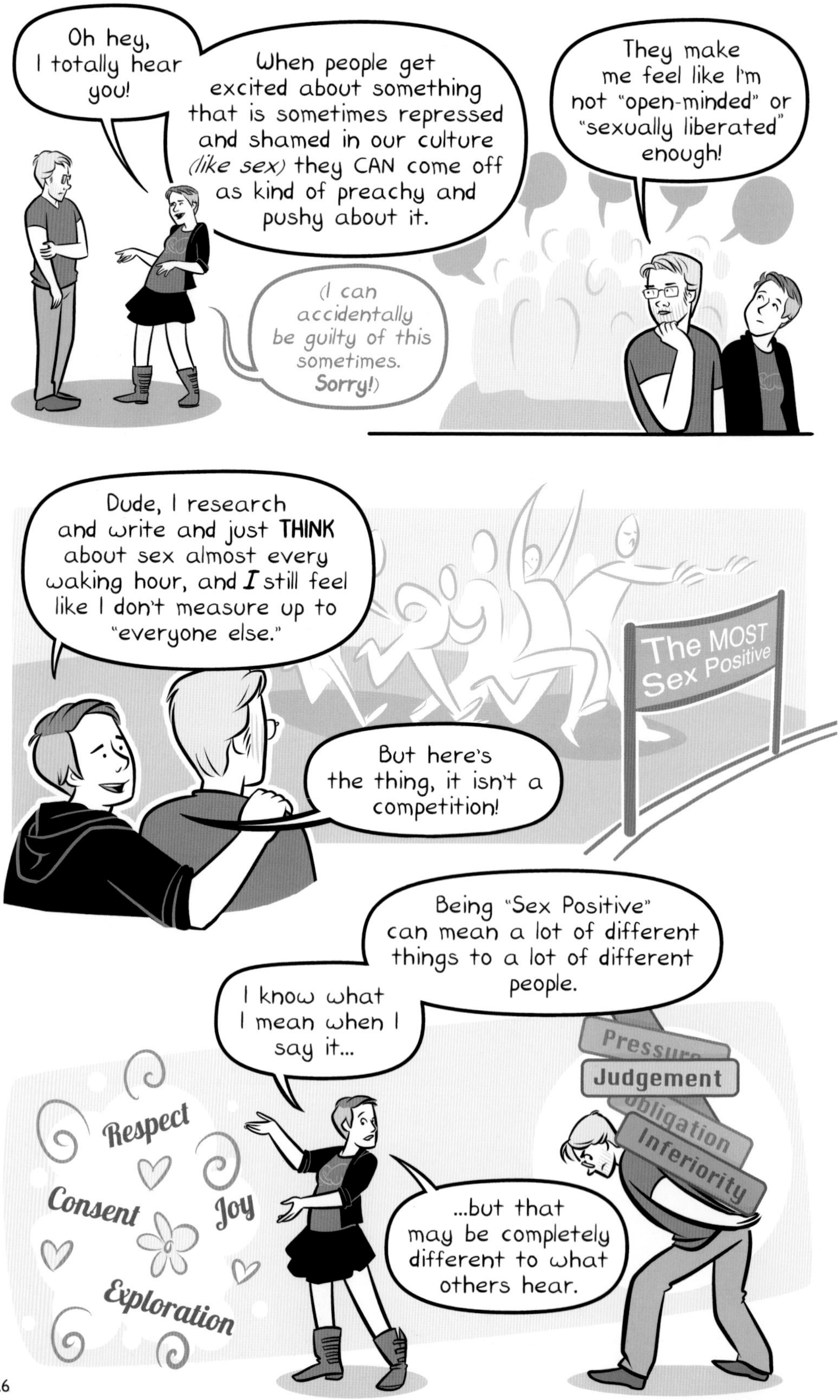

Oh hey, I totally hear you!
When people get excited about something that is sometimes repressed and shamed in our culture *(like sex)* they CAN come off as kind of preachy and pushy about it.
(I can accidentally be guilty of this sometimes. **Sorry!**)
They make me feel like I'm not "open-minded" or "sexually liberated" enough!
Dude, I research and write and just **THINK** about sex almost every waking hour, and *I* still feel like I don't measure up to "everyone else."
The MOST Sex Positive
But here's the thing, it isn't a competition!
Being "Sex Positive" can mean a lot of different things to a lot of different people.
I know what I mean when I say it...
Respect
Consent
Joy
Exploration
Judgement
Obligation
Inferiority
...but that may be completely different to what others hear.

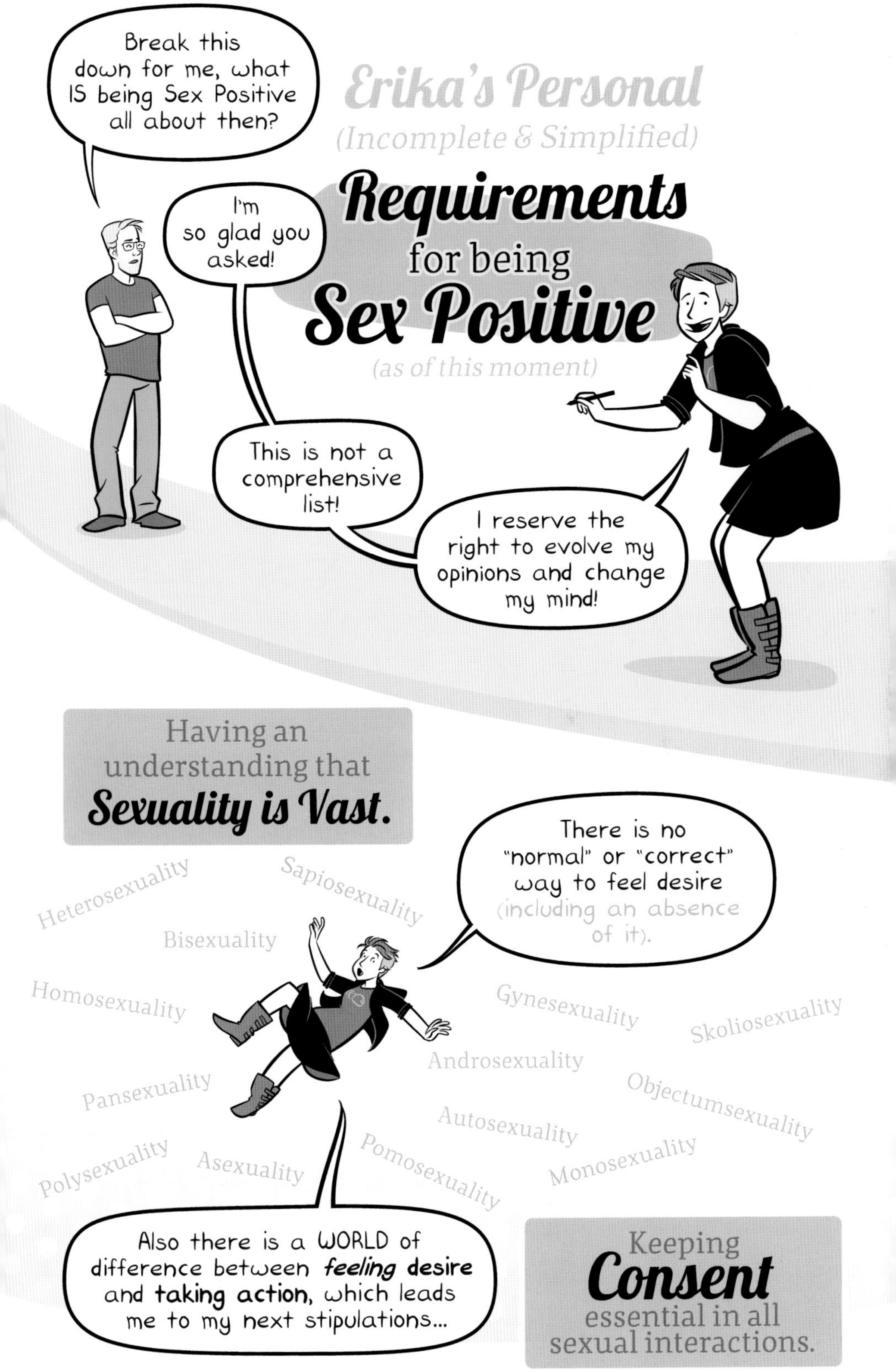

Break this down for me, what IS being Sex Positive all about then?
Erika's Personal
(Incomplete & Simplified)
Requirements for being Sex Positive
(as of this moment)
I'm so glad you asked!
This is not a comprehensive list!
I reserve the right to evolve my opinions and change my mind!
Having an understanding that Sexuality is Vast.
There is no "normal" or "correct" way to feel desire (including an absence of it).
Heterosexuality
Sapiosexuality
Bisexuality
Homosexuality
Gynesexuality
Skoliosexuality
Androsexuality
Pansexuality
Objectumsexuality
Autosexuality
Polysexuality
Asexuality
Pomosexuality
Monosexuality
Also there is a WORLD of difference between *feeling* **desire** and **taking action**, which leads me to my next stipulations...
Keeping Consent essential in all sexual interactions.

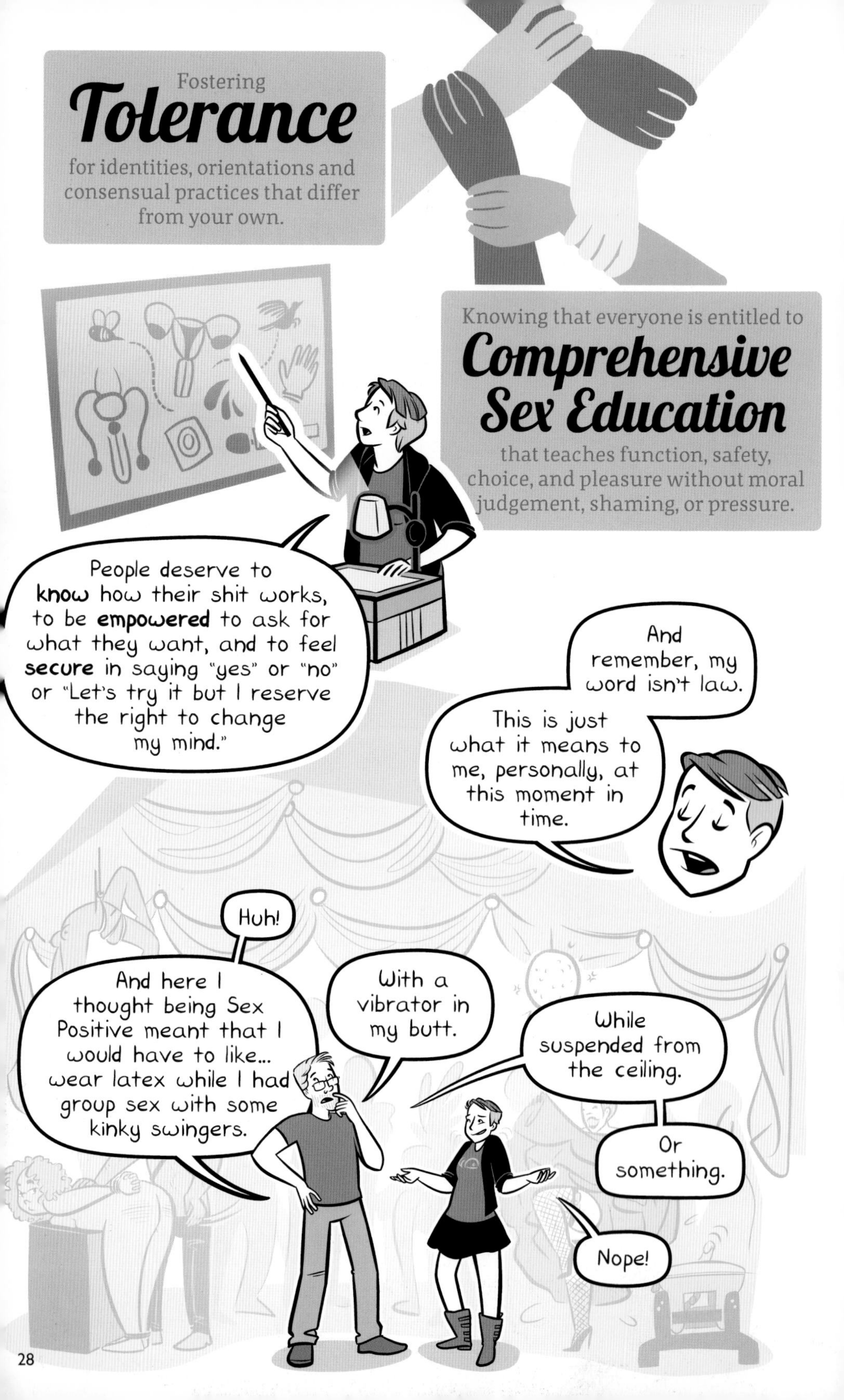
Fostering
Tolerance
for identities, orientations and consensual practices that differ from your own.
Knowing that everyone is entitled to
Comprehensive Sex Education
that teaches function, safety, choice, and pleasure without moral judgement, shaming, or pressure.
People deserve to **know** how their shit works, to be **empowered** to ask for what they want, and to feel **secure** in saying "yes" or "no" or "Let's try it but I reserve the right to change my mind."
And remember, my word isn't law.
This is just what it means to me, personally, at this moment in time.
Huh!
And here I thought being Sex Positive meant that I would have to like... wear latex while I had group sex with some kinky swingers.
With a vibrator in my butt.
While suspended from the ceiling.
Or something.
Nope!

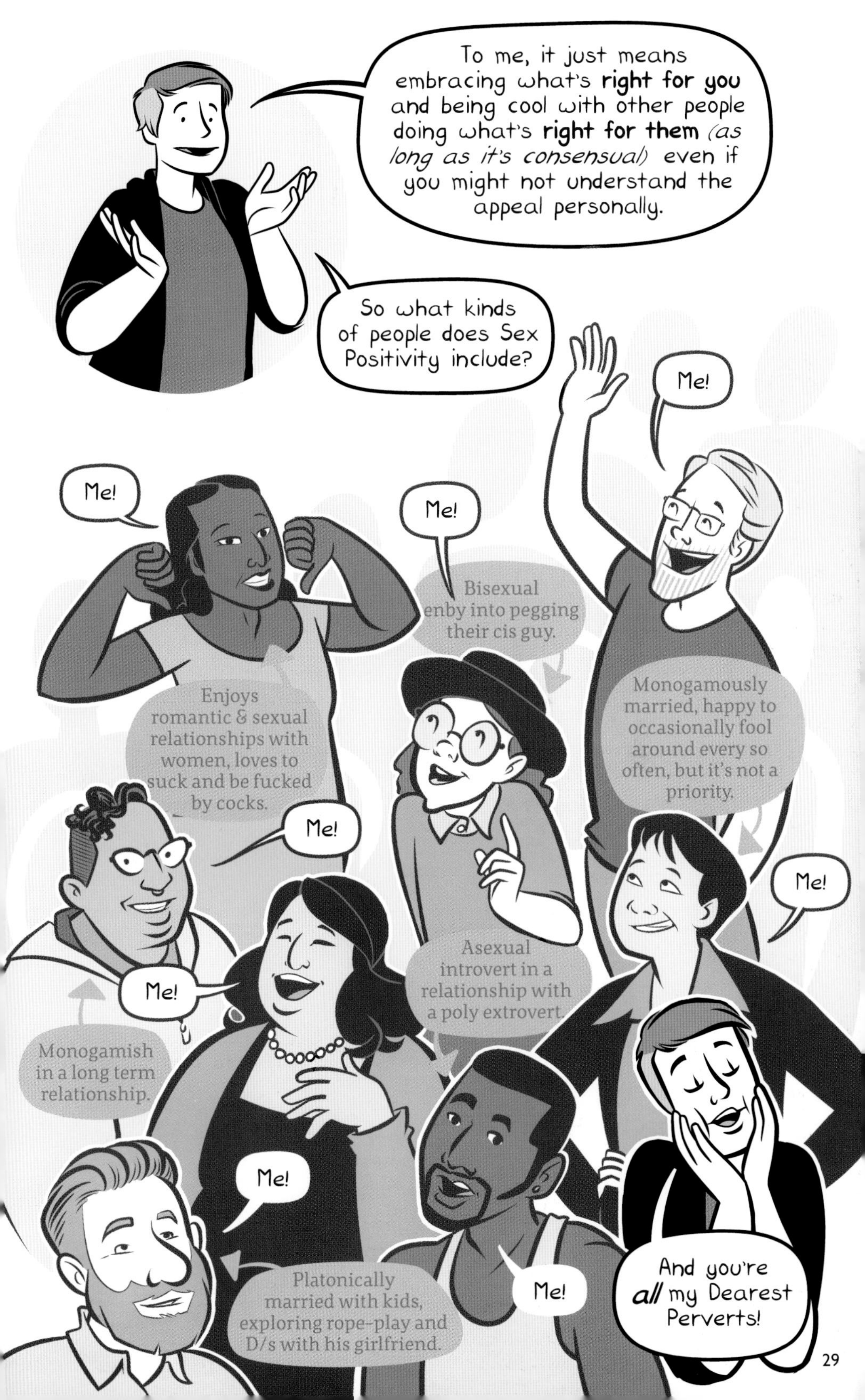
To me, it just means embracing what's **right for you** and being cool with other people doing what's **right for them** *(as long as it's consensual)* even if you might not understand the appeal personally.
So what kinds of people does Sex Positivity include?
Me!
Me!
Me!
Bisexual enby into pegging their cis guy.
Enjoys romantic & sexual relationships with women, loves to suck and be fucked by cocks.
Monogamously married, happy to occasionally fool around every so often, but it's not a priority.
Me!
Me!
Me!
Asexual introvert in a relationship with a poly extrovert.
Monogamish in a long term relationship.
Me!
Platonically married with kids, exploring rope-play and D/s with his girlfriend.
Me!
And you're *all* my Dearest Perverts!

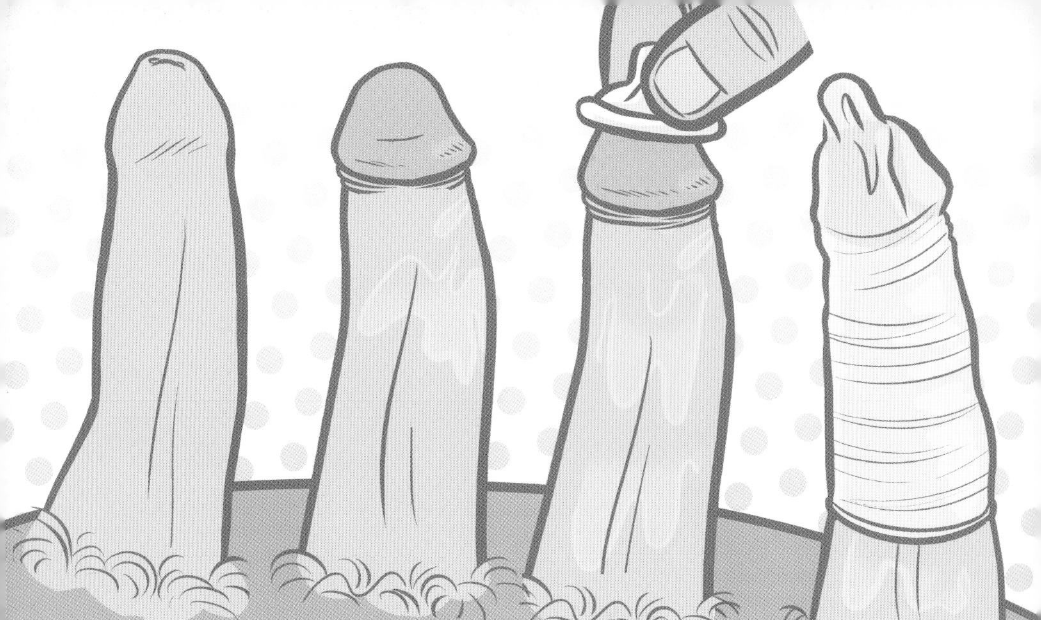

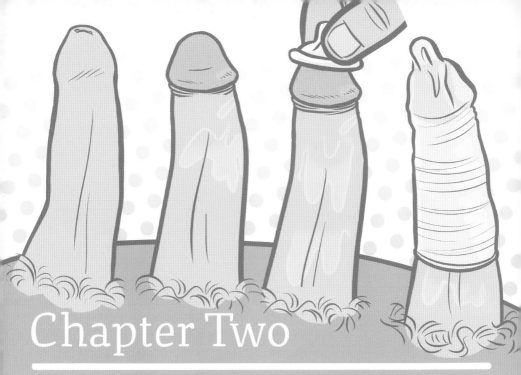

Chapter Two

Doin' It Safely

Dancing! Fencing! Rowing! Tandem bicycling! Building! Bobsledding... and SEX!

Just like all group physical activities, sex can be a fun, rewarding, and bonding experience. With the right people and the right mindset, sexual intimacy can be a great time. But just like with all these activities, sex also comes with some risks to your health and safety. In this chapter we'll go over some best practices and advice to keep yourself and your partner(s) as safe as possible.

Sexually transmitted infections and diseases (STIs and STDs) and pregnancy are all possible when you take a sexy tumble with another person, and we're here to tell you not to be frightened about this stuff or ashamed if it happens. Our culture acts as if somebody picking up an STI or unintended pregnancy is an anomaly, but all of these things are SO freaking common!

That being said, there's no reason to be irresponsible and, as these comics will show you, there's a HUGE arsenal of precautions out there for you to make use of! From warding off pregnancy-making sperm to avoiding nasty germs, there are tons of options out there to help you play safer!

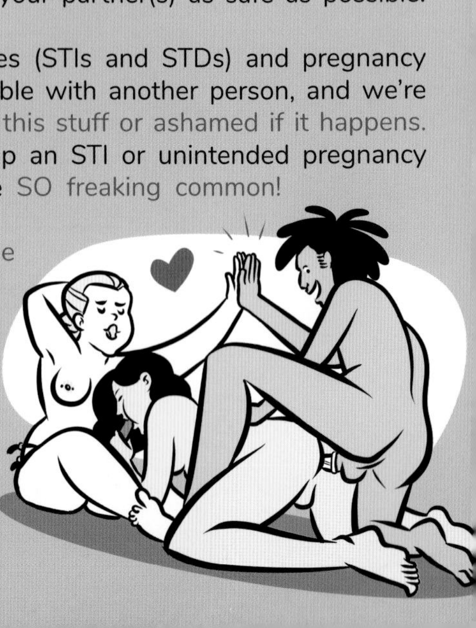

Study up, play safe, and make some fond memories!

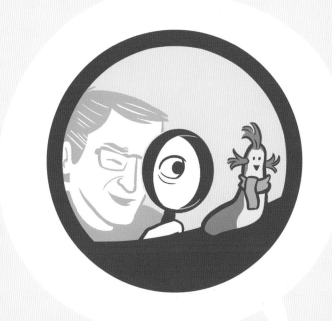

STI Testing

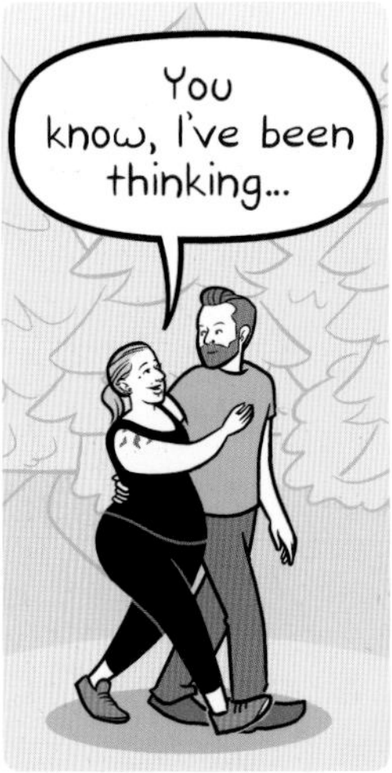
You know, I've been thinking...

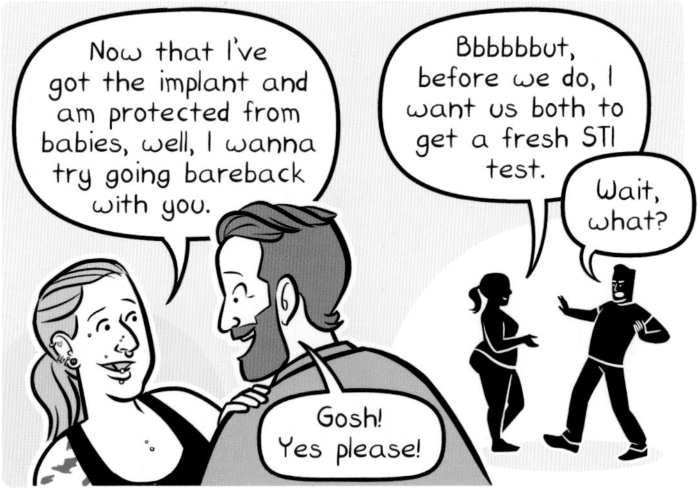
Now that I've got the implant and am protected from babies, well, I wanna try going bareback with you.
Gosh! Yes please!
Bbbbbbut, before we do, I want us both to get a fresh STI test.
Wait, what?

An STI is a **Sexually Transmitted Infection**: they're little bug-a-boos that can be picked up when you're swapping fluids with someone else.

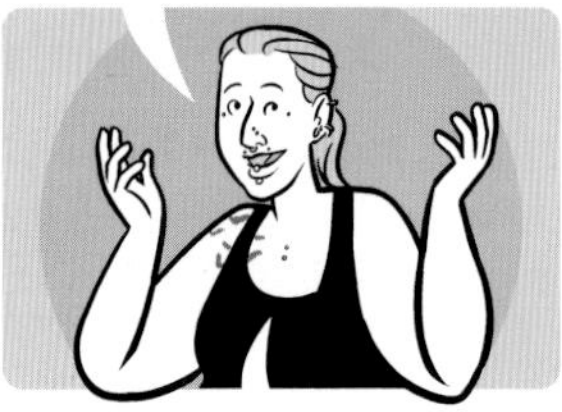

Stuff like HPV, herpes, chlamydia, gonorrhea, HIV...

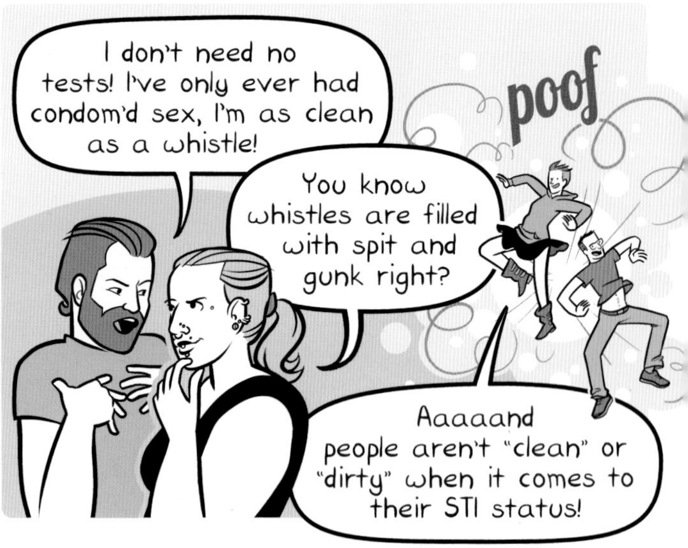
I don't need no tests! I've only ever had condom'd sex, I'm as clean as a whistle!
You know whistles are filled with spit and gunk right?
poof
Aaaaand people aren't "clean" or "dirty" when it comes to their STI status!

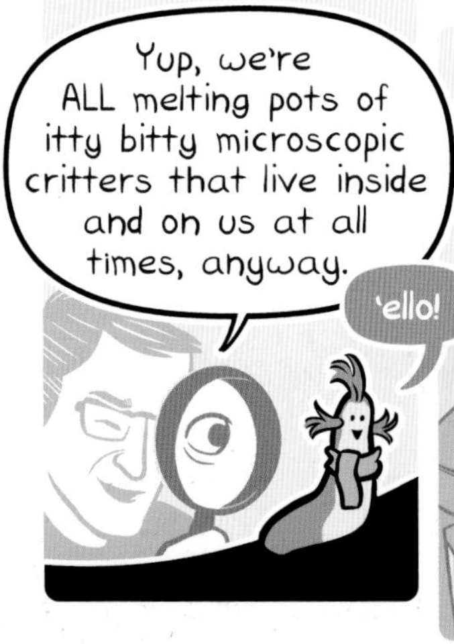
Yup, we're ALL melting pots of itty bitty microscopic critters that live inside and on us at all times, anyway.
'ello!

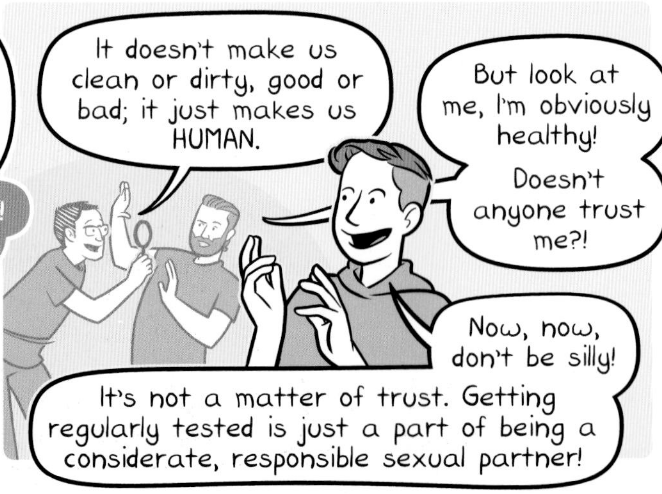
It doesn't make us clean or dirty, good or bad; it just makes us HUMAN.
But look at me, I'm obviously healthy!
Doesn't anyone trust me?!
Now, now, don't be silly!
It's not a matter of trust. Getting regularly tested is just a part of being a considerate, responsible sexual partner!

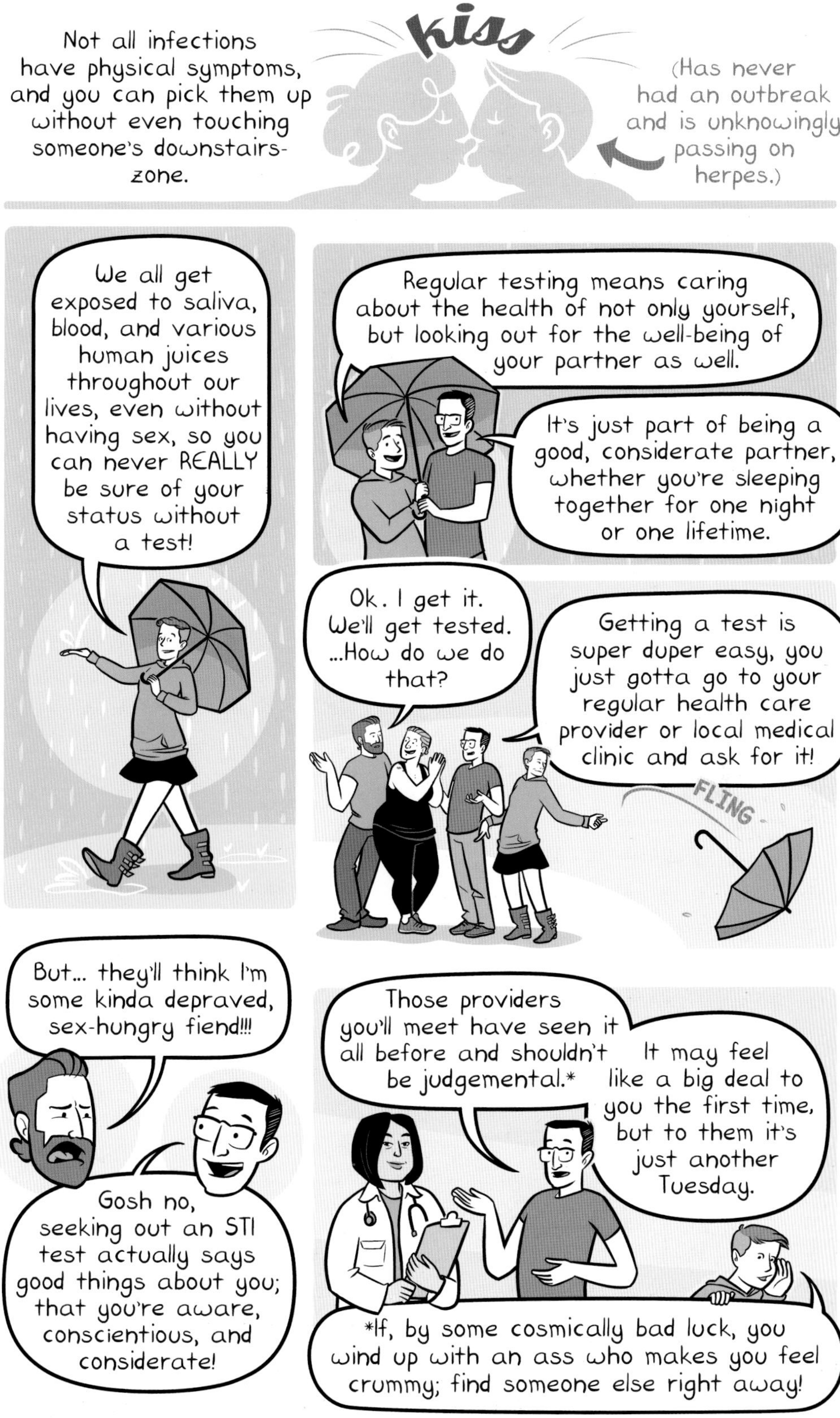
Not all infections have physical symptoms, and you can pick them up without even touching someone's downstairs-zone.
Kiss
(Has never had an outbreak and is unknowingly passing on herpes.)
We all get exposed to saliva, blood, and various human juices throughout our lives, even without having sex, so you can never REALLY be sure of your status without a test!
Regular testing means caring about the health of not only yourself, but looking out for the well-being of your partner as well.
It's just part of being a good, considerate partner, whether you're sleeping together for one night or one lifetime.
Ok. I get it. We'll get tested. ...How do we do that?
Getting a test is super duper easy, you just gotta go to your regular health care provider or local medical clinic and ask for it!
FLING
But... they'll think I'm some kinda depraved, sex-hungry fiend!!!
Gosh no, seeking out an STI test actually says good things about you; that you're aware, conscientious, and considerate!
Those providers you'll meet have seen it all before and shouldn't be judgemental.*
It may feel like a big deal to you the first time, but to them it's just another Tuesday.
*If, by some cosmically bad luck, you wind up with an ass who makes you feel crummy; find someone else right away!

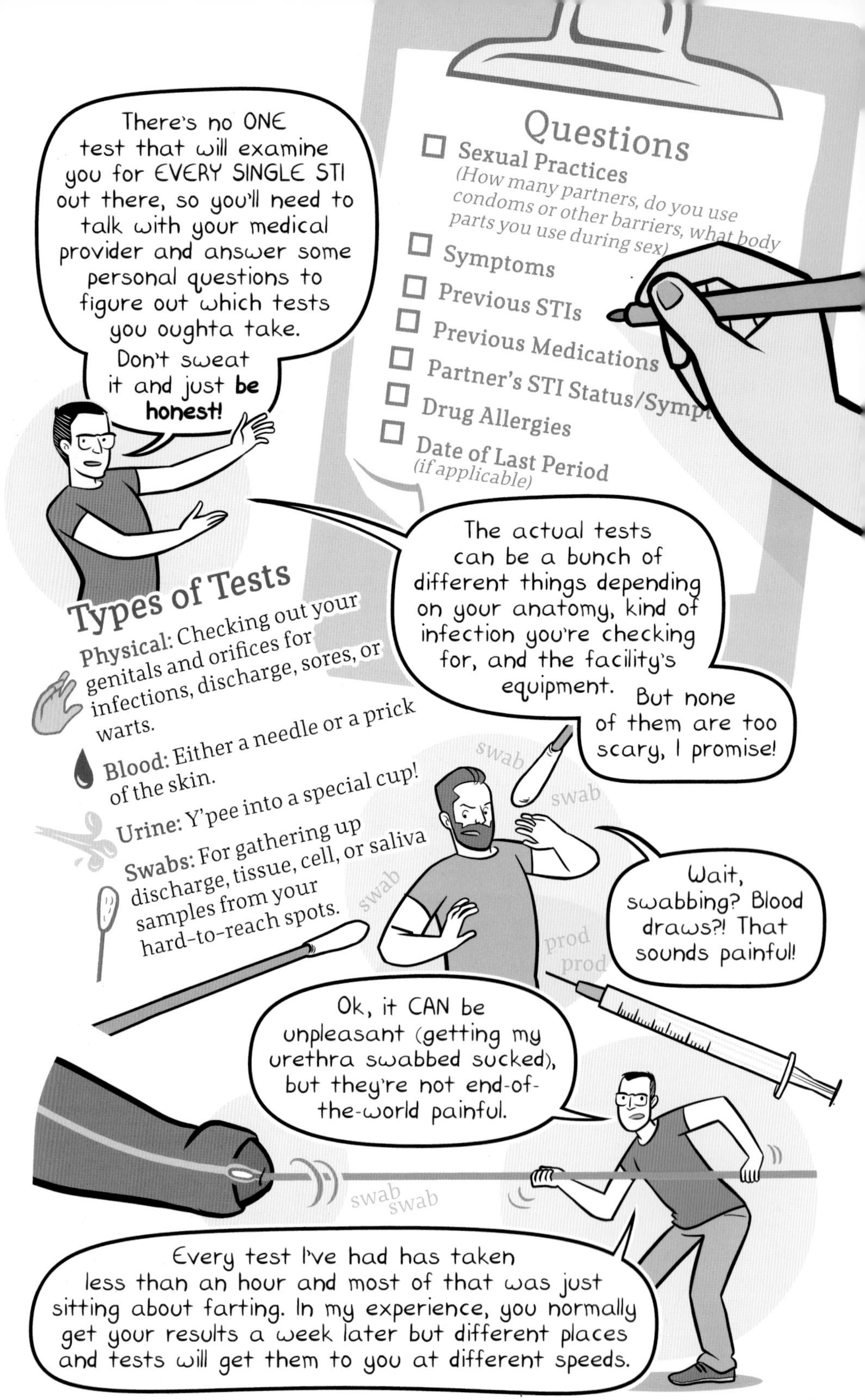
There's no ONE test that will examine you for EVERY SINGLE STI out there, so you'll need to talk with your medical provider and answer some personal questions to figure out which tests you oughta take.
Don't sweat it and just **be honest!**
Questions
Sexual Practices (How many partners, do you use condoms or other barriers, what body parts you use during sex)
Symptoms
Previous STIs
Previous Medications
Partner's STI Status/Sympt
Drug Allergies
Date of Last Period (if applicable)
The actual tests can be a bunch of different things depending on your anatomy, kind of infection you're checking for, and the facility's equipment.
But none of them are too scary, I promise!
Types of Tests
Physical: Checking out your genitals and orifices for infections, discharge, sores, or warts.
Blood: Either a needle or a prick of the skin.
Urine: Y'pee into a special cup!
Swabs: For gathering up discharge, tissue, cell, or saliva samples from your hard-to-reach spots.
swab
swab
swab
prod
prod
Wait, swabbing? Blood draws?! That sounds painful!
Ok, it CAN be unpleasant (getting my urethra swabbed sucked), but they're not end-of-the-world painful.
swab
swab
Every test I've had has taken less than an hour and most of that was just sitting about farting. In my experience, you normally get your results a week later but different places and tests will get them to you at different speeds.

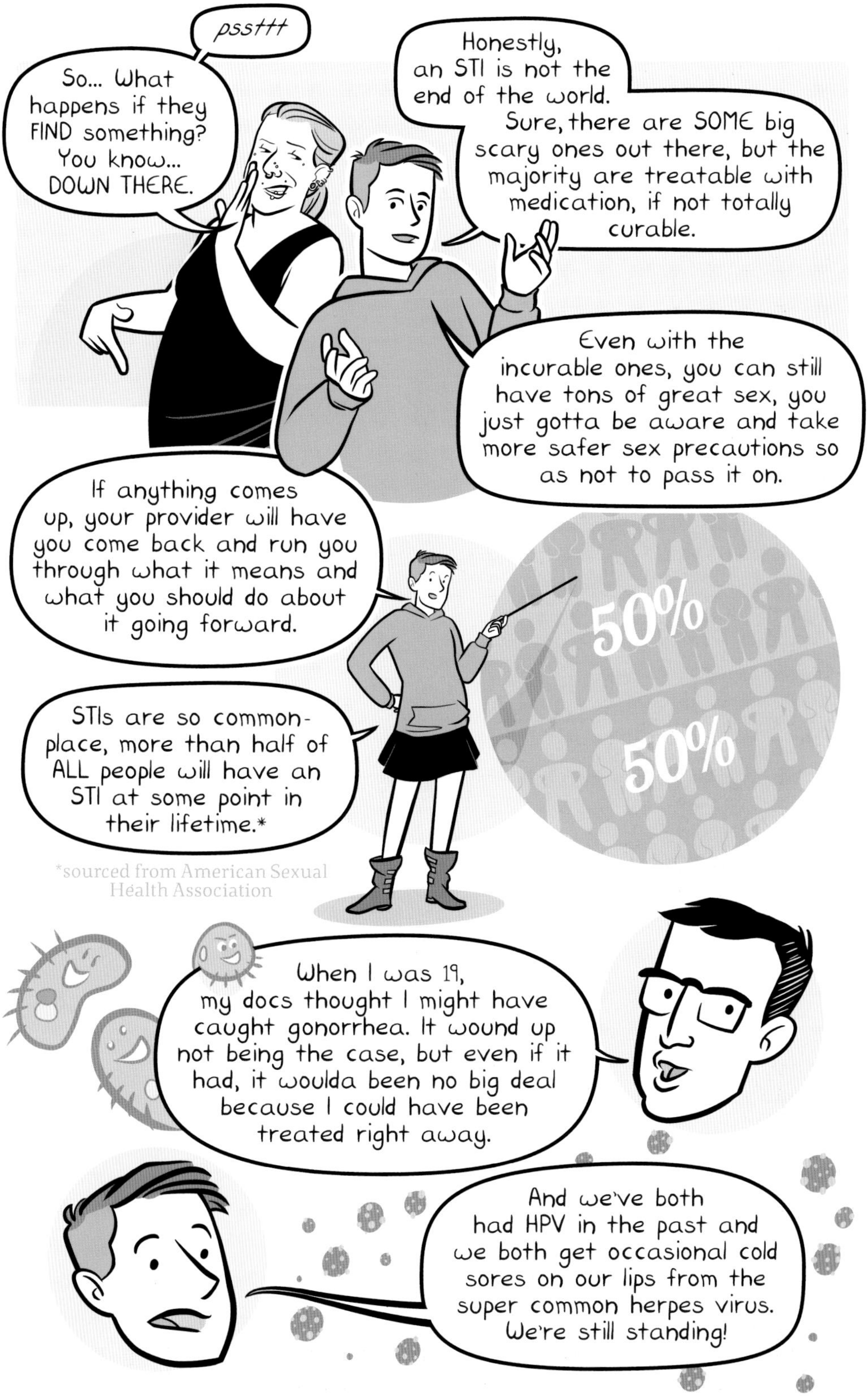
psssttt
So... What happens if they FIND something? You know... DOWN THERE.
Honestly, an STI is not the end of the world.
Sure, there are SOME big scary ones out there, but the majority are treatable with medication, if not totally curable.
Even with the incurable ones, you can still have tons of great sex, you just gotta be aware and take more safer sex precautions so as not to pass it on.
If anything comes up, your provider will have you come back and run you through what it means and what you should do about it going forward.
50%
50%
STIs are so common-place, more than half of ALL people will have an STI at some point in their lifetime.*
*sourced from American Sexual Health Association
When I was 19, my docs thought I might have caught gonorrhea. It wound up not being the case, but even if it had, it woulda been no big deal because I could have been treated right away.
And we've both had HPV in the past and we both get occasional cold sores on our lips from the super common herpes virus. We're still standing!

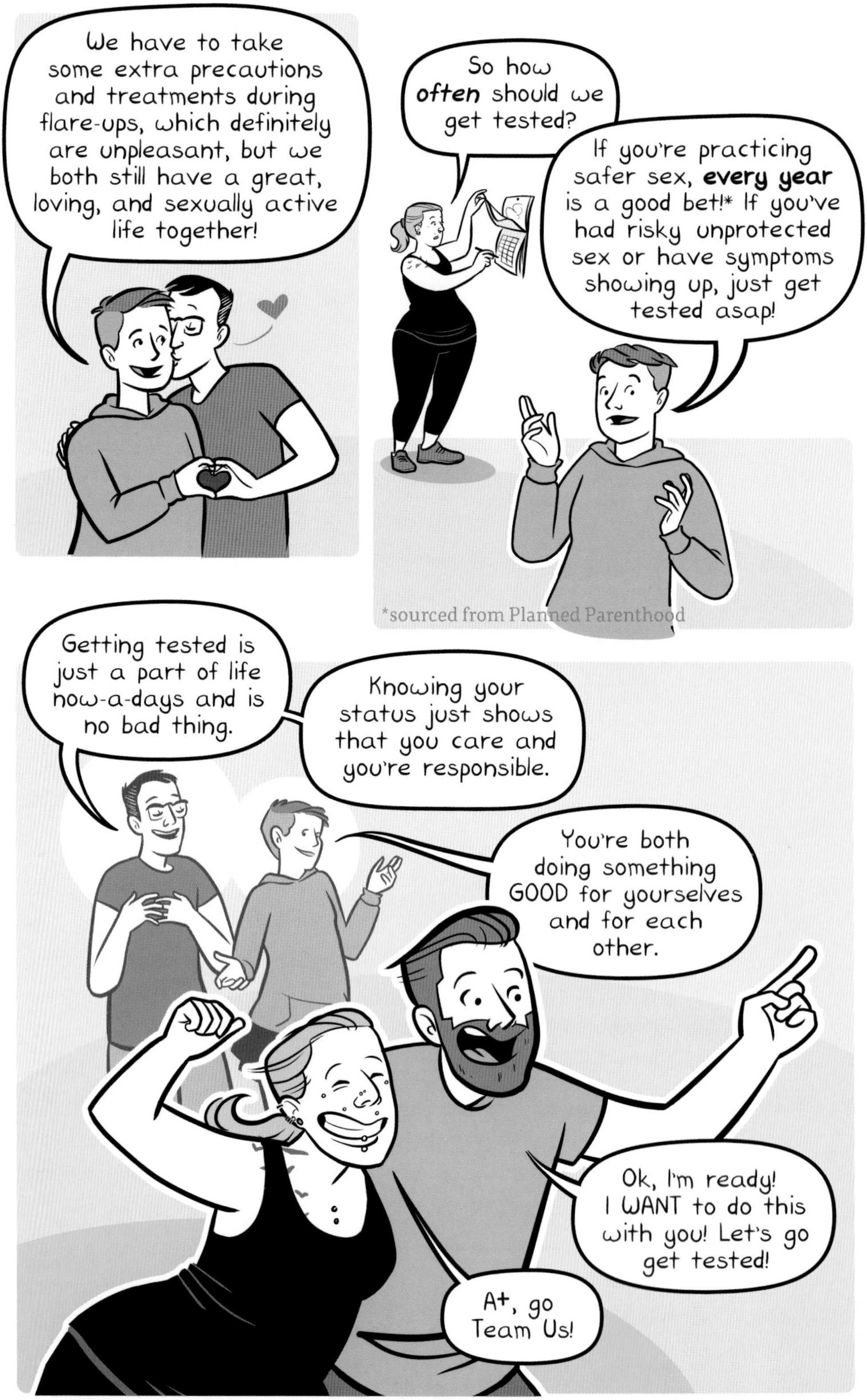
We have to take some extra precautions and treatments during flare-ups, which definitely are unpleasant, but we both still have a great, loving, and sexually active life together!
So how **often** should we get tested?
If you're practicing safer sex, **every year** is a good bet!* If you've had risky unprotected sex or have symptoms showing up, just get tested asap!
*sourced from Planned Parenthood
Getting tested is just a part of life now-a-days and is no bad thing.
Knowing your status just shows that you care and you're responsible.
You're both doing something GOOD for yourselves and for each other.
Ok, I'm ready! I WANT to do this with you! Let's go get tested!
A+, go Team Us!

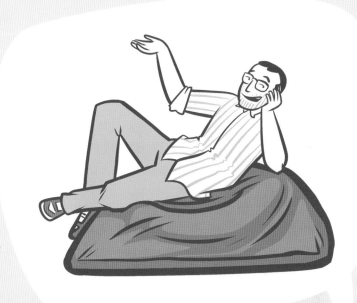

Condoms

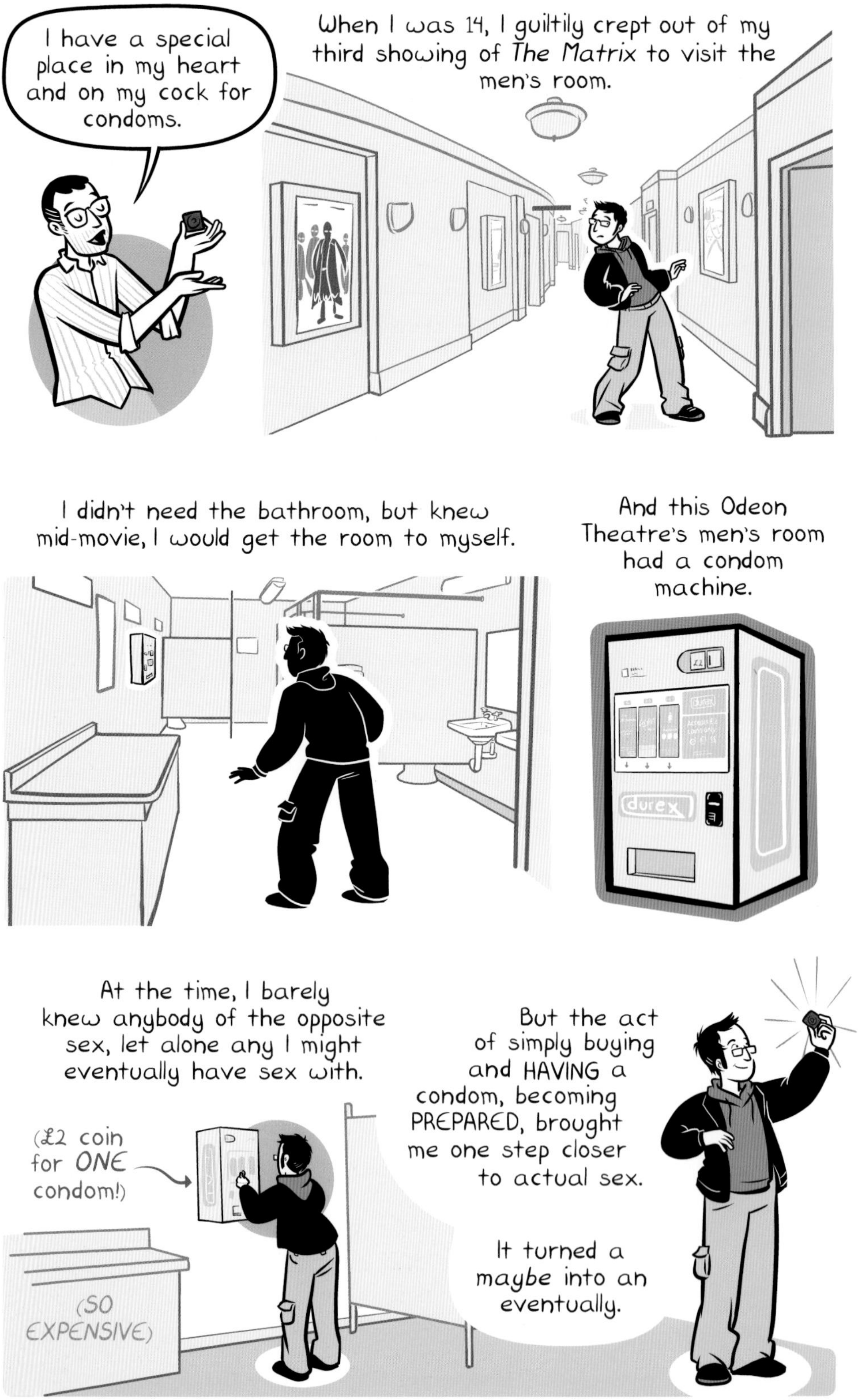
I have a special place in my heart and on my cock for condoms.
When I was 14, I guiltily crept out of my third showing of *The Matrix* to visit the men's room.
I didn't need the bathroom, but knew mid-movie, I would get the room to myself.
And this Odeon Theatre's men's room had a condom machine.
durex
At the time, I barely knew anybody of the opposite sex, let alone any I might eventually have sex with.
(£2 coin for ONE condom!)
(SO EXPENSIVE)
But the act of simply buying and HAVING a condom, becoming PREPARED, brought me one step closer to actual sex.
It turned a *maybe* into an eventually.

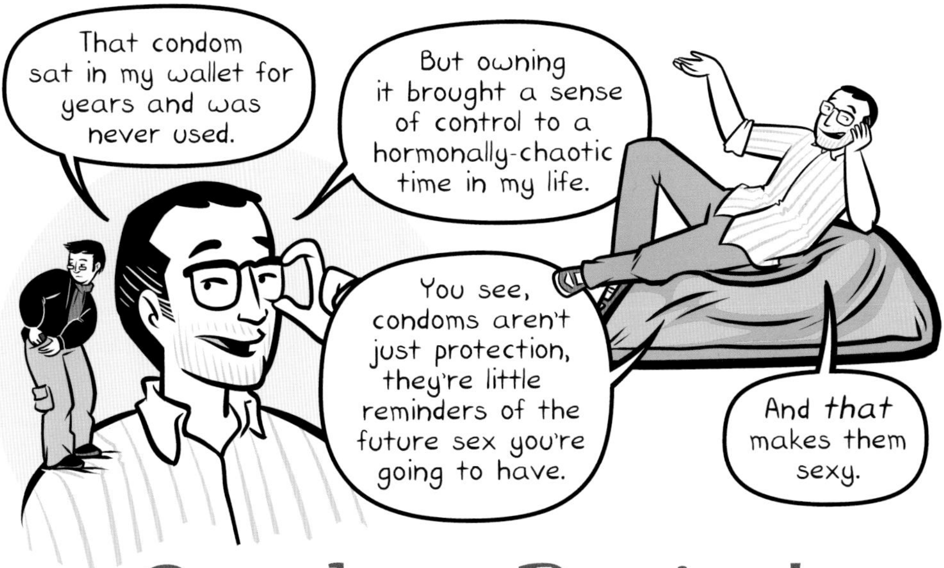
That condom sat in my wallet for years and was never used.
But owning it brought a sense of control to a hormonally-chaotic time in my life.
You see, condoms aren't just protection, they're little reminders of the future sex you're going to have.
And *that* makes them sexy.

Condom Basics!

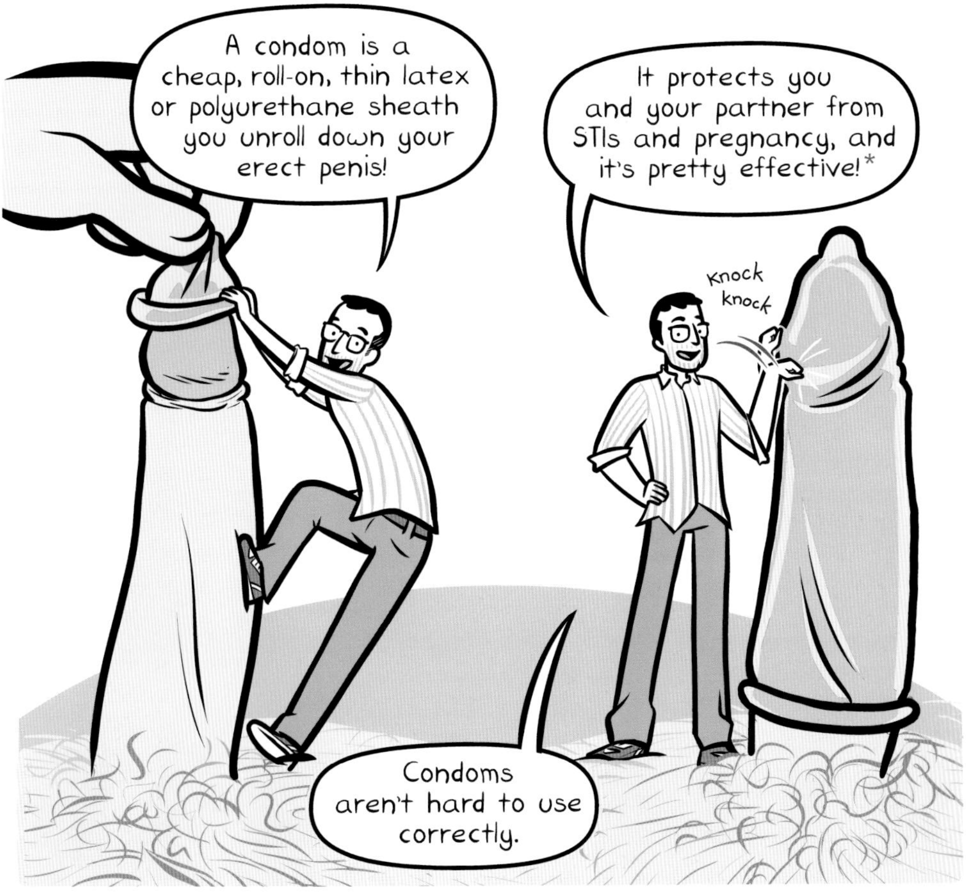
A condom is a cheap, roll-on, thin latex or polyurethane sheath you unroll down your erect penis!
It protects you and your partner from STIs and pregnancy, and it's pretty effective!*
Knock knock
Condoms aren't hard to use correctly.

*sourced from Planned Parenthood

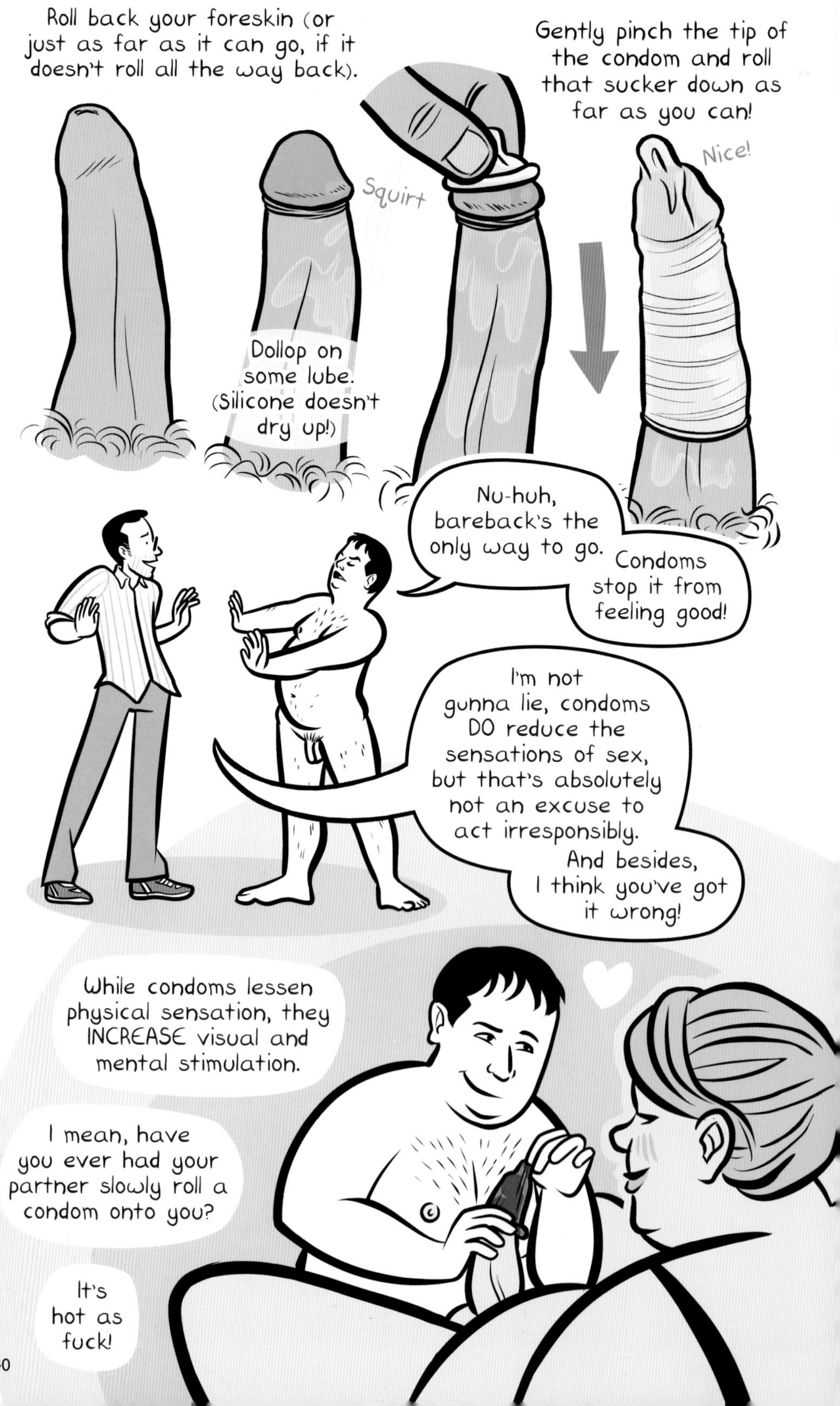

Roll back your foreskin (or just as far as it can go, if it doesn't roll all the way back).
Dollop on some lube. (Silicone doesn't dry up!)
Squirt
Gently pinch the tip of the condom and roll that sucker down as far as you can!
Nice!
Nu-huh, bareback's the only way to go.
Condoms stop it from feeling good!
I'm not gunna lie, condoms DO reduce the sensations of sex, but that's absolutely not an excuse to act irresponsibly.
And besides, I think you've got it wrong!
While condoms lessen physical sensation, they INCREASE visual and mental stimulation.
I mean, have you ever had your partner slowly roll a condom onto you?
It's hot as fuck!

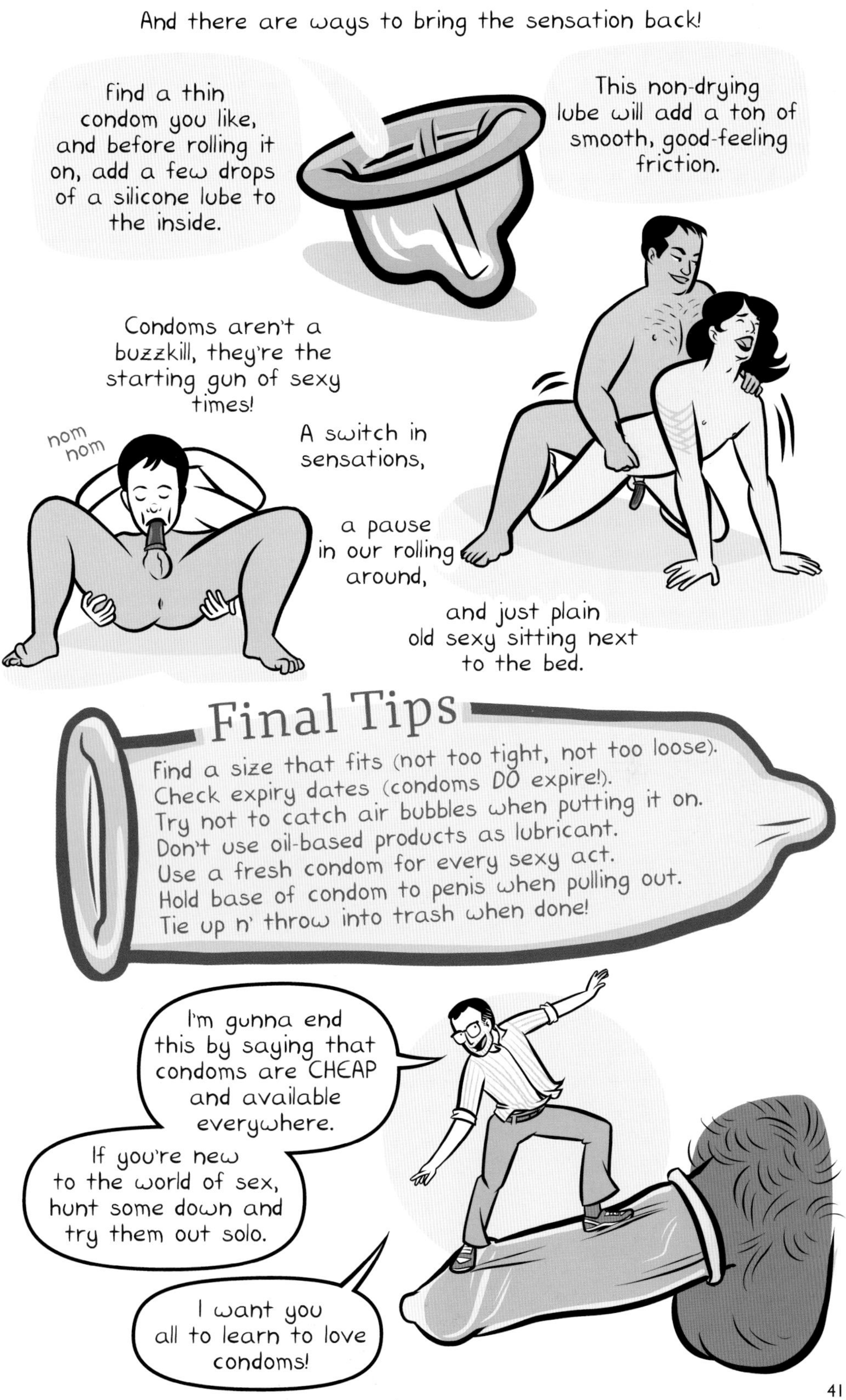
And there are ways to bring the sensation back!
find a thin condom you like, and before rolling it on, add a few drops of a silicone lube to the inside.
This non-drying lube will add a ton of smooth, good-feeling friction.
Condoms aren't a buzzkill, they're the starting gun of sexy times!
nom nom
A switch in sensations,
a pause in our rolling around,
and just plain old sexy sitting next to the bed.
Final Tips
Find a size that fits (not too tight, not too loose).
Check expiry dates (condoms DO expire!).
Try not to catch air bubbles when putting it on.
Don't use oil-based products as lubricant.
Use a fresh condom for every sexy act.
Hold base of condom to penis when pulling out.
Tie up n' throw into trash when done!
I'm gunna end this by saying that condoms are CHEAP and available everywhere.
If you're new to the world of sex, hunt some down and try them out solo.
I want you all to learn to love condoms!

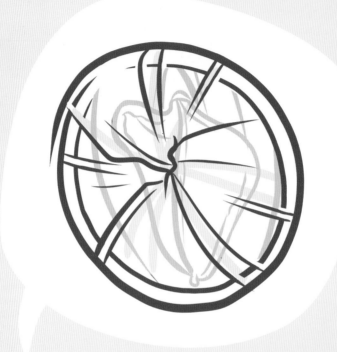

Internal Condoms

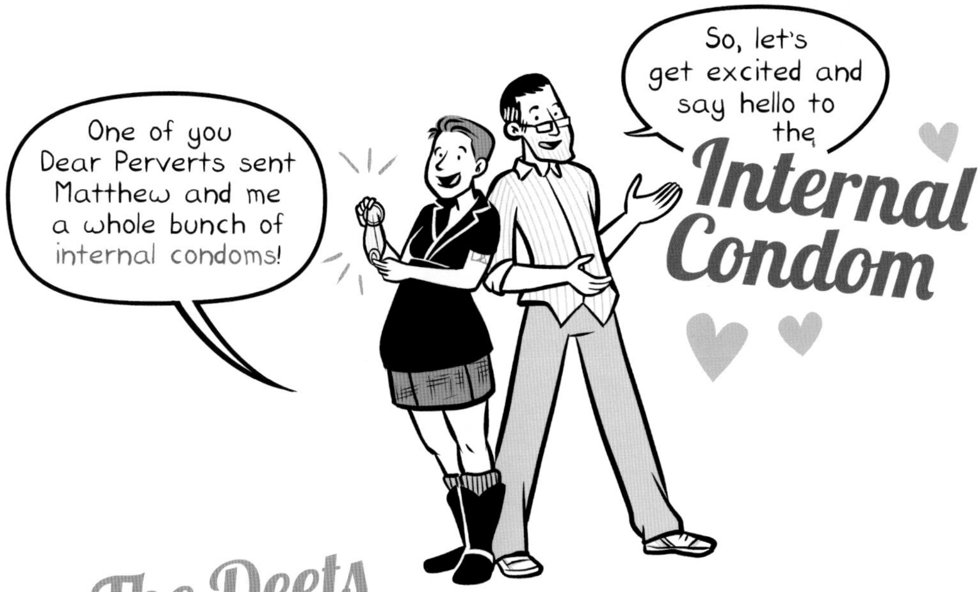
One of you Dear Perverts sent Matthew and me a whole bunch of internal condoms!
So, let's get excited and say hello to the
Internal Condom

The Deets

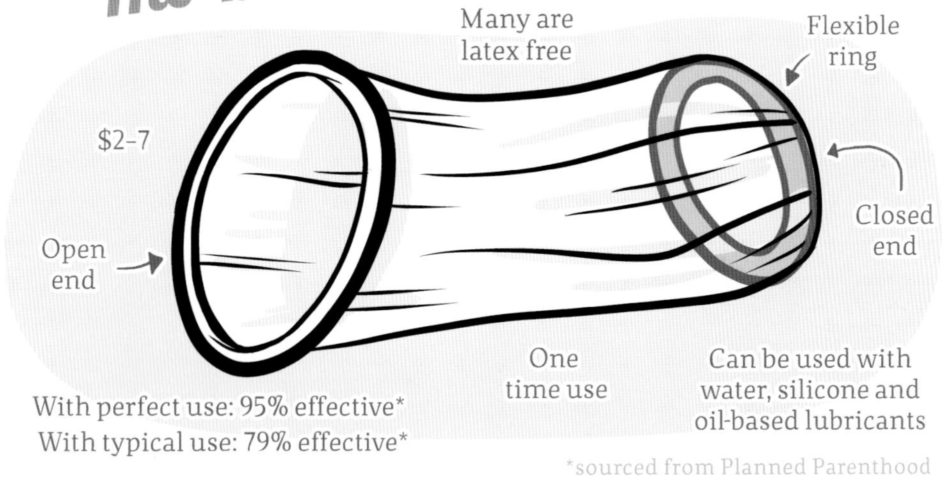
Many are latex free
Flexible ring
$2-7
Closed end
Open end
One time use
Can be used with water, silicone and oil-based lubricants
With perfect use: 95% effective*
With typical use: 79% effective*
*sourced from Planned Parenthood

How does it work?

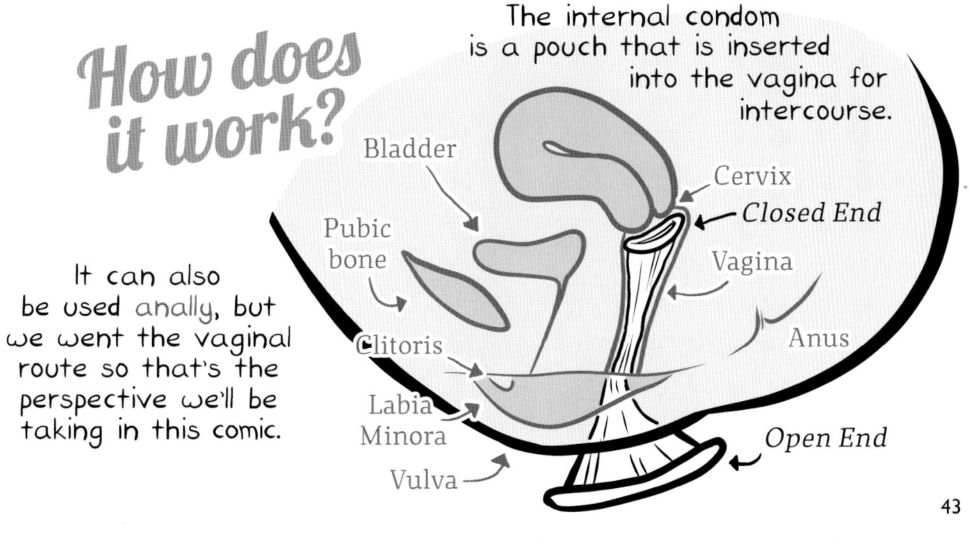
The internal condom is a pouch that is inserted into the vagina for intercourse.
Bladder
Cervix
Closed End
Pubic bone
Vagina
It can also be used anally, but we went the vaginal route so that's the perspective we'll be taking in this comic.
Clitoris
Anus
Labia Minora
Open End
Vulva

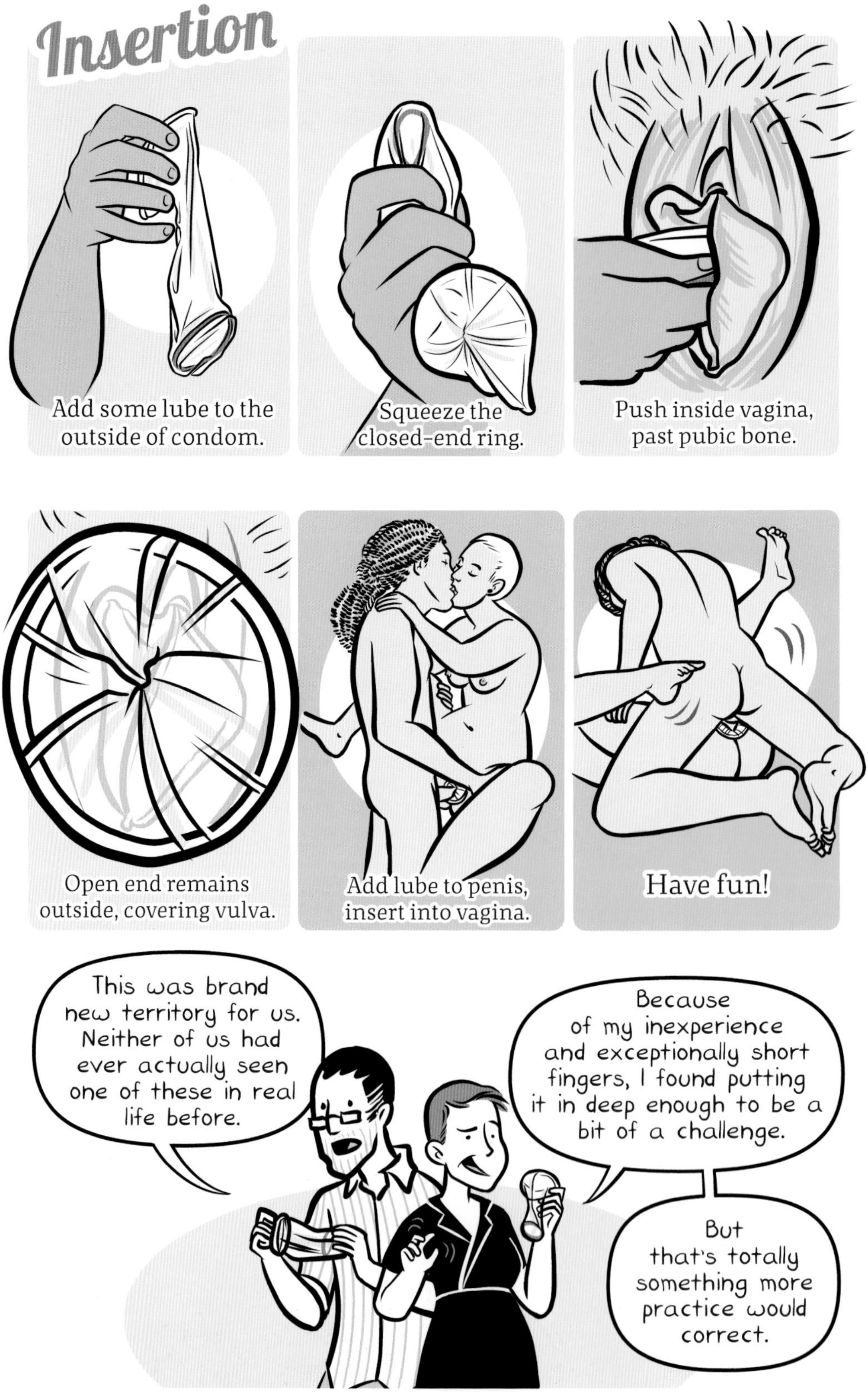
Insertion
Add some lube to the outside of condom.
Squeeze the closed-end ring.
Push inside vagina, past pubic bone.
Open end remains outside, covering vulva.
Add lube to penis, insert into vagina.
Have fun!
This was brand new territory for us. Neither of us had ever actually seen one of these in real life before.
Because of my inexperience and exceptionally short fingers, I found putting it in deep enough to be a bit of a challenge.
But that's totally something more practice would correct.

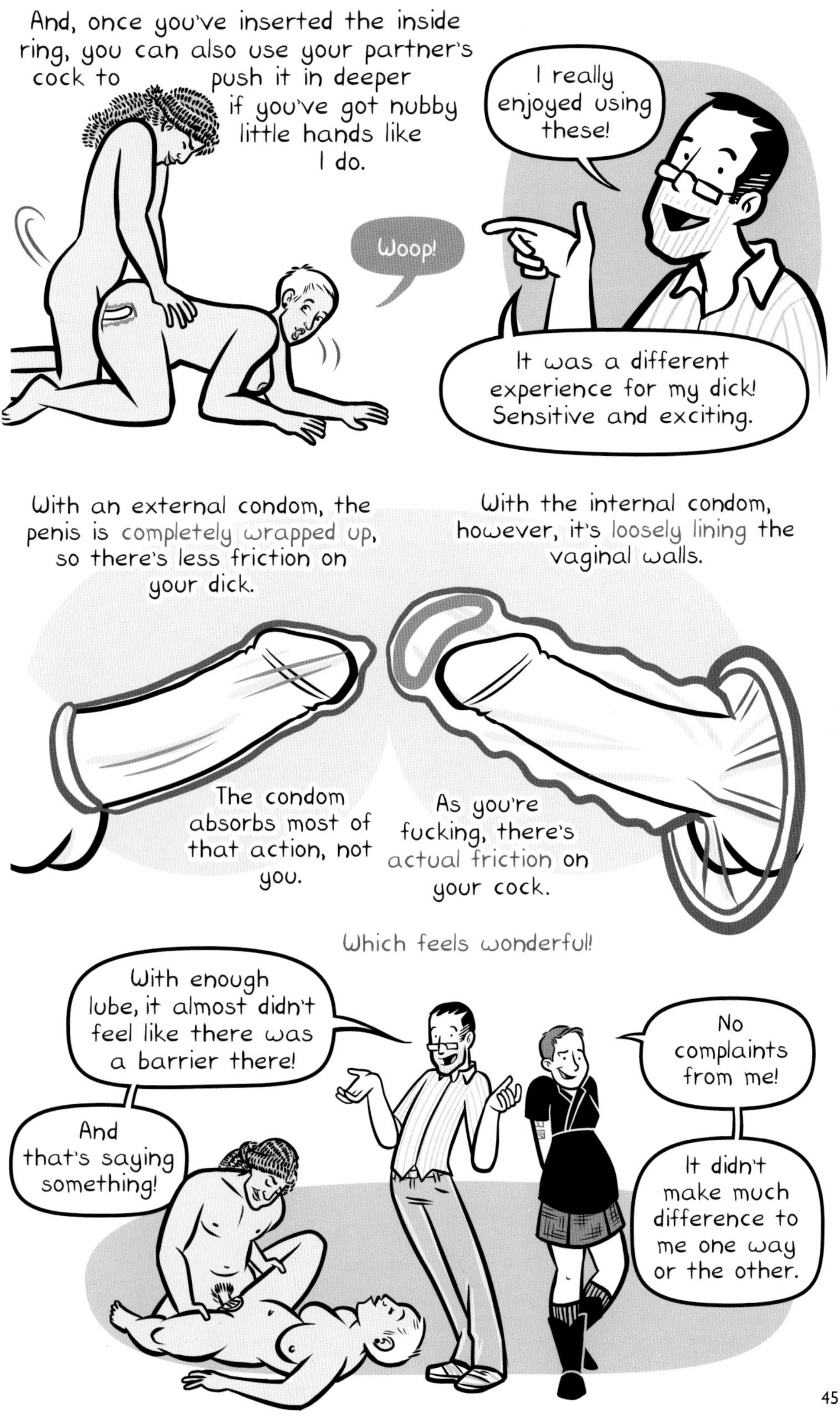

And, once you've inserted the inside ring, you can also use your partner's cock to push it in deeper if you've got nubby little hands like I do.
Woop!
I really enjoyed using these!
It was a different experience for my dick! Sensitive and exciting.
With an external condom, the penis is completely wrapped up, so there's less friction on your dick.
With the internal condom, however, it's loosely lining the vaginal walls.
The condom absorbs most of that action, not you.
As you're fucking, there's actual friction on your cock.
Which feels wonderful!
With enough lube, it almost didn't feel like there was a barrier there!
And that's saying something!
No complaints from me!
It didn't make much difference to me one way or the other.

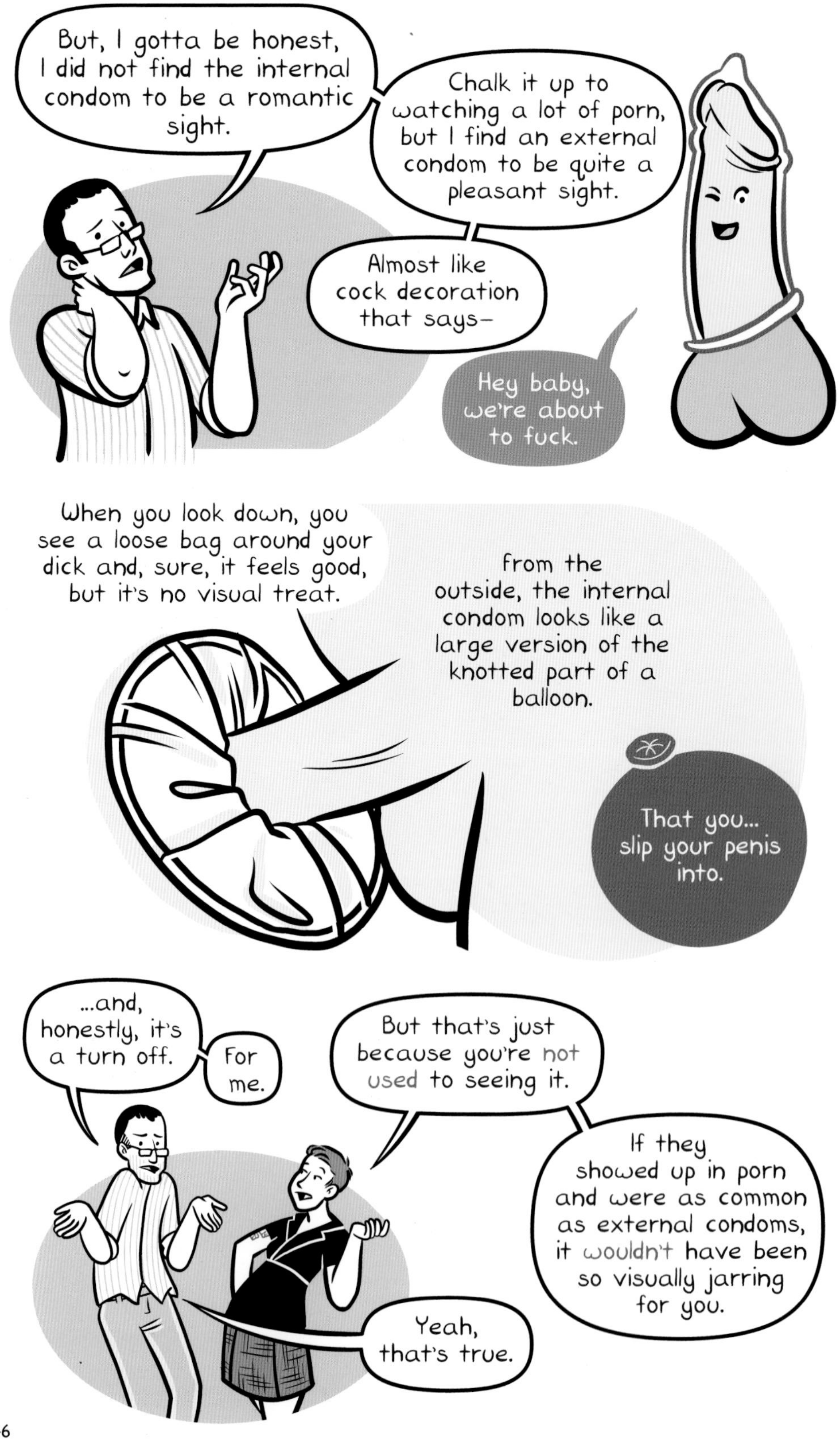
But, I gotta be honest, I did not find the internal condom to be a romantic sight.
Chalk it up to watching a lot of porn, but I find an external condom to be quite a pleasant sight.
Almost like cock decoration that says–
Hey baby, we're about to fuck.
When you look down, you see a loose bag around your dick and, sure, it feels good, but it's no visual treat.
from the outside, the internal condom looks like a large version of the knotted part of a balloon.
That you... slip your penis into.
...and, honestly, it's a turn off.
For me.
But that's just because you're not used to seeing it.
If they showed up in porn and were as common as external condoms, it wouldn't have been so visually jarring for you.
Yeah, that's true.

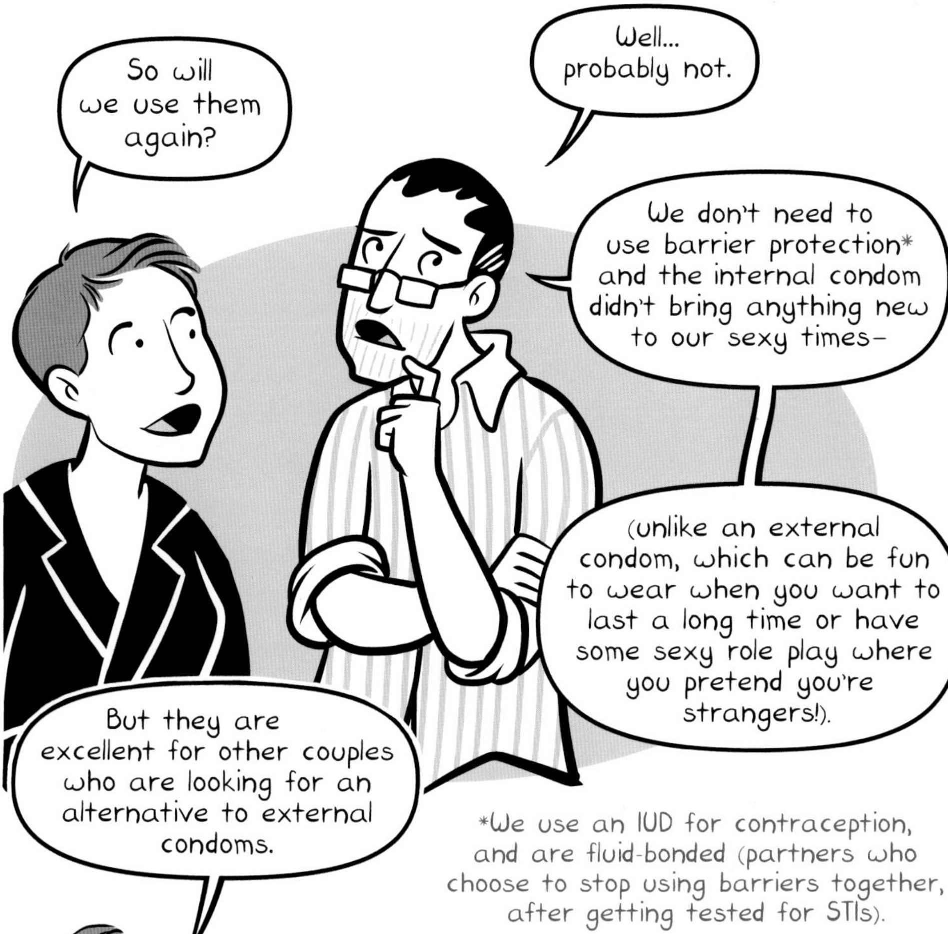
So will we use them again?
Well... probably not.
We don't need to use barrier protection* and the internal condom didn't bring anything new to our sexy times–
(unlike an external condom, which can be fun to wear when you want to last a long time or have some sexy role play where you pretend you're strangers!).
But they are excellent for other couples who are looking for an alternative to external condoms.
*We use an IUD for contraception, and are fluid-bonded (partners who choose to stop using barriers together, after getting tested for STIs).

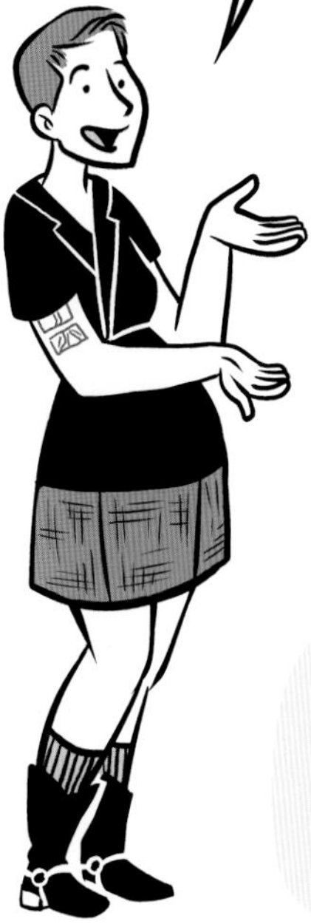

Positives

Increased sensation for the penis-haver

Can be inserted long before any sexy times start, so you don't need to interrupt anything to put on protection

Empowers the vagina-haver to be in charge of protecting themselves, not dependent on the other partner to use protection

Penis does not need to be erect for the condom to be effective (good option for people who have trouble maintaining erections)

Can be used during menstruation

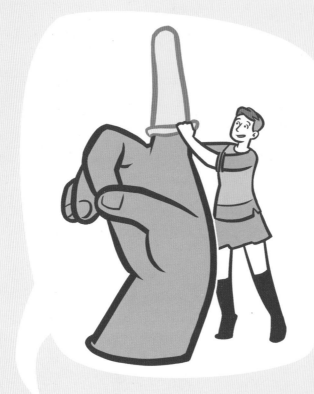

Other Barriers

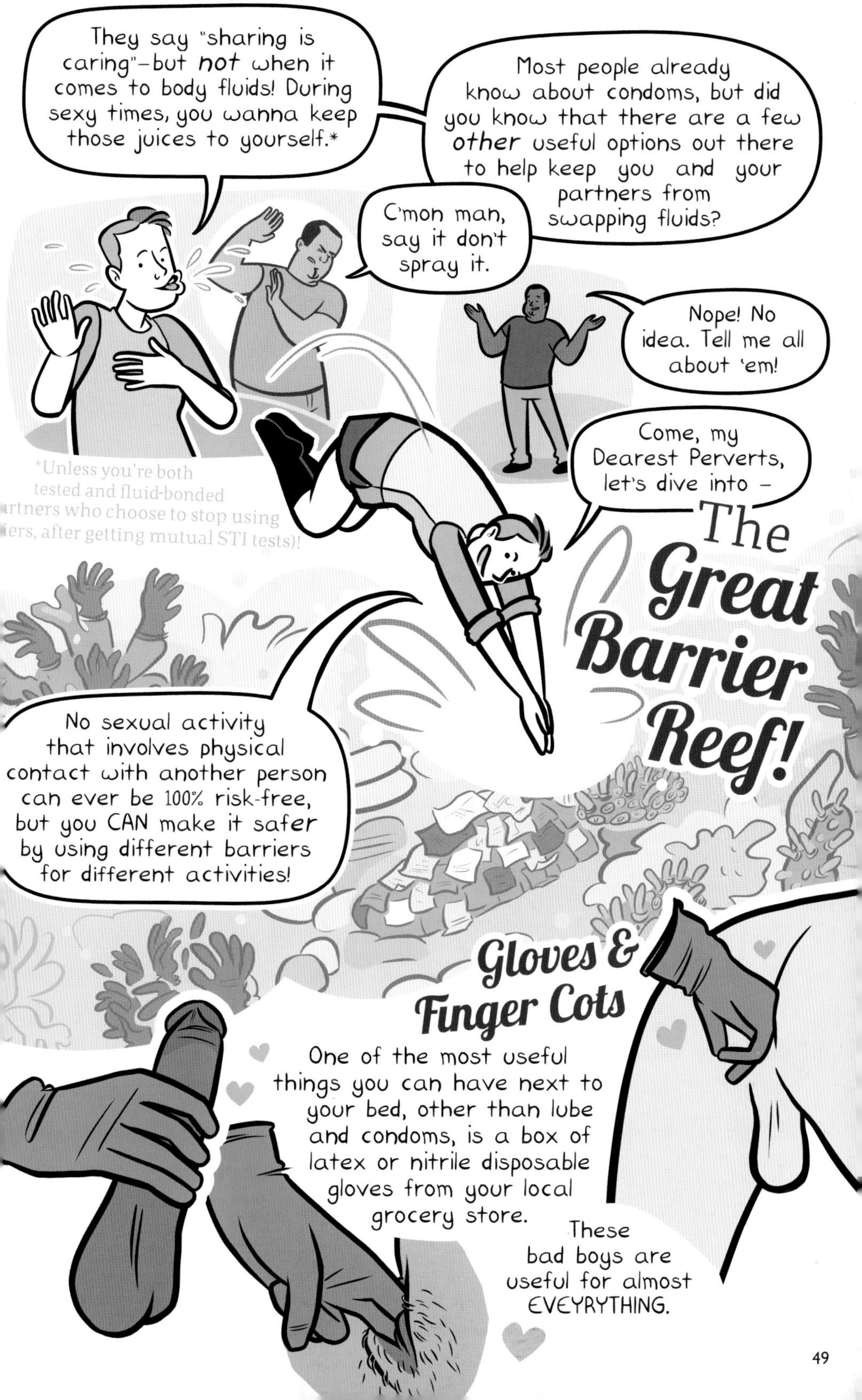

They say "sharing is caring"—but not when it comes to body fluids! During sexy times, you wanna keep those juices to yourself.*
Most people already know about condoms, but did you know that there are a few other useful options out there to help keep you and your partners from swapping fluids?
C'mon man, say it don't spray it.
Nope! No idea. Tell me all about 'em!
Come, my Dearest Perverts, let's dive into –
The Great Barrier Reef!
*Unless you're both tested and fluid-bonded
rtners who choose to stop using
iers, after getting mutual STI tests)!
No sexual activity that involves physical contact with another person can ever be 100% risk-free, but you CAN make it safer by using different barriers for different activities!
Gloves & Finger Cots
One of the most useful things you can have next to your bed, other than lube and condoms, is a box of latex or nitrile disposable gloves from your local grocery store.
These bad boys are useful for almost EVEYRYTHING.

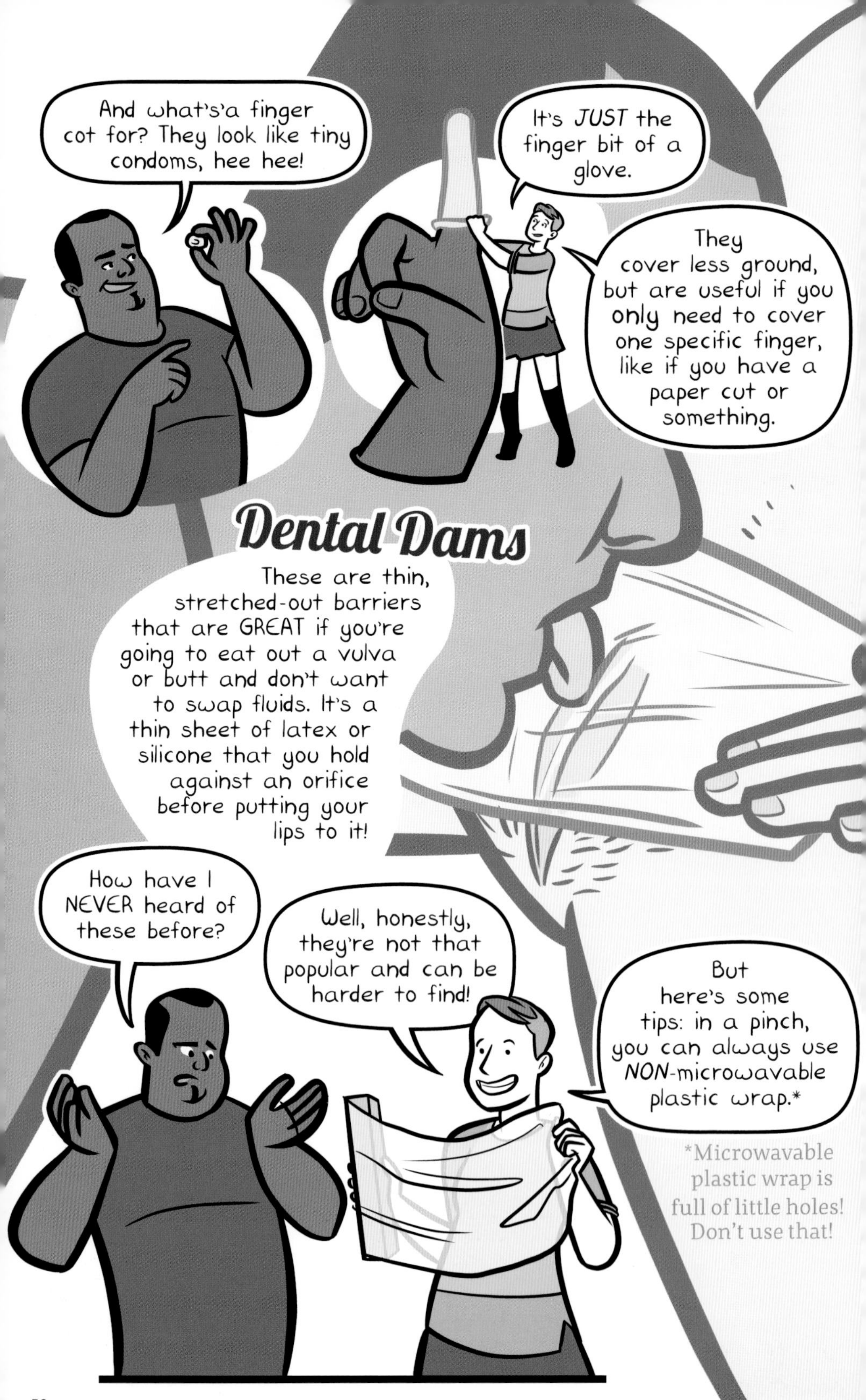
And what's'a finger cot for? They look like tiny condoms, hee hee!
It's *JUST* the finger bit of a glove.
They cover less ground, but are useful if you only need to cover one specific finger, like if you have a paper cut or something.
Dental Dams
These are thin, stretched-out barriers that are GREAT if you're going to eat out a vulva or butt and don't want to swap fluids. It's a thin sheet of latex or silicone that you hold against an orifice before putting your lips to it!
How have I NEVER heard of these before?
Well, honestly, they're not that popular and can be harder to find!
But here's some tips: in a pinch, you can always use *NON*-microwavable plastic wrap.*
*Microwavable plastic wrap is full of little holes! Don't use that!

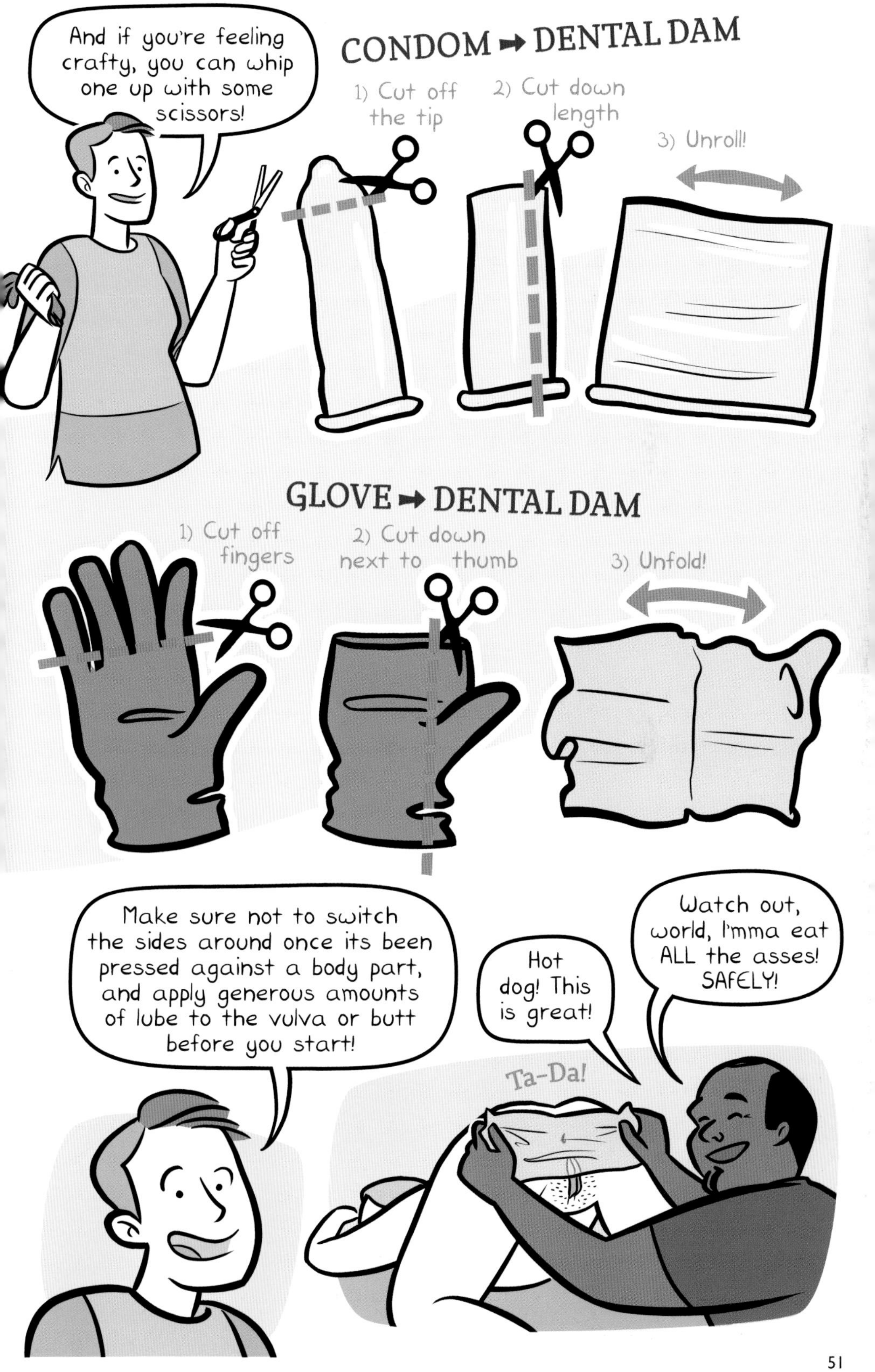

And if you're feeling crafty, you can whip one up with some scissors!
CONDOM ➡ DENTAL DAM
1) Cut off the tip
2) Cut down length
3) Unroll!
GLOVE ➡ DENTAL DAM
1) Cut off fingers
2) Cut down next to thumb
3) Unfold!
Make sure not to switch the sides around once its been pressed against a body part, and apply generous amounts of lube to the vulva or butt before you start!
Hot dog! This is great!
Watch out, world, I'mma eat ALL the asses! SAFELY!
Ta-Da!

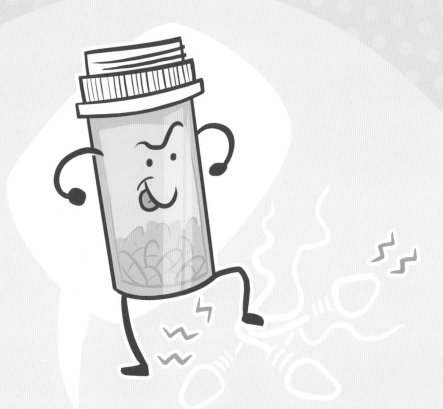

The Pill

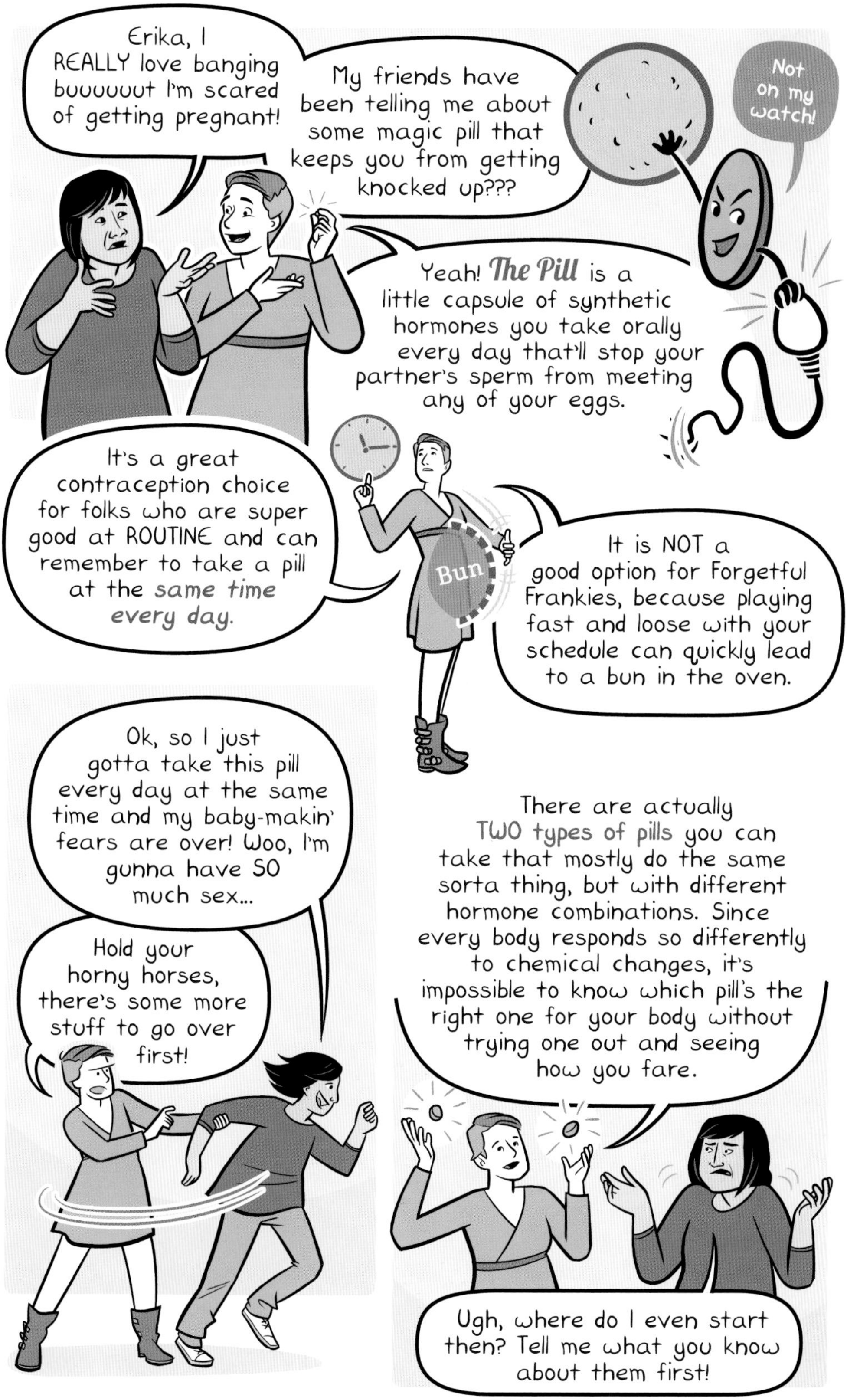

Erika, I REALLY love banging buuuuuut I'm scared of getting pregnant!
My friends have been telling me about some magic pill that keeps you from getting knocked up???
Not on my watch!
Yeah! The Pill is a little capsule of synthetic hormones you take orally every day that'll stop your partner's sperm from meeting any of your eggs.
It's a great contraception choice for folks who are super good at ROUTINE and can remember to take a pill at the same time every day.
Bun
It is NOT a good option for Forgetful Frankies, because playing fast and loose with your schedule can quickly lead to a bun in the oven.
Ok, so I just gotta take this pill every day at the same time and my baby-makin' fears are over! Woo, I'm gunna have SO much sex...
Hold your horny horses, there's some more stuff to go over first!
There are actually TWO types of pills you can take that mostly do the same sorta thing, but with different hormone combinations. Since every body responds so differently to chemical changes, it's impossible to know which pill's the right one for your body without trying one out and seeing how you fare.
Ugh, where do I even start then? Tell me what you know about them first!

Keep in mind this is surface-level information, so you should definitely go do more in-depth research at PlannedParenthood.org and Scarleteen.com annnnnd hella talk with your doc!

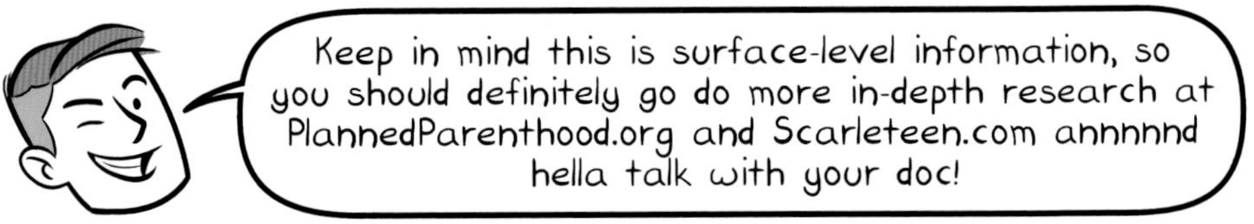

Combination Pill
(Estrogen and progestin hormones)

Taken orally every day, ***roughly*** around the same time.

12 hour grace period before the pill is late

Minipill
(Progestin-Only)

Taken orally every day ***at the same time.***

3 hour grace period before the pill is late.

Effectiveness:

Combination Pill

Perfect Use:
99.7%
(Less than 1 out of 100 folks will get pregnant in a year)

Typical Use:
91%
(9 out of 100 folks will get pregnant in a year)

Minipill

Typical Use:
90%
(10 out of 100 folks will get pregnant in a year)

Perfect Use:
99+%
(Less than 1 out of 100 folks will get pregnant in a year)

*Sourced from Scarleteen

How it Works:

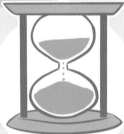

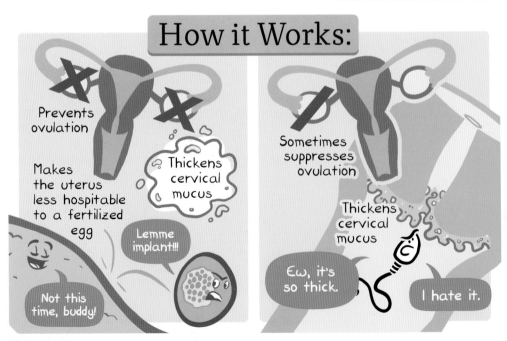

Prevents ovulation
Thickens cervical mucus
Makes the uterus less hospitable to a fertilized egg
Lemme implant!!!
Not this time, buddy!

Sometimes suppresses ovulation
Thickens cervical mucus
Ew, it's so thick.
I hate it.

Possible Side Effects:

Combination Pill

More regulated monthly bleeding, lighter periods, less cramping, decreased PMS symptoms, vaginal dryness, skin changes, spotting, nausea, headaches, tender breasts, mood changes, decreased sexual desire, weight gain, possibly more yeast infections, and it can take longer to conceive after quitting the pill.

Minipill

Reduced or straight up absent periods, unpredictable spotting, less cramping, decreased PMS symptoms, weight gain, more yeast infections, and an increased risk of ovarian cysts.

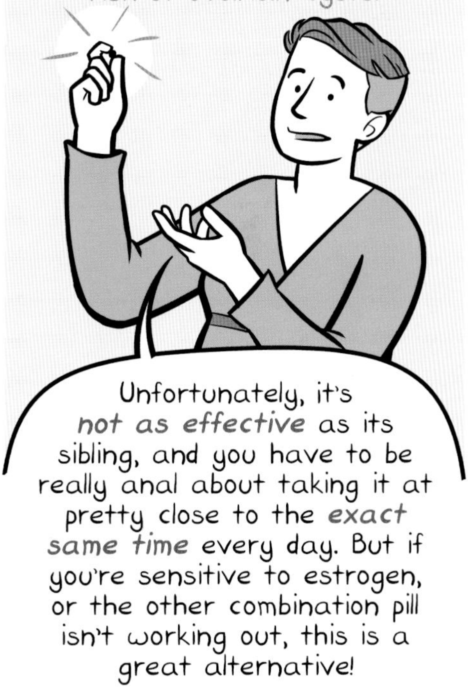
Unfortunately, it's *not as effective* as its sibling, and you have to be really anal about taking it at pretty close to the *exact same time* every day. But if you're sensitive to estrogen, or the other combination pill isn't working out, this is a great alternative!

The combination pill is NOT for you if you...

Smoke and are over 35, get migraines, breastfeed, know you are sensitive to estrogens, have had bad experiences on hormonal birth control that contained estrogen.

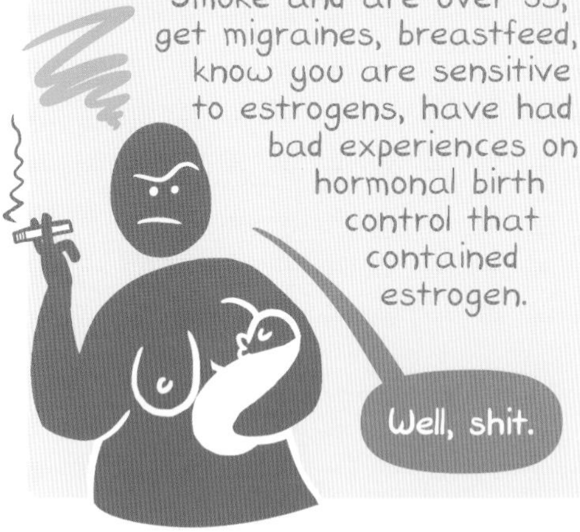
Well, shit.

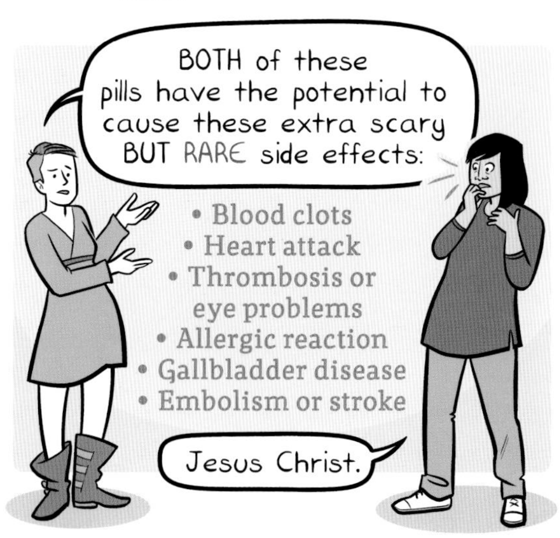
BOTH of these pills have the potential to cause these extra scary BUT RARE side effects:
• Blood clots
• Heart attack
• Thrombosis or eye problems
• Allergic reaction
• Gallbladder disease
• Embolism or stroke
Jesus Christ.

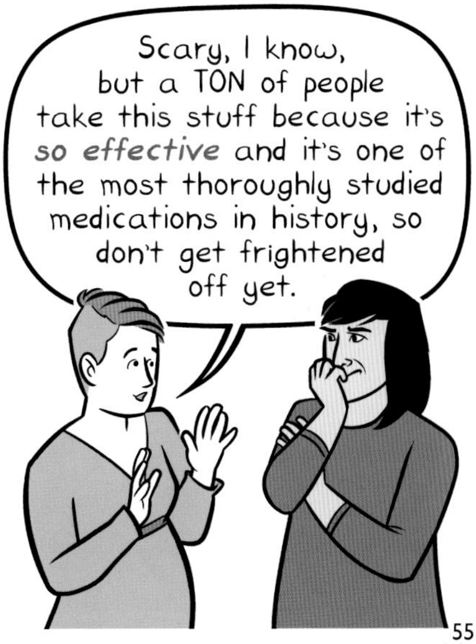
Scary, I know, but a TON of people take this stuff because it's *so effective* and it's one of the most thoroughly studied medications in history, so don't get frightened off yet.

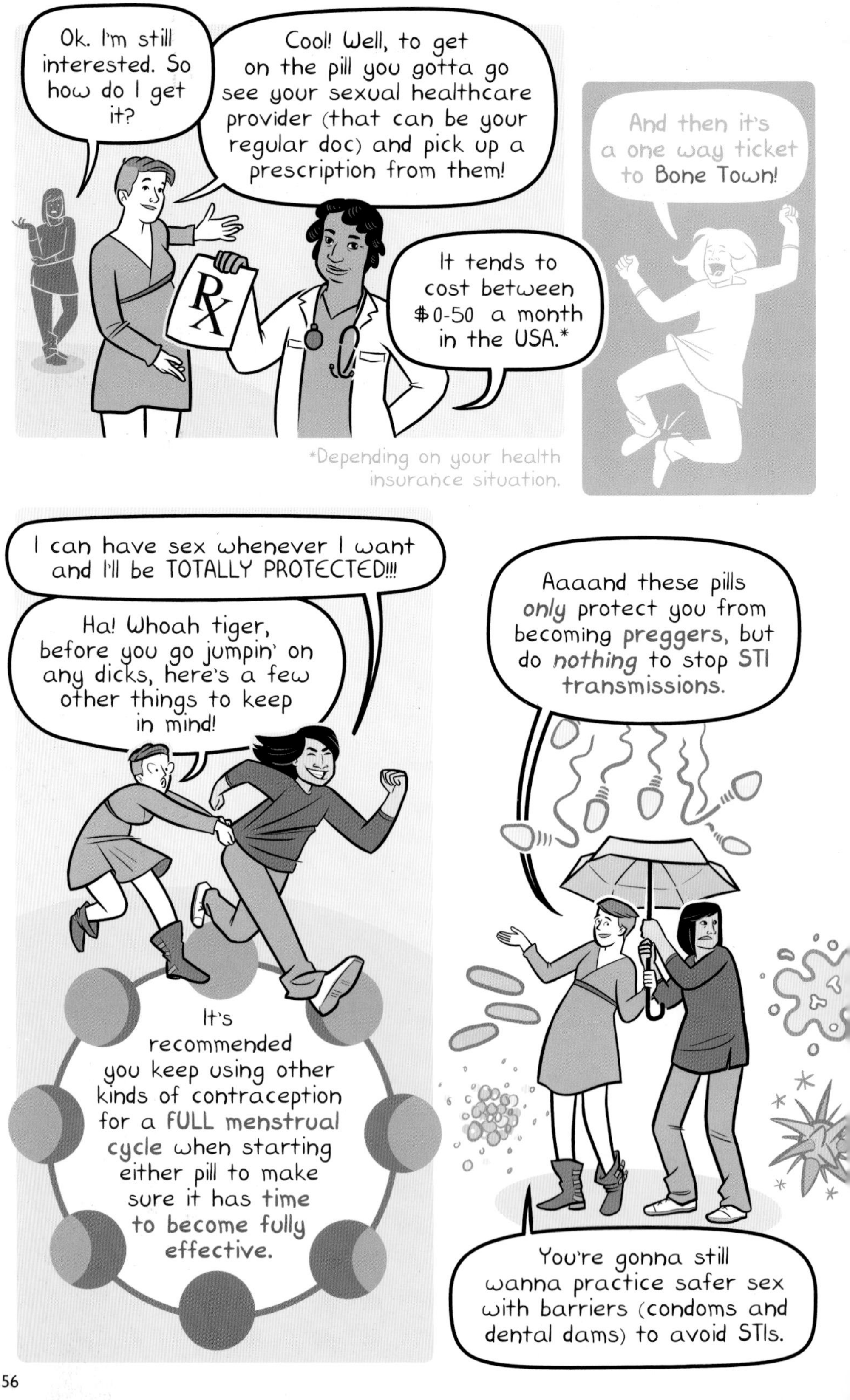
Ok. I'm still interested. So how do I get it?
Cool! Well, to get on the pill you gotta go see your sexual healthcare provider (that can be your regular doc) and pick up a prescription from them!
RX
It tends to cost between $0-50 a month in the USA.*
*Depending on your health insurance situation.
And then it's a one way ticket to Bone Town!
I can have sex whenever I want and I'll be TOTALLY PROTECTED!!!
Ha! Whoah tiger, before you go jumpin' on any dicks, here's a few other things to keep in mind!
It's recommended you keep using other kinds of contraception for a FULL menstrual cycle when starting either pill to make sure it has time to become fully effective.
Aaaand these pills only protect you from becoming preggers, but do nothing to stop STI transmissions.
You're gonna still wanna practice safer sex with barriers (condoms and dental dams) to avoid STIs.

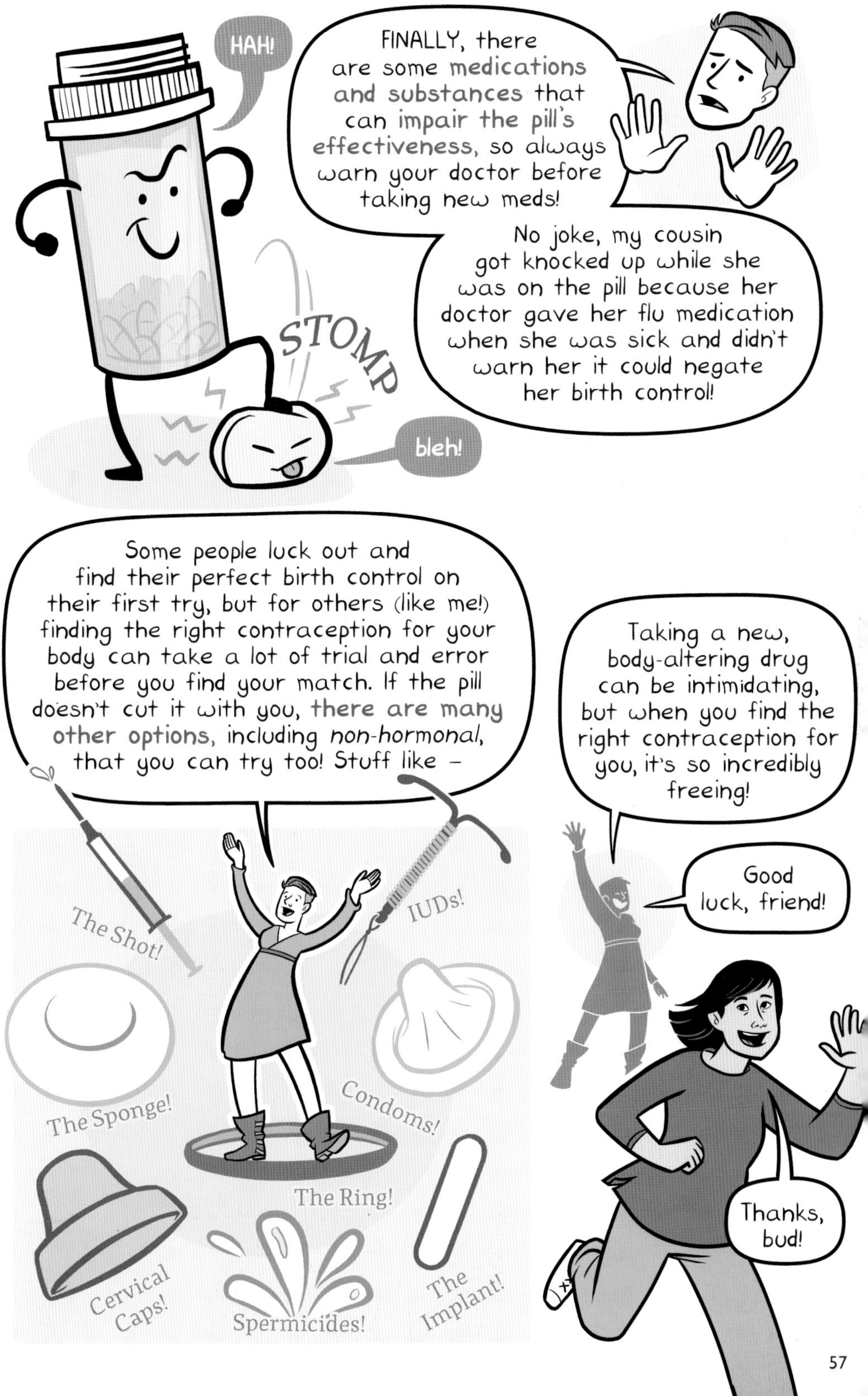
HAH!
FINALLY, there are some medications and substances that can impair the pill's effectiveness, so always warn your doctor before taking new meds!
No joke, my cousin got knocked up while she was on the pill because her doctor gave her flu medication when she was sick and didn't warn her it could negate her birth control!
STOMP
bleh!
Some people luck out and find their perfect birth control on their first try, but for others (like me!) finding the right contraception for your body can take a lot of trial and error before you find your match. If the pill doesn't cut it with you, there are many other options, including non-hormonal, that you can try too! Stuff like –
The Shot!
IUDs!
The Sponge!
Condoms!
The Ring!
Cervical Caps!
Spermicides!
The Implant!
Taking a new, body-altering drug can be intimidating, but when you find the right contraception for you, it's so incredibly freeing!
Good luck, friend!
Thanks, bud!

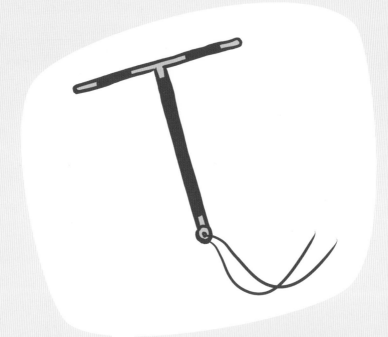

Copper IUD

For many years, I only dated folks with vaginas, which meant the only things I had to worry about were STIs and squeezing boobs too hard.

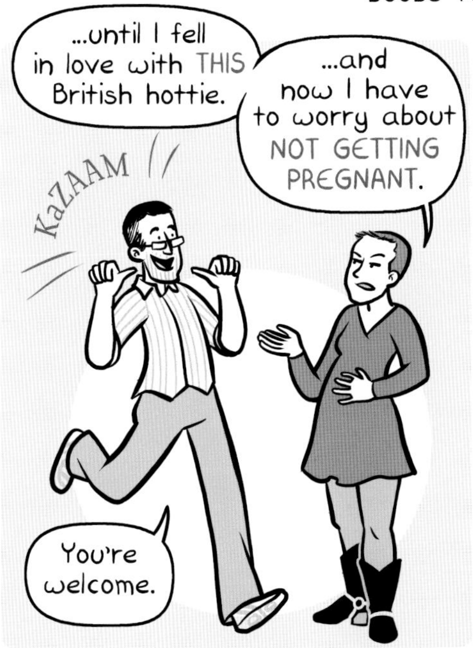
...until I fell in love with THIS British hottie.
...and now I have to worry about NOT GETTING PREGNANT.
KaZAAM
You're welcome.

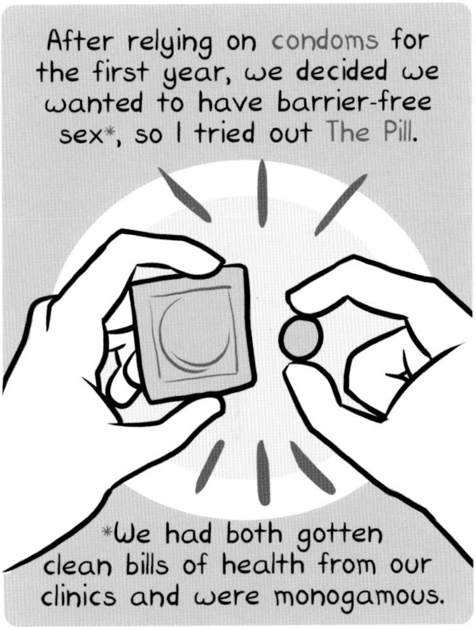
After relying on condoms for the first year, we decided we wanted to have barrier-free sex*, so I tried out The Pill.
*We had both gotten clean bills of health from our clinics and were monogamous.

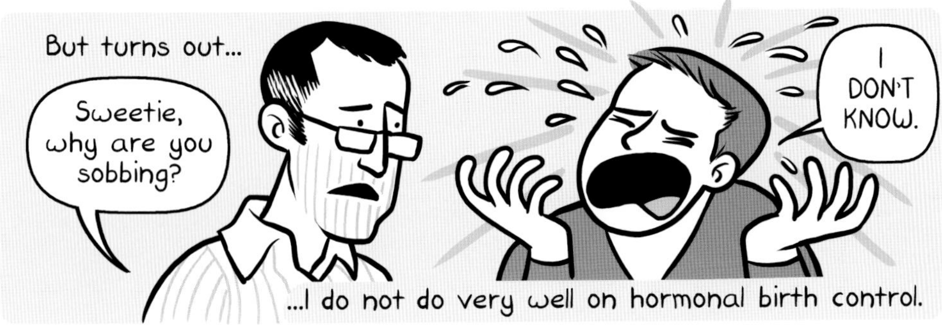
But turns out...
Sweetie, why are you sobbing?
I DON'T KNOW.
...I do not do very well on hormonal birth control.

So in 2006, I decided to try out a...

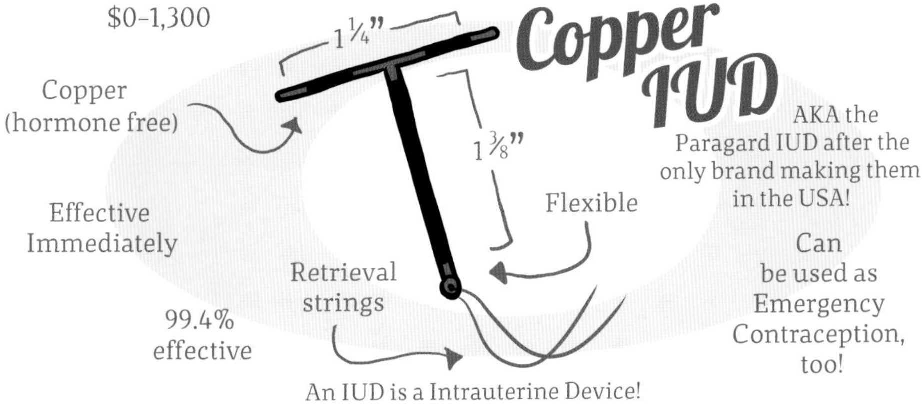
Copper IUD
$0-1,300
1¼"
1⅜"
Copper (hormone free)
Effective Immediately
99.4% effective
Retrieval strings
Flexible
AKA the Paragard IUD after the only brand making them in the USA!
Can be used as Emergency Contraception, too!
An IUD is a Intrauterine Device!

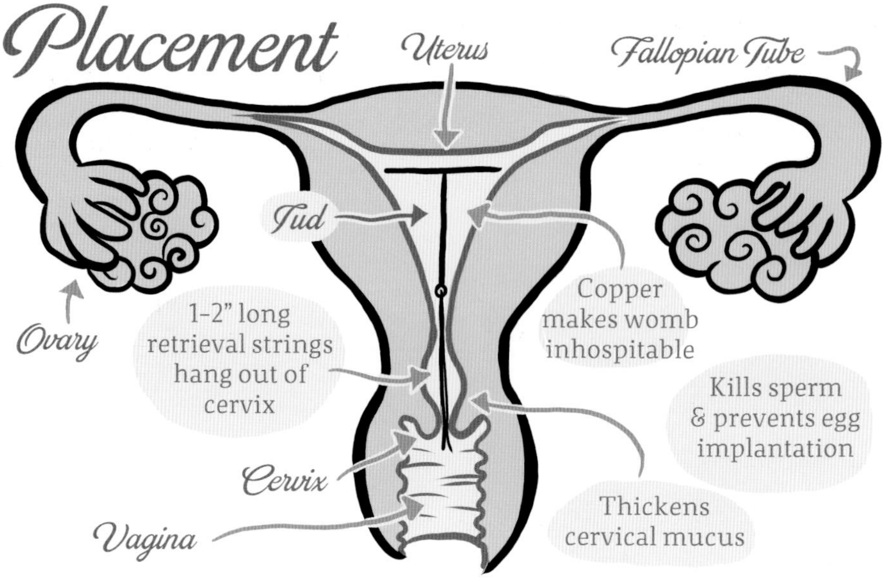
Placement
Uterus
Fallopian Tube
Iud
Ovary
1-2" long retrieval strings hang out of cervix
Copper makes womb inhospitable
Kills sperm & prevents egg implantation
Cervix
Vagina
Thickens cervical mucus

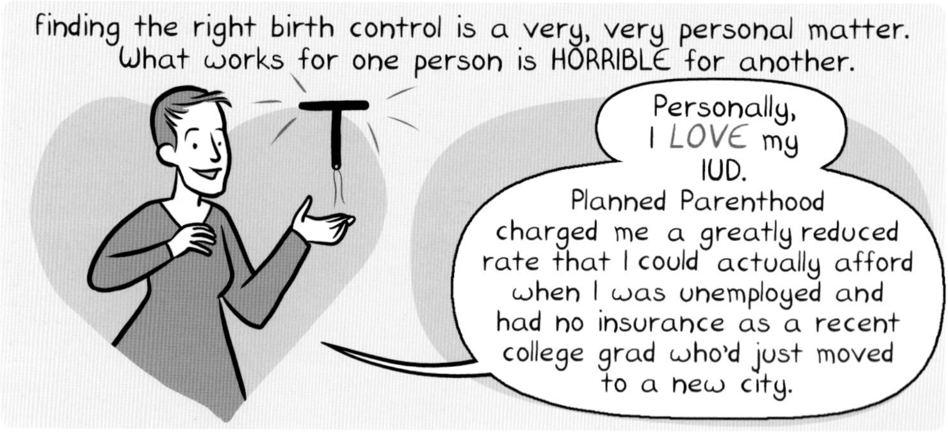
finding the right birth control is a very, very personal matter. What works for one person is HORRIBLE for another.
Personally, I LOVE my IUD. Planned Parenthood charged me a greatly reduced rate that I could actually afford when I was unemployed and had no insurance as a recent college grad who'd just moved to a new city.

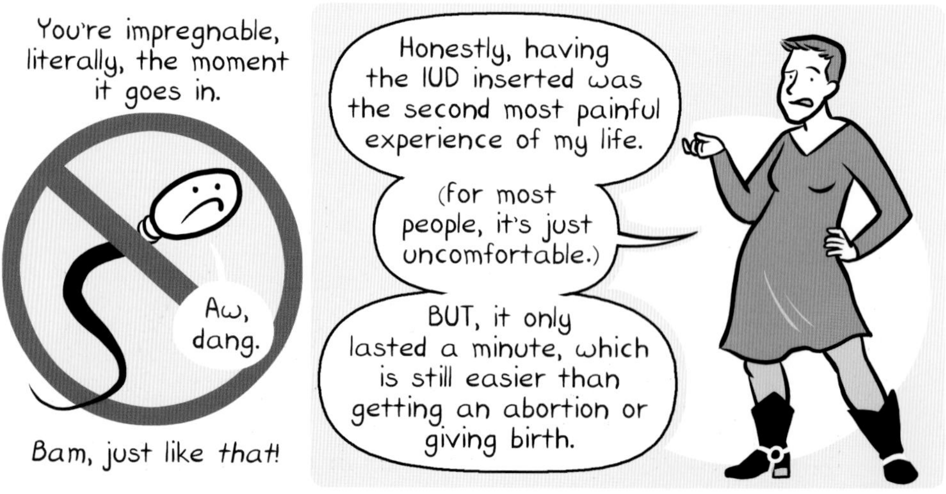
You're impregnable, literally, the moment it goes in.
Aw, dang.
Bam, just like that!
Honestly, having the IUD inserted was the second most painful experience of my life.
(for most people, it's just uncomfortable.)
BUT, it only lasted a minute, which is still easier than getting an abortion or giving birth.

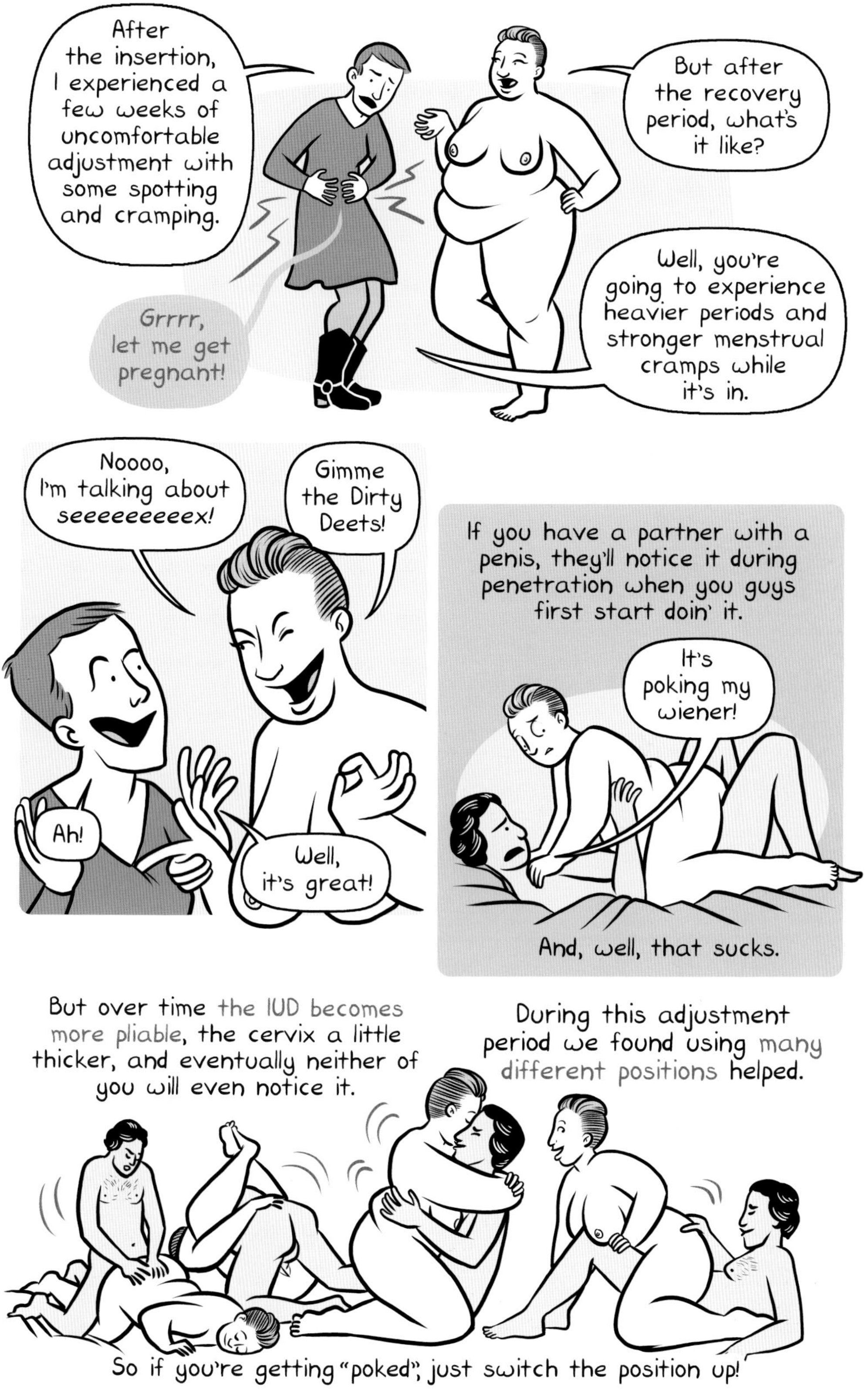

After the insertion, I experienced a few weeks of uncomfortable adjustment with some spotting and cramping.
But after the recovery period, what's it like?
Grrrr, let me get pregnant!
Well, you're going to experience heavier periods and stronger menstrual cramps while it's in.
Noooo, I'm talking about seeeeeeeeex!
Gimme the Dirty Deets!
Ah!
Well, it's great!
If you have a partner with a penis, they'll notice it during penetration when you guys first start doin' it.
It's poking my wiener!
And, well, that sucks.
But over time the IUD becomes more pliable, the cervix a little thicker, and eventually neither of you will even notice it.
During this adjustment period we found using many different positions helped.
So if you're getting "poked", just switch the position up!

Is there a faster way to speed up softening it that won't poke my penis?
Time to BREAK OUT THE DILDOS, my friend!
Wobble Wobble
That's your solution to *everything*, Erika.

How do I know if a copper IUD is right for me?
Well, let's look at the pros and cons.

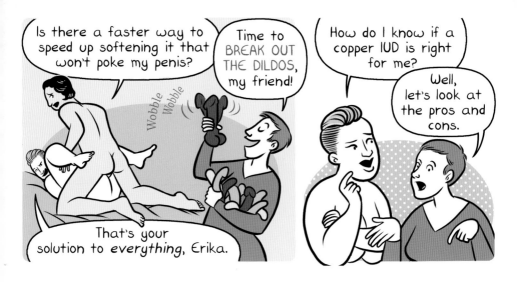

Pros

ULTRA effective at preventing pregnancy (99.4% with perfect & typical use)

One insertion lasts 10-12 years, don't have to worry about administrating daily / weekly / monthly dosages

SUPER cost-effective: long-term it's *the* cheapest contraceptive option

Hormone-free, good for the biologically sensitive

No maintenance. It's in, forget about it

Totally reversible, you're fertile as soon as it's out

Cons

Up-front cost is expensive (But it's the *only* payment you'll make on it)

Doctor needed to insert & remove it

Uncomfortable / painful insertion

More difficult periods

IUD strings might poke partner's penis during intercourse at first (they soften up over time)

Higher chance of rejection if you've never been pregnant before

If the IUD breaks or fails, it's a horror show (ectopic pregnancy, torn womb)

Sourced from Planned Parenthood & Paragard

Is it the right birth control for me?
Yes!
My Paragard IUD has made my life so easy and stress-free.
Will it be right for you?
Maybe!
Talk with your doc and do what feels right for you.

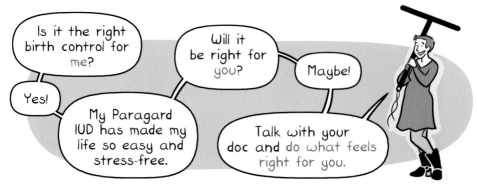

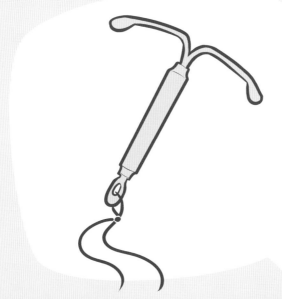

Hormonal IUD

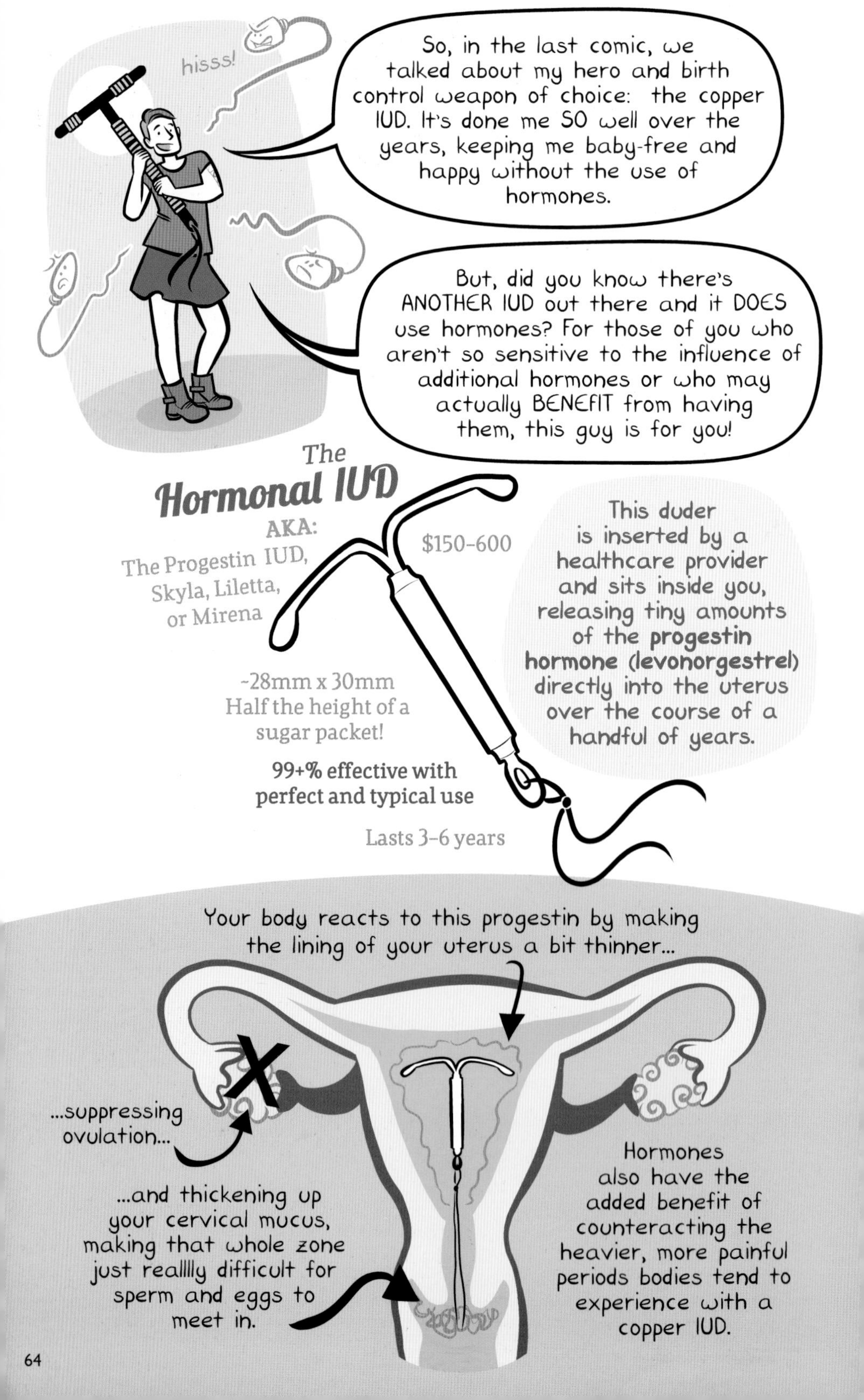
hisss!
So, in the last comic, we talked about my hero and birth control weapon of choice: the copper IUD. It's done me SO well over the years, keeping me baby-free and happy without the use of hormones.
But, did you know there's ANOTHER IUD out there and it DOES use hormones? For those of you who aren't so sensitive to the influence of additional hormones or who may actually BENEFIT from having them, this guy is for you!
The Hormonal IUD
AKA:
The Progestin IUD, Skyla, Liletta, or Mirena
$150–600
This duder is inserted by a healthcare provider and sits inside you, releasing tiny amounts of the **progestin hormone (levonorgestrel)** directly into the uterus over the course of a handful of years.
~28mm x 30mm
Half the height of a sugar packet!
99+% effective with perfect and typical use
Lasts 3–6 years
Your body reacts to this progestin by making the lining of your uterus a bit thinner...
...suppressing ovulation...
...and thickening up your cervical mucus, making that whole zone just realllly difficult for sperm and eggs to meet in.
Hormones also have the added benefit of counteracting the heavier, more painful periods bodies tend to experience with a copper IUD.

Because it has NO estrogen and the hormone release is localized to your uterus and not into your blood (like the pill does), folks using it typically experience fewer side effects than other hormonal birth controls.

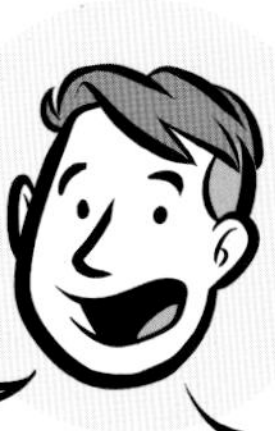

Even tiny doses of hormones can have significant good and bad side effects, so let's go over them!

Pro

–Can reduce menstrual pain and cramping!
–Will reduce menstrual bleeding (great if you suffer from anemia!)
–Can reduce your risk of getting pelvic infections and endometrial cancer
–Cost effective (over long term)
–Constant coverage for years
–Easily reversible

Pro/Con?

–Can decrease or stop periods over time, but can also make them really inconsistent and hard to track, which can be scary for some (About 20% of people stop having periods after one year of using a Mirena – neato!)
–Immediately effective if implanted during a menstrual period, otherwise it takes a week to come online
–Thins your uterus lining which can be good if you have thicker than usual lining or abnormal growth, but bad if your uterus lining is too thin already

Con

–Headaches
–Acne
–Breast tenderness
–Irregular bleeding (which tends to improve after six months of use)
–Mood changes
–Cramping or pelvic pain
–Doesn't protect against STIs
–First few weeks can be very uncomfortable while it settles in
–Potential for scary things like perforation during implant, and if you DO get pregnant it'll be more than likely epicly bad (like an ectopic pregnancy)
–Uncomfortable implantation for small cervix or shallow wombs havers - like in younger folk, and those who've not ever been pregnant

And finally, you probably should **avoid it** if you have breast, uterine or cervical cancer (past or present), vaginal not-menstrual-related bleeding, liver disease, an abortion in the last three months, allergies or sensitivity to levonorgestrel/progestin.

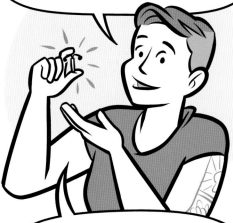

Do some more research on your own and talk with your healthcare provider to figure out if this may be the right BC for you! Good luck!

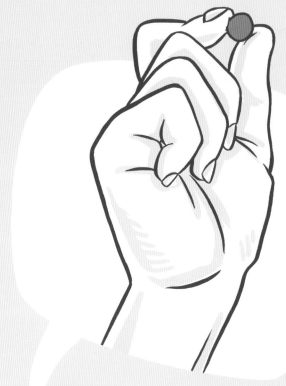

Emergency
Contraception

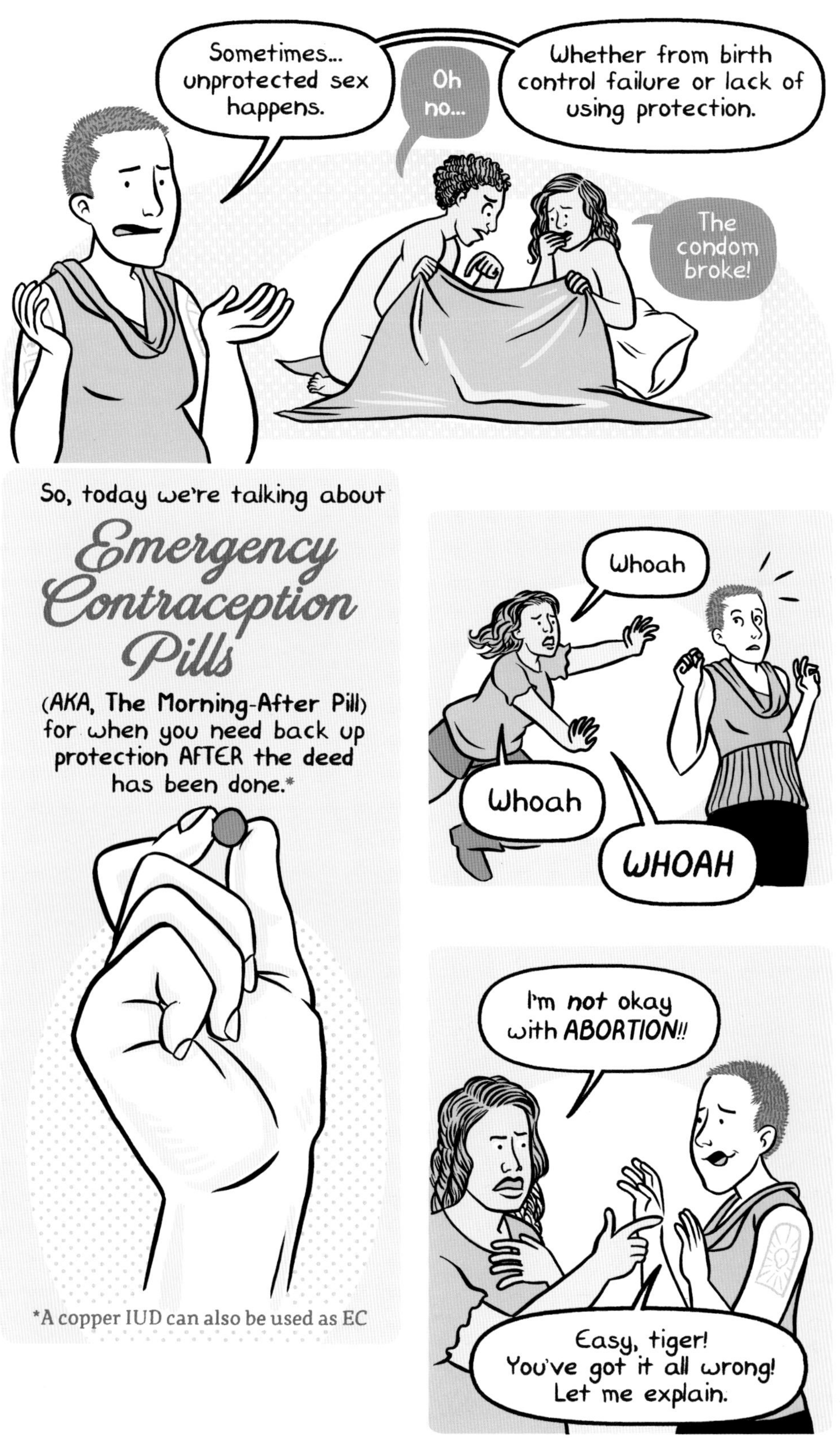
Sometimes... unprotected sex happens.
Oh no...
Whether from birth control failure or lack of using protection.
The condom broke!
So, today we're talking about
Emergency Contraception Pills
(AKA, The Morning-After Pill) for when you need back up protection AFTER the deed has been done.*
Whoah
Whoah
WHOAH
I'm not okay with ABORTION!!
Easy, tiger! You've got it all wrong! Let me explain.

*A copper IUD can also be used as EC

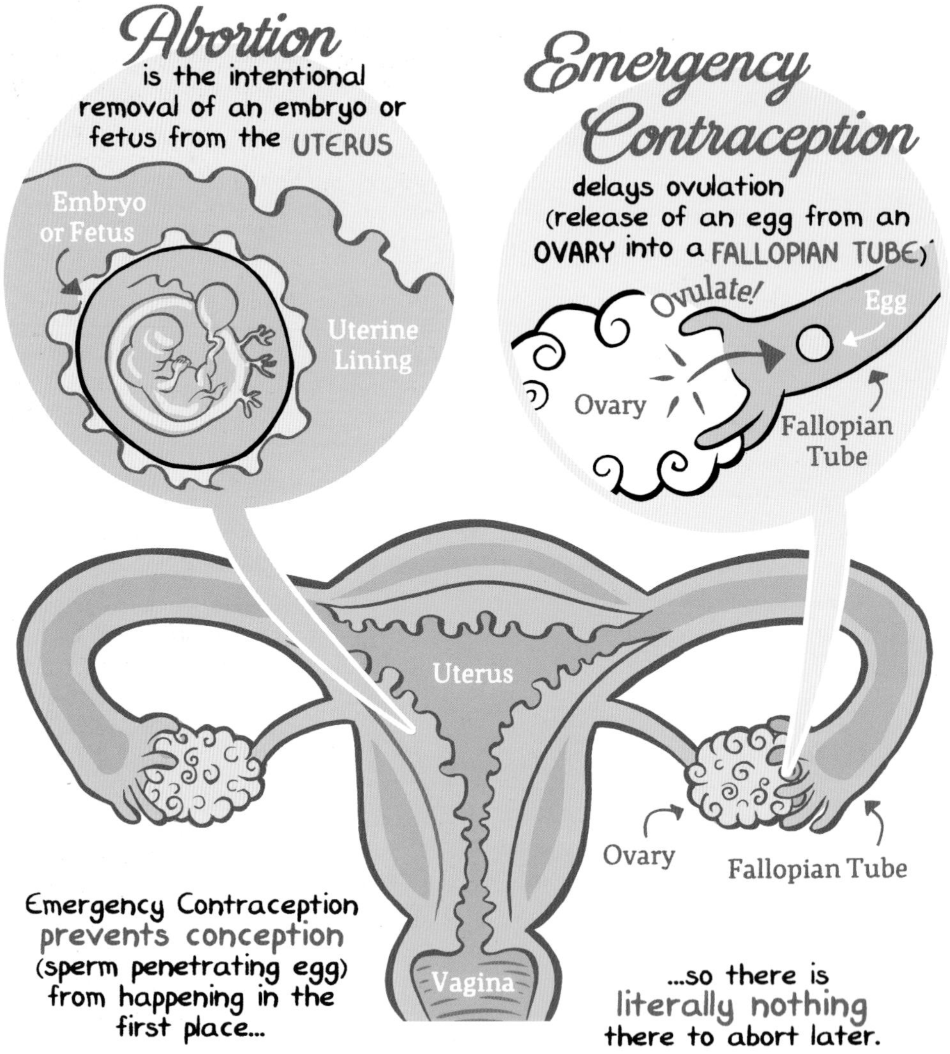
Abortion
is the intentional removal of an embryo or fetus from the UTERUS
Embryo or Fetus
Uterine Lining
Emergency Contraception
delays ovulation (release of an egg from an OVARY into a FALLOPIAN TUBE)
Ovulate!
Egg
Ovary
Fallopian Tube
Uterus
Ovary
Fallopian Tube
Vagina
Emergency Contraception prevents conception (sperm penetrating egg) from happening in the first place...
...so there is literally nothing there to abort later.

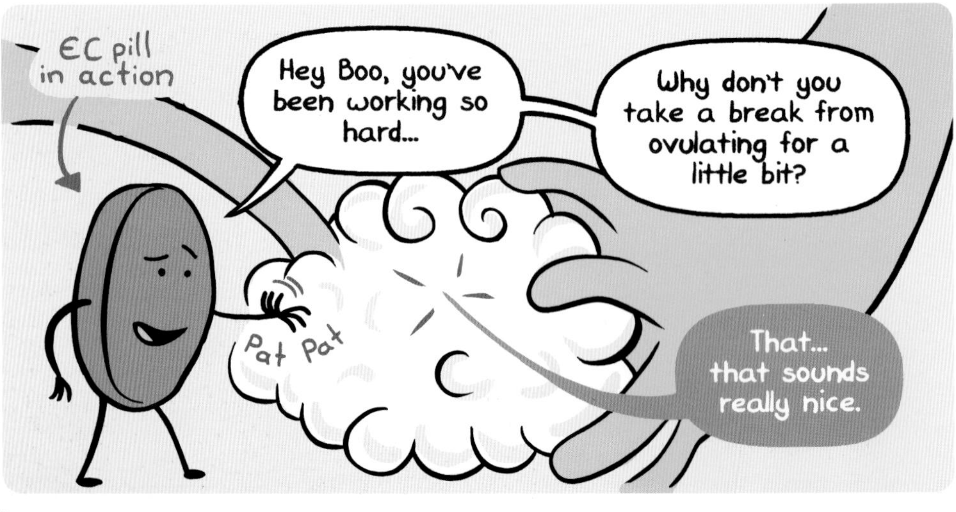
EC pill in action
Hey Boo, you've been working so hard...
Why don't you take a break from ovulating for a little bit?
Pat Pat
That... that sounds really nice.

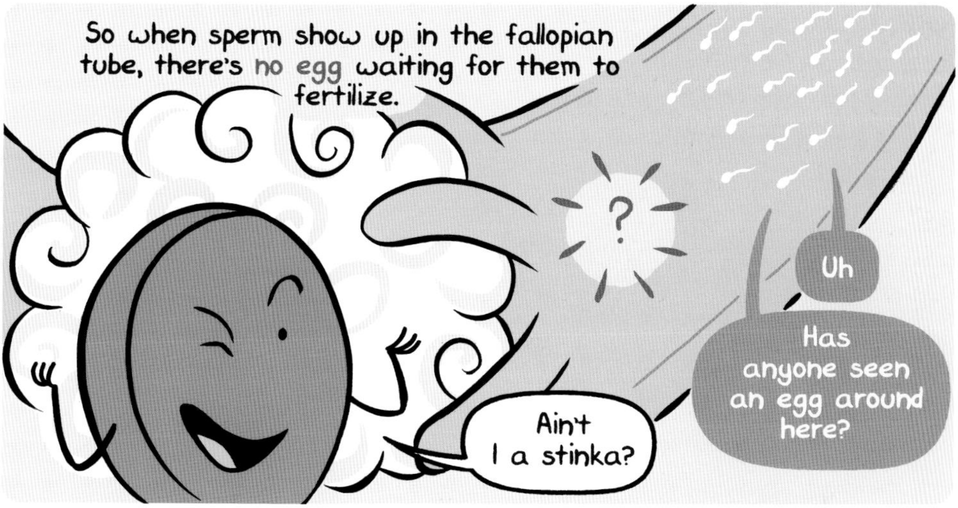
So when sperm show up in the fallopian tube, there's no egg waiting for them to fertilize.
?
Ain't I a stinka?
Uh
Has anyone seen an egg around here?

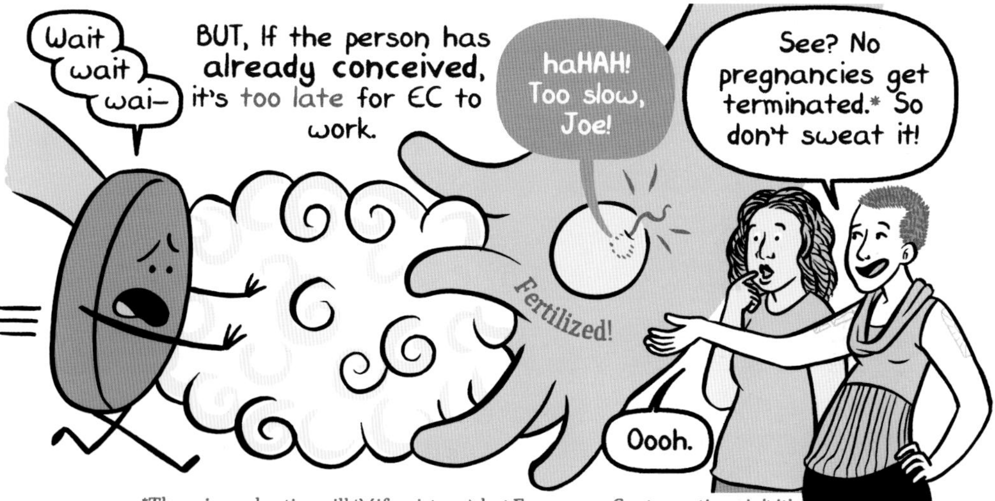
Wait wait wai–
BUT, If the person has already conceived, it's too late for EC to work.
haHAH! Too slow, Joe!
See? No pregnancies get terminated.* So don't sweat it!
Fertilized!
Oooh.

*There *is* an abortion pill (Mifepristone), but Emergency Contraception ain't it!

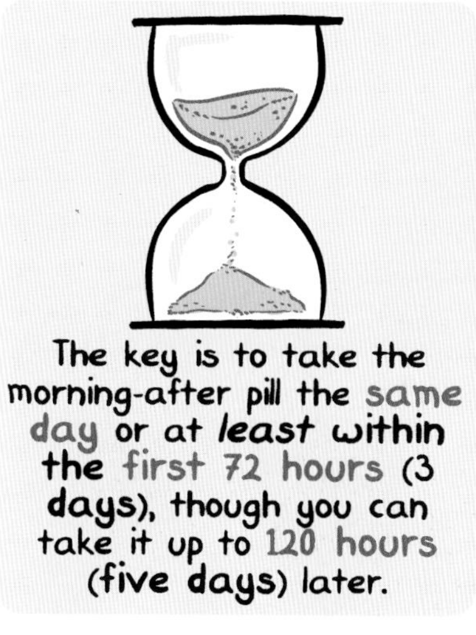
The key is to take the morning-after pill the same day or at *least* within the first 72 hours (3 days), though you can take it up to 120 hours (five days) later.

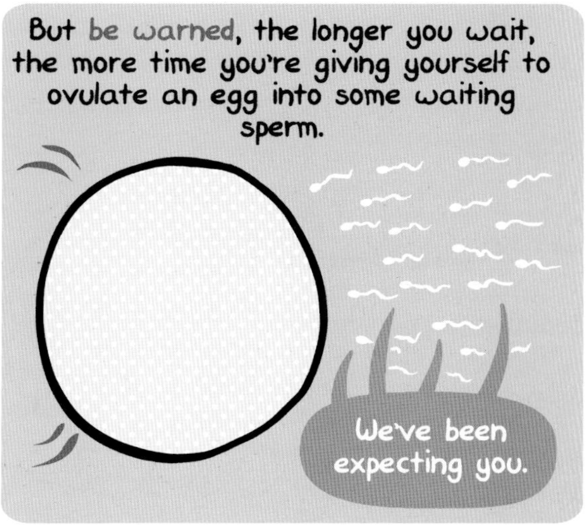
But be warned, the longer you wait, the more time you're giving yourself to ovulate an egg into some waiting sperm.
We've been expecting you.

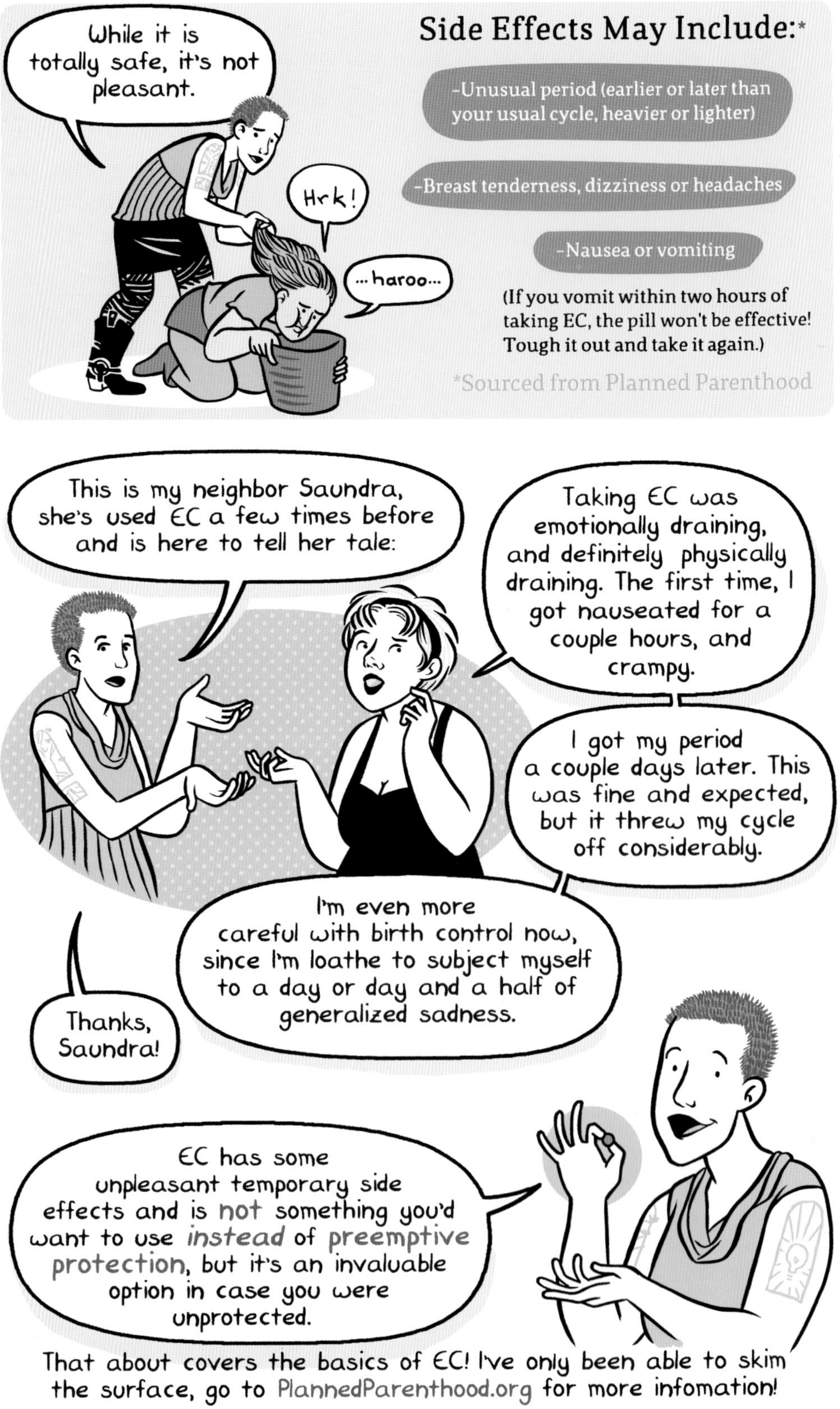
While it is totally safe, it's not pleasant.
Side Effects May Include:*
-Unusual period (earlier or later than your usual cycle, heavier or lighter)
-Breast tenderness, dizziness or headaches
Hrk!
-Nausea or vomiting
...haroo...
(If you vomit within two hours of taking EC, the pill won't be effective! Tough it out and take it again.)
*Sourced from Planned Parenthood
This is my neighbor Saundra, she's used EC a few times before and is here to tell her tale:
Taking EC was emotionally draining, and definitely physically draining. The first time, I got nauseated for a couple hours, and crampy.
I got my period a couple days later. This was fine and expected, but it threw my cycle off considerably.
I'm even more careful with birth control now, since I'm loathe to subject myself to a day or day and a half of generalized sadness.
Thanks, Saundra!
EC has some unpleasant temporary side effects and is not something you'd want to use instead of preemptive protection, but it's an invaluable option in case you were unprotected.
That about covers the basics of EC! I've only been able to skim the surface, go to PlannedParenthood.org for more infomation!

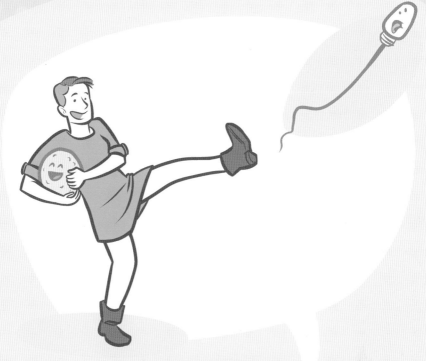

Other
Contraception
Methods

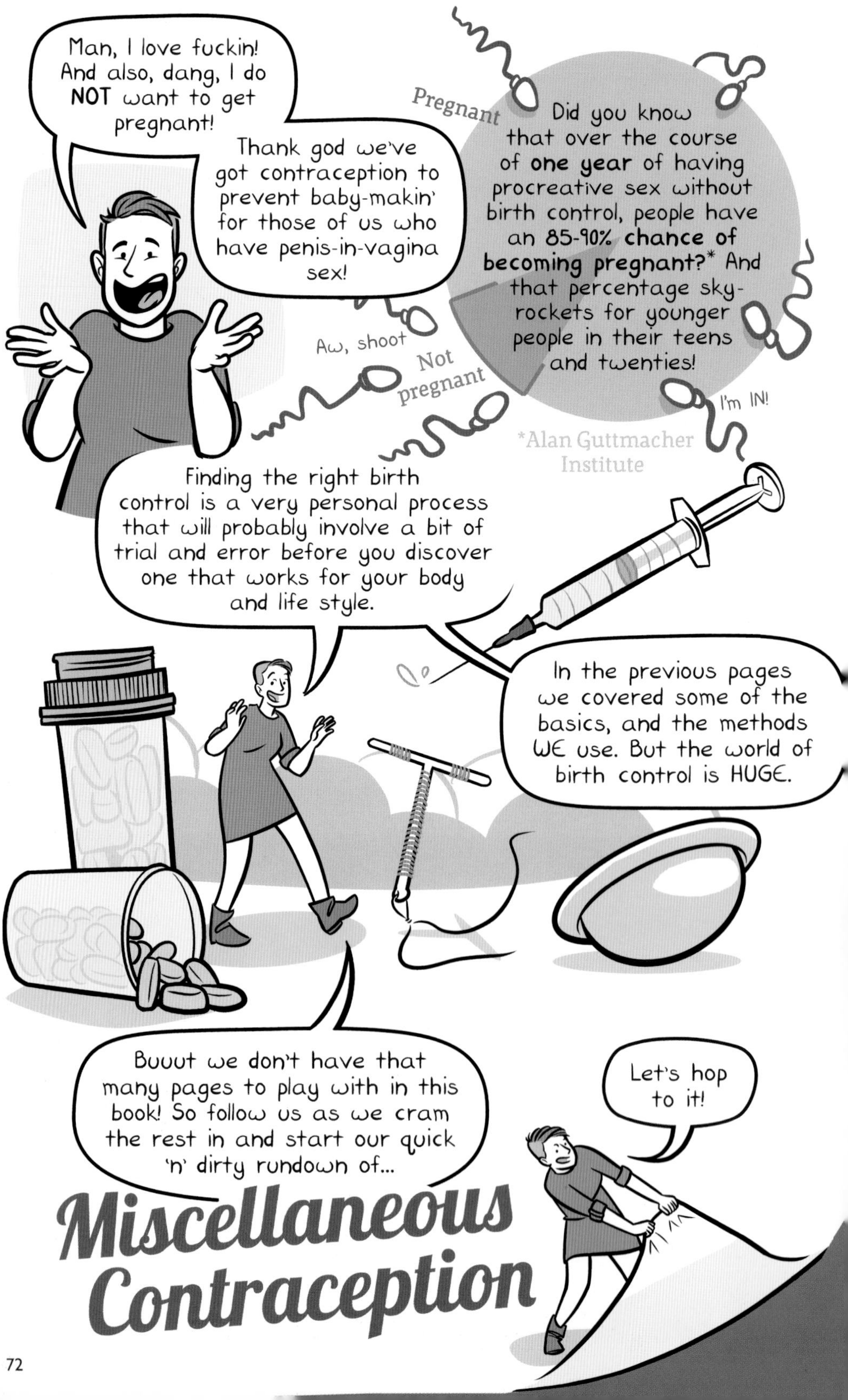
Man, I love fuckin! And also, dang, I do NOT want to get pregnant!
Thank god we've got contraception to prevent baby-makin' for those of us who have penis-in-vagina sex!
Pregnant
Did you know that over the course of one year of having procreative sex without birth control, people have an 85-90% chance of becoming pregnant?* And that percentage sky-rockets for younger people in their teens and twenties!
Aw, shoot
Not pregnant
I'm IN!
*Alan Guttmacher Institute
Finding the right birth control is a very personal process that will probably involve a bit of trial and error before you discover one that works for your body and life style.
In the previous pages we covered some of the basics, and the methods WE use. But the world of birth control is HUGE.
Buuut we don't have that many pages to play with in this book! So follow us as we cram the rest in and start our quick 'n' dirty rundown of...
Let's hop to it!
Miscellaneous Contraception

Cervical Barriers

$50–70 for the device, plus the recurring cost of spermicide

Latex or silicone

Reusable for several years

Hormone-free!

Diaphragm

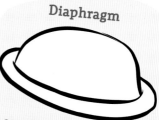

94% effective w/ perfect use, 86% w/ typical use

CAN be used during menstruation

Cervical Cap

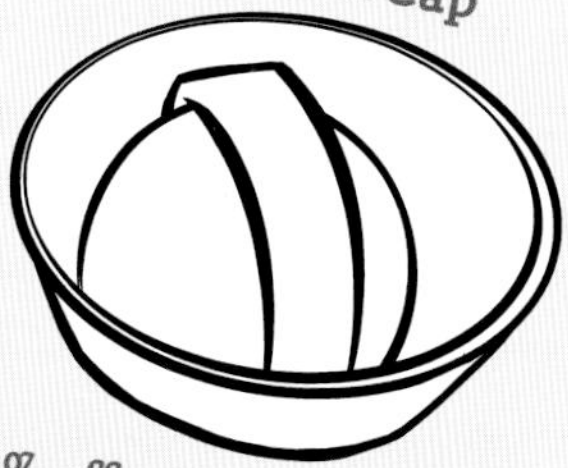

91% effective w/ perfect use, 84% w/ typical use

CANNOT be used during menstruation

Sizing is initially determined by your healthcare provider, but then your barrier is reusable for several years. Fill barrier with spermicide and insert into vagina up to two hours before intercourse and then leave in 6-8 hours afterwards. These things block access to the cervix, either obstructing or even killing the little spermies who swim that way.

Cautions: Not recommended for people who are sensitive or allergic to spermicides or have had TSS, and some people have more frequent bladder or urinary tract infections from using them. New size may be required if your body changes significantly, either from giving birth or changing weight.

The Implant

99+% effective

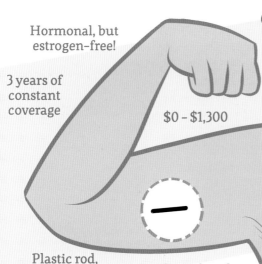

Hormonal, but estrogen-free!

3 years of constant coverage

$0 – $1,300

Plastic rod, size of matchstick

Implanted under skin

Become a CYBORG! A healthcare provider inserts this little plastic stick into your non-dominant arm and it releases a small amount of the hormone progestin. It's a great hormonal option for people who don't do well on estrogen, plus you don't have to think twice about your birth control for several years because it's just ALWAYS in you! You can't fuck it up by forgetting to take a pill or using it incorrectly!

Cautions:
It can change what kind of period you have and cause extra surprise spotting or bleeding. All the downsides that come from hormonal BC* plus there may be issues with your body accepting a foreign object into it.

The Patch

Hormonal

Prescription

$30 – $35/month

99% effective w/ perfect use, 92% with w/typical use

Kinda like a Nicotine patch! Except you're quitting being fertile, not ciggies! Once a week, you stick a fresh patch onto your body and let it release birth control hormones into your skin. The fourth week you leave it off, but you'll still be protected. May make your period lighter with less PMS – neat!

Cautions:

No smokers, people over 35, breastfeeders, diabetics, or people with a history of high blood pressure, cardiovascular disorders, or high cholesterol. May not be as effective for people over 198 lbs. All the downsides that come from hormonal BC*

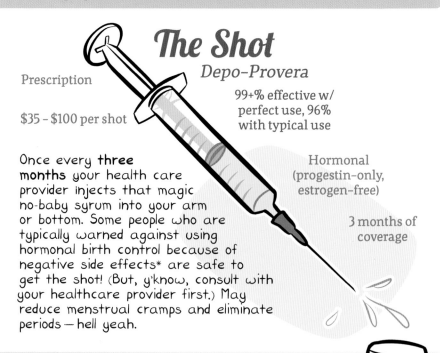

The Shot
Depo-Provera

Prescription

$35 – $100 per shot

99+% effective w/ perfect use, 96% with typical use

Once every **three months** your health care provider injects that magic no-baby syrum into your arm or bottom. Some people who are typically warned against using hormonal birth control because of negative side effects* are safe to get the shot! (But, y'know, consult with your healthcare provider first.) May reduce menstrual cramps and eliminate periods – hell yeah.

Hormonal (progestin-only, estrogen-free)

3 months of coverage

Cautions:

It is associated with bone loss, especially for adolescents and young adults who are still growing. Remains in your body for at least three months, so if you have a bad reaction to these hormones you are s-t-u-c-k with them for that time, and side effects may even last years. May not be a good match for people with Cushing's Syndrome, breast cancer, or mysterious vaginal bleeding.

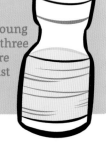

*See page 77!

Spermicides

83% effective w/perfect use, 72% w/typical use

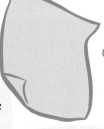

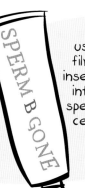

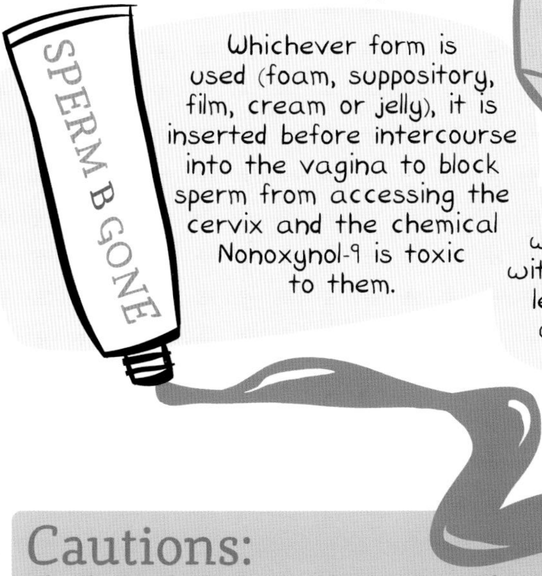

Whichever form is used (foam, suppository, film, cream or jelly), it is inserted before intercourse into the vagina to block sperm from accessing the cervix and the chemical Nonoxynol-9 is toxic to them.

Works best when paired up with a barrier, it's least effective when used on its own.

Over the counter

Use with a barrier

$7 - $18

Hormone free

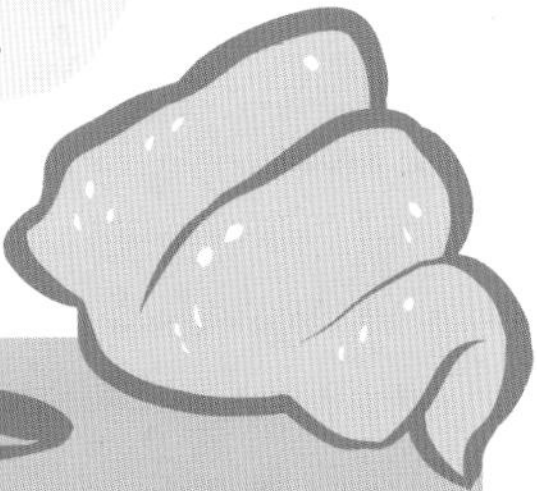

Cautions:

The chemicals in it can cause irritation and contribute to micro-abrasions in your vagina which can increase the risk of catching an STI.

Sponge

91% effective w/ perfect use, 86% w/ typical use

Hormone-free

$0 - $15 for pack of three, plus the recurring cost of spermicide

Over the counter

Up to 24 hours before intercourse, insert the spermicide foam-soaked sponge deep inside the vagina to block the cervix. Leave in for six hours after fucking, but make sure you've pulled it out before twenty-four hours is up.

Cautions:

Sponges work most effectively for people who have never given birth, not so much for folks who have. Don't use if you've had TSS or have any sensitivities or allergies to spermicides, polyurethane or sulfa drugs. Don't use during menstruation.

Vaginal Ring

99.7% effective w/ perfect use, 92% w/ typical use.

One of these suckers is inserted into the vagina and left there for three weeks at a time, where it releases estrogen and progestin hormones into the walls of your pussy.

Hormonal

$15-50 per ring

Prescription

It is removed for one week at the end of its cycle, but you will still be protected from pregnancy by the left-over hormones still in your system.

It has the lowest dose of estrogen out of all the other methods, so if you've struggled on a full dose and want to see how you handle a lighter one, this is a good baby step. Can also make lighter, shorter periods with fewer cramps and PMS symptoms.

Cautions:

The ring can cause irritation, odor, and other effects in the vagina and vulva area, including more frequent infections and imbalances. All the downsides that come with hormonal BC*.

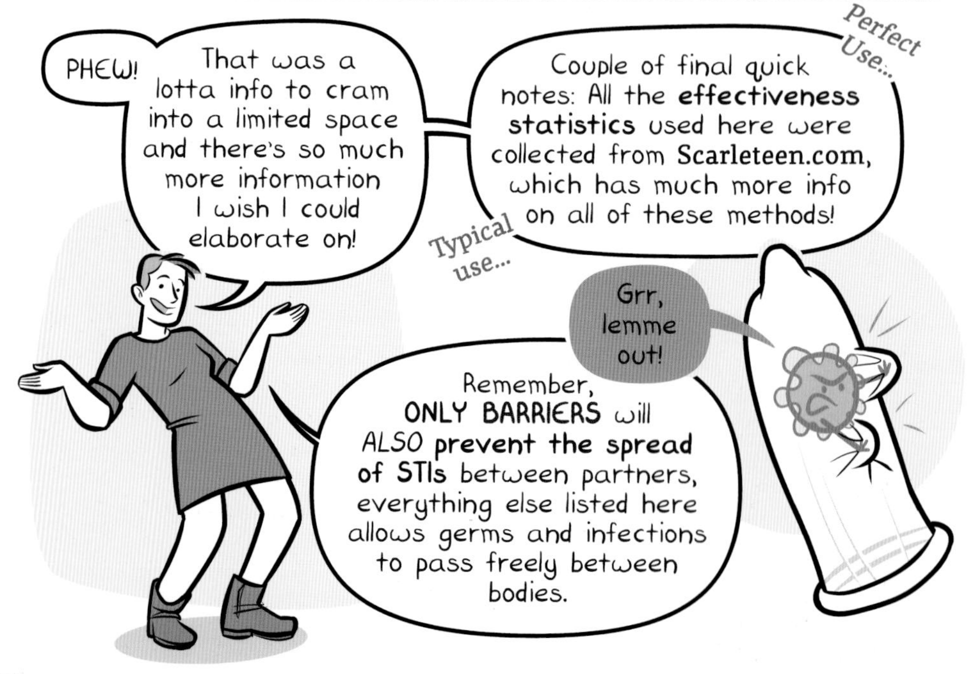

PHEW! That was a lotta info to cram into a limited space and there's so much more information I wish I could elaborate on!

Couple of final quick notes: All the **effectiveness statistics** used here were collected from Scarleteen.com, which has much more info on all of these methods!

Perfect Use:..

Typical use...

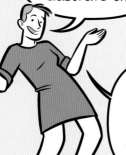

Grr, lemme out!

Remember, **ONLY BARRIERS** will ALSO **prevent the spread of STIs** between partners, everything else listed here allows germs and infections to pass freely between bodies.

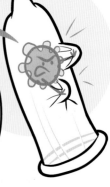

*Potential Downsides of Hormonal Birth Control:

Headaches, bloating, nausea, breast tenderness, vaginal dryness, mood changes, increased anxiety or depression, lessened desire for sex, weight gain, skin irritation, more frequent yeast infections, allergic reactions, blood clots, embolism or stroke, and just, like, a laundry list of other bummers.

Certain medications will decrease the effectiveness of hormonal BC or just straight up render them useless, so always consult with your healthcare provider before starting something new.

$$$ Birth control is **free or low cost** on most health insurance plans, Medicaid, and some government programs, so if any of these prices look out of your budget, **consult with your health clinic** to find out what **affordable options** may exist for you! $$$

(That last bit is just for us Americans, if you live in a country that actually takes care of its citizens... uh... THAT SOUNDS COOL.)

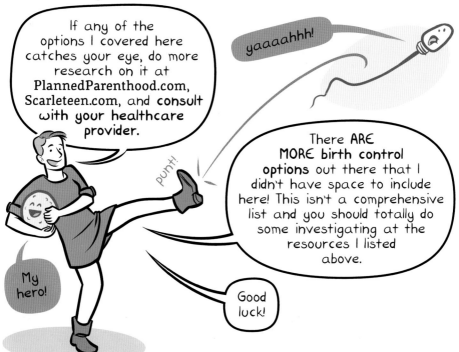

If any of the options I covered here catches your eye, do more research on it at PlannedParenthood.com, Scarleteen.com, and **consult with your healthcare provider.**

yaaaahhh!

punt!

My hero!

Good luck!

There ARE MORE birth control options out there that I didn't have space to include here! This isn't a comprehensive list and you should totally do some investigating at the resources I listed above.

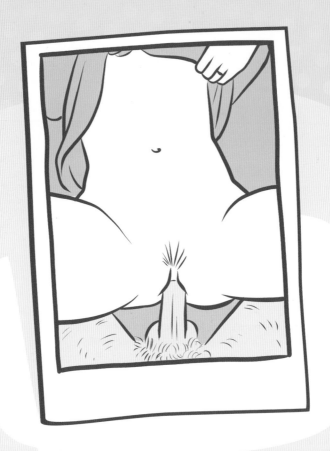

Sexting

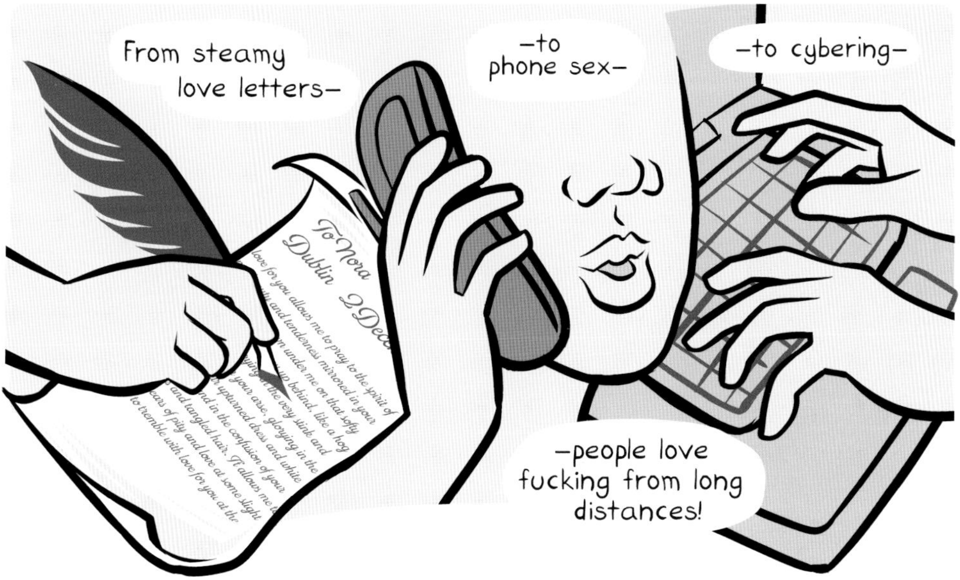

From steamy love letters—
To Nora
Dublin
—to phone sex—
—to cybering—
—people love fucking from long distances!

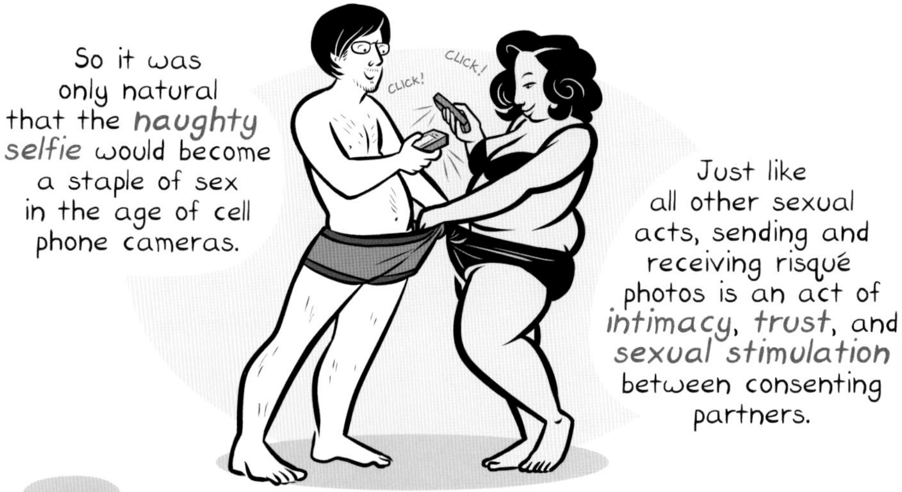

So it was only natural that the naughty selfie would become a staple of sex in the age of cell phone cameras.
CLICK!
CLICK!
Just like all other sexual acts, sending and receiving risqué photos is an act of intimacy, trust, and sexual stimulation between consenting partners.

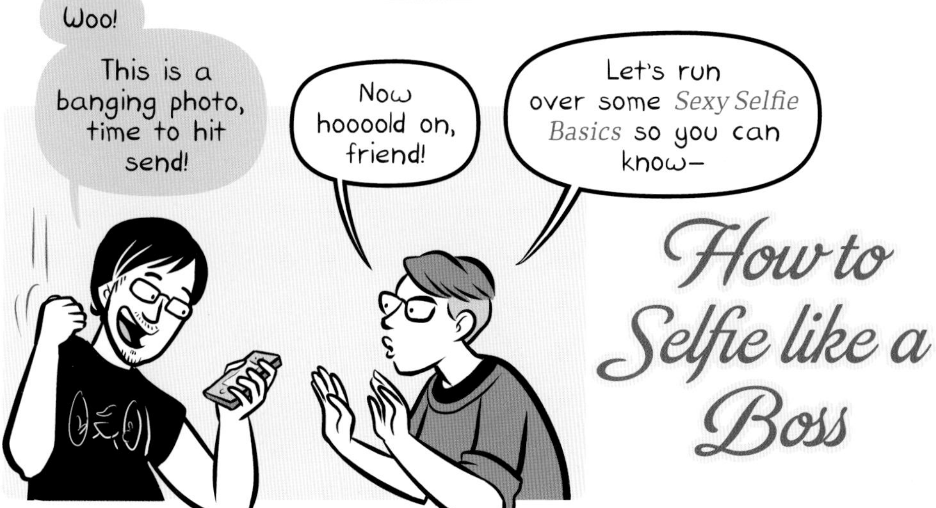

Woo!
This is a banging photo, time to hit send!
Now hoooold on, friend!
Let's run over some Sexy Selfie Basics so you can know—
How to Selfie like a Boss

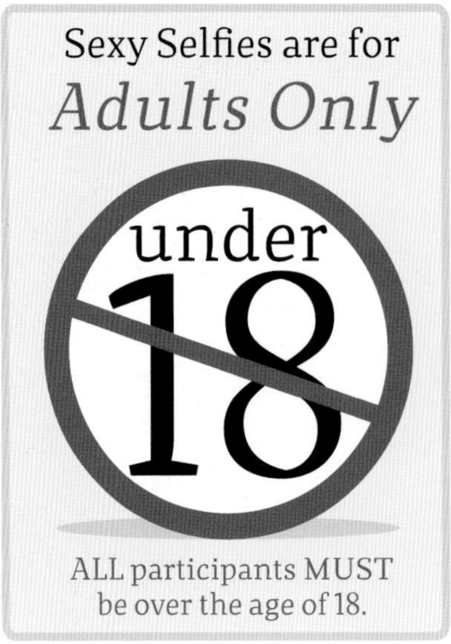
Sexy Selfies are for
Adults Only
under
18
ALL participants MUST
be over the age of 18.

There are *serious legal consequences* for any naked photos that are exchanged between people where anyone is under 18.

Creating/sharing/possessing any photos of a minor is legally *CHILD PORNOGRAPHY*, a *felony*!

(Even if it's consensually from one 17-and-a-half year old to another.)

Don't get incarcerated or have to register as a sex offender because you swapped naughty pictures with your high school sweetie!

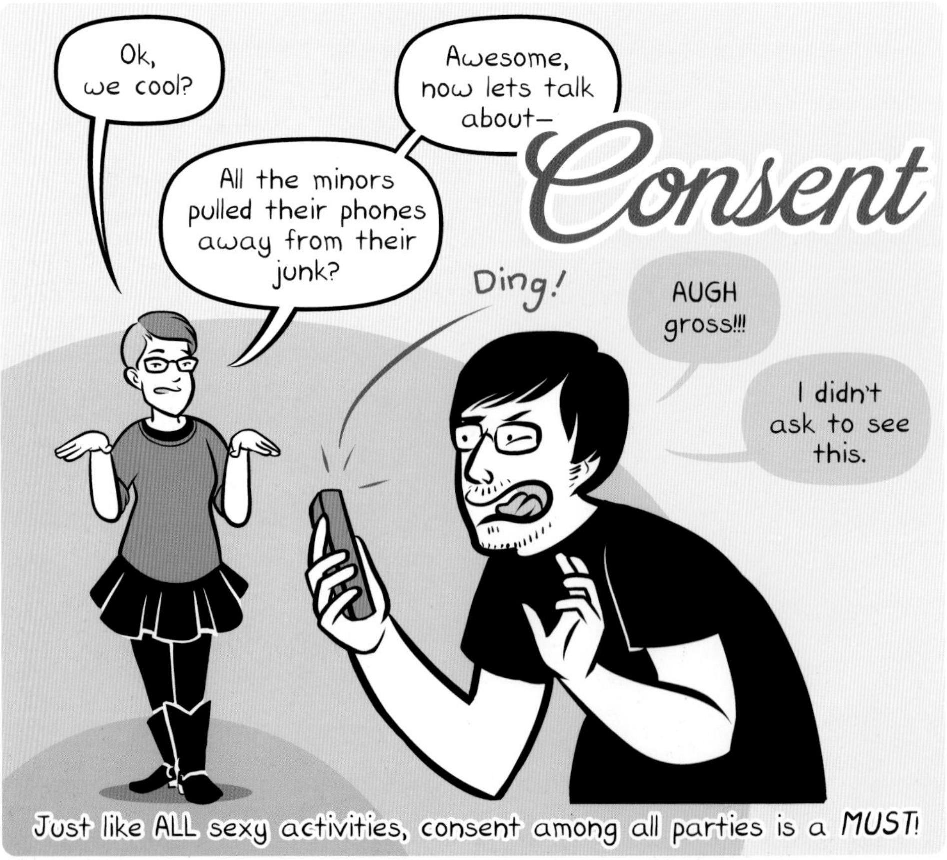
Ok, we cool?
Awesome, now lets talk about–
Consent
All the minors pulled their phones away from their junk?
Ding!
AUGH gross!!!
I didn't ask to see this.
Just like ALL sexy activities, consent among all parties is a MUST!

You want that special someone to be *HAPPY* when they get a picture of your goods—

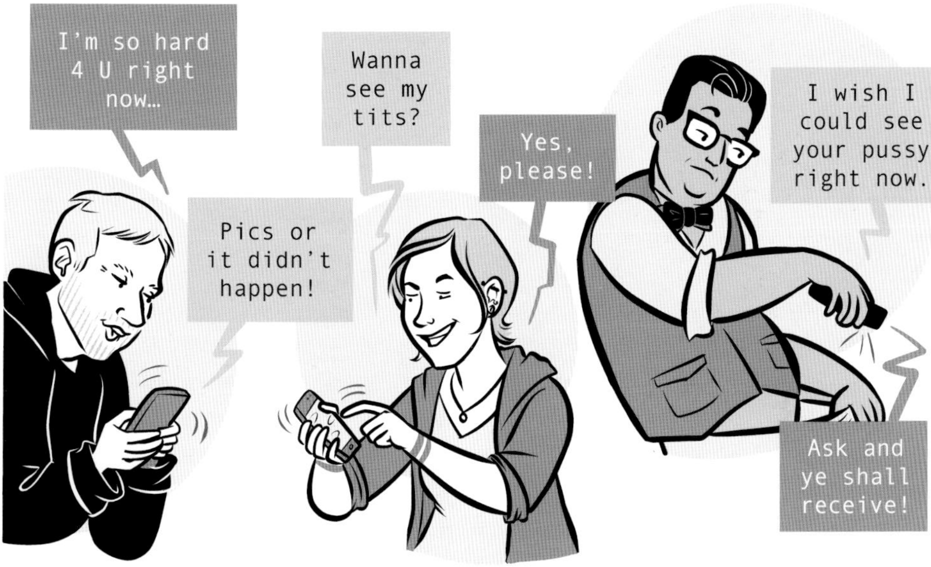

I'm so hard 4 U right now...
Pics or it didn't happen!
Wanna see my tits?
Yes, please!
I wish I could see your pussy right now.
Ask and ye shall receive!

—so you need to get confirmation that they want to see 'em before you send 'em.

NO SHARING

NEVER EVER share a naked photo that you received consensually unless you have explicit permission.

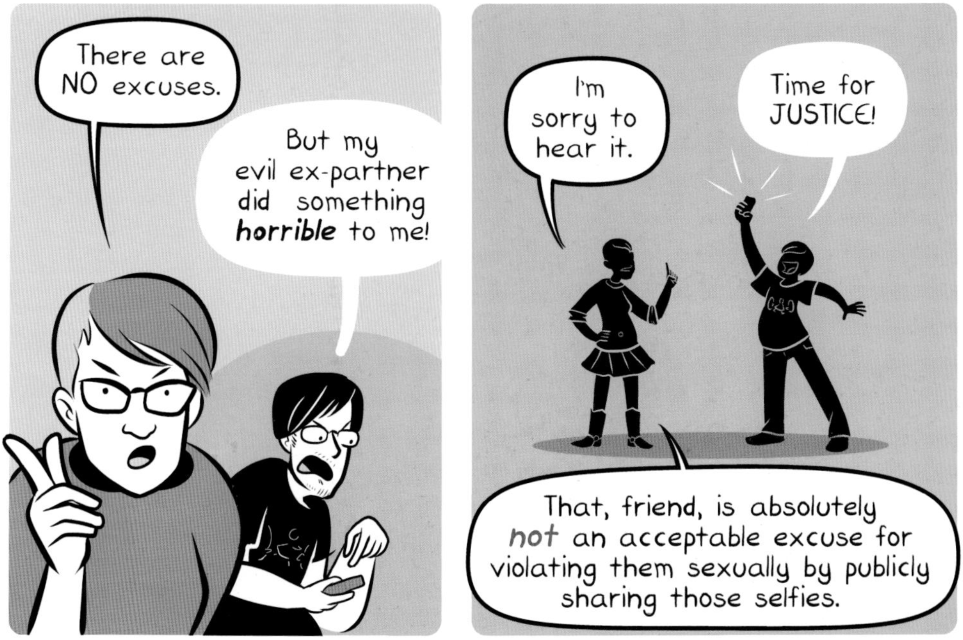

There are NO excuses.
But my evil ex-partner did something *horrible* to me!
I'm sorry to hear it.
Time for JUSTICE!
That, friend, is absolutely *not* an acceptable excuse for violating them sexually by publicly sharing those selfies.

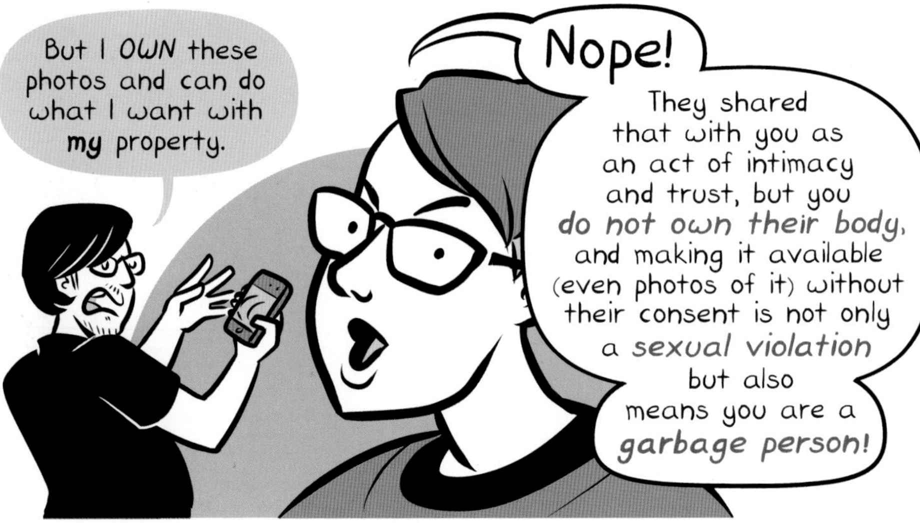
But I OWN these photos and can do what I want with my property.
Nope!
They shared that with you as an act of intimacy and trust, but you do not own their body, and making it available (even photos of it) without their consent is not only a sexual violation but also means you are a garbage person!

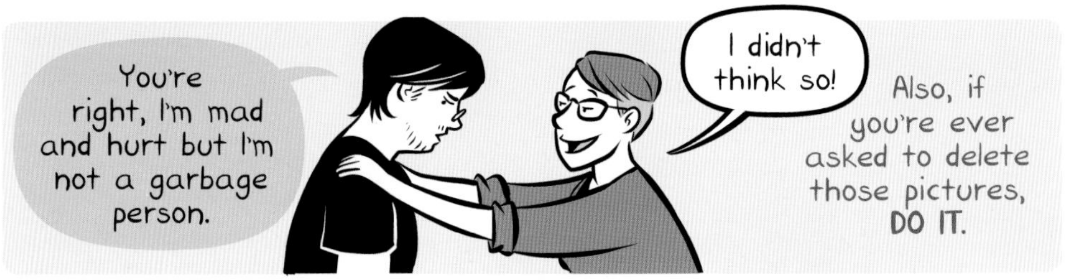
You're right, I'm mad and hurt but I'm not a garbage person.
I didn't think so!
Also, if you're ever asked to delete those pictures, DO IT.

Use your noggin and take *Precautions*

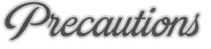

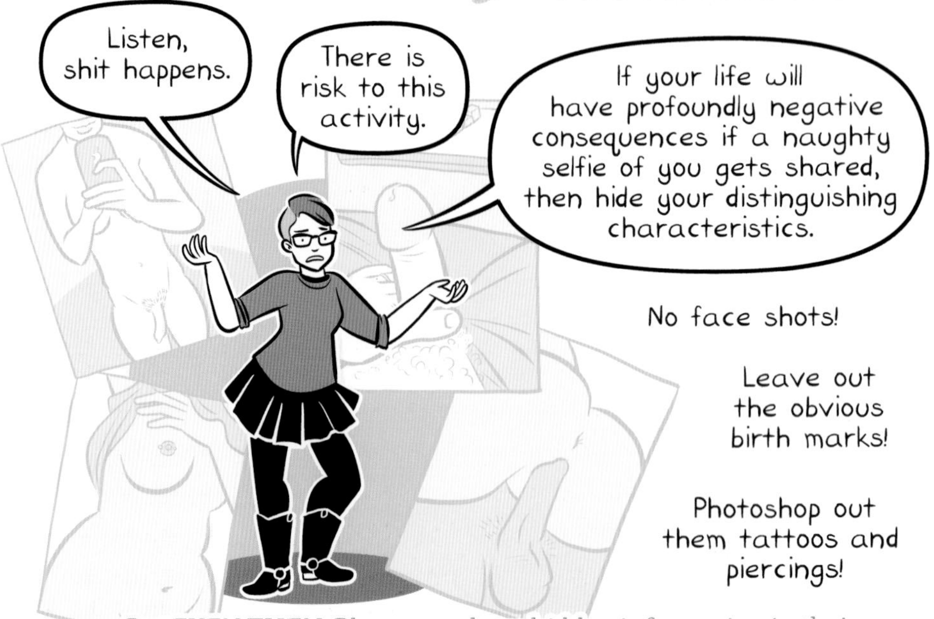
Listen, shit happens.
There is risk to this activity.
If your life will have profoundly negative consequences if a naughty selfie of you gets shared, then hide your distinguishing characteristics.
No face shots!
Leave out the obvious birth marks!
Photoshop out them tattoos and piercings!

But EVEN THEN. Photos can have hidden information in their data that may still lead back to you, so realize there's ALWAYS gonna be risk.

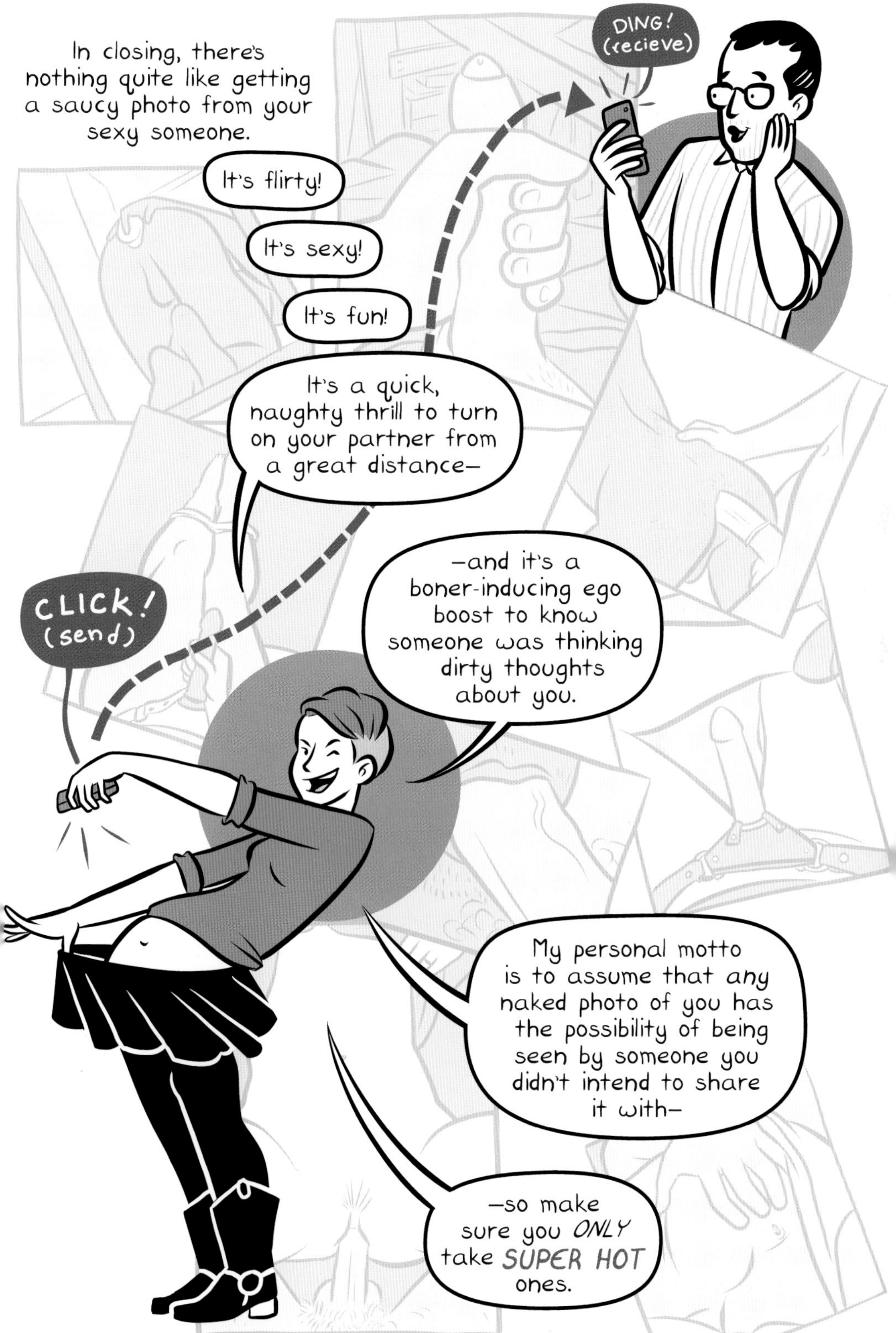

In closing, there's nothing quite like getting a saucy photo from your sexy someone.
It's flirty!
It's sexy!
It's fun!
It's a quick, naughty thrill to turn on your partner from a great distance–
DING! (recieve)
CLICK! (send)
–and it's a boner-inducing ego boost to know someone was thinking dirty thoughts about you.
My personal motto is to assume that *any* naked photo of you has the possibility of being seen by someone you didn't intend to share it with–
–so make sure you *ONLY* take SUPER HOT ones.

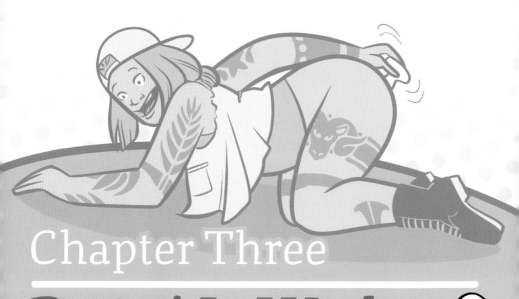

Chapter Three

Doin' It With Yourself

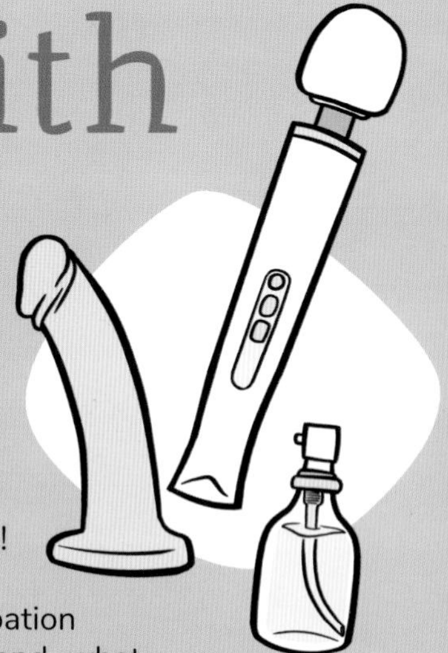

You gotta walk before you can run, and the same goes with becoming sexual! In this section we're going over having sex... with yourself. Which might sound like an impossible thing, but it's totally not. We're talking about your sexual imagination, how your body responds to arousal, and how to masturbate!

Way back in the day, I had HEARD masturbation and orgasms felt great but I just didn't understand what my body needed to get there. I tried and tried to clumsily touch myself with my hands but... nothing. It wasn't until I used a tiny, cheap vibrator for the very first time that I had an orgasm and my whole life changed.

Learning to masturbate put me in touch with a part of me that I didn't know existed. My body woke up and showed me I could love myself in a way I never imagined before.

Of course, masturbation and orgasming are not mandatory and they're not for everyone! Not having a desire to mess around with your bits or not especially enjoying it is also perfectly normal and there are so many people out there who have happy lives and relationships that don't include this stuff. We're all built differently, with different wants and needs! The most important sexual relationship you'll have is with yourself, in whatever form that takes, so get to know yourself and find what feels right for you. Good luck!

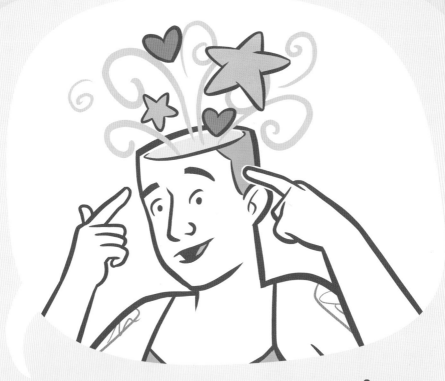

Sexual Fantasies

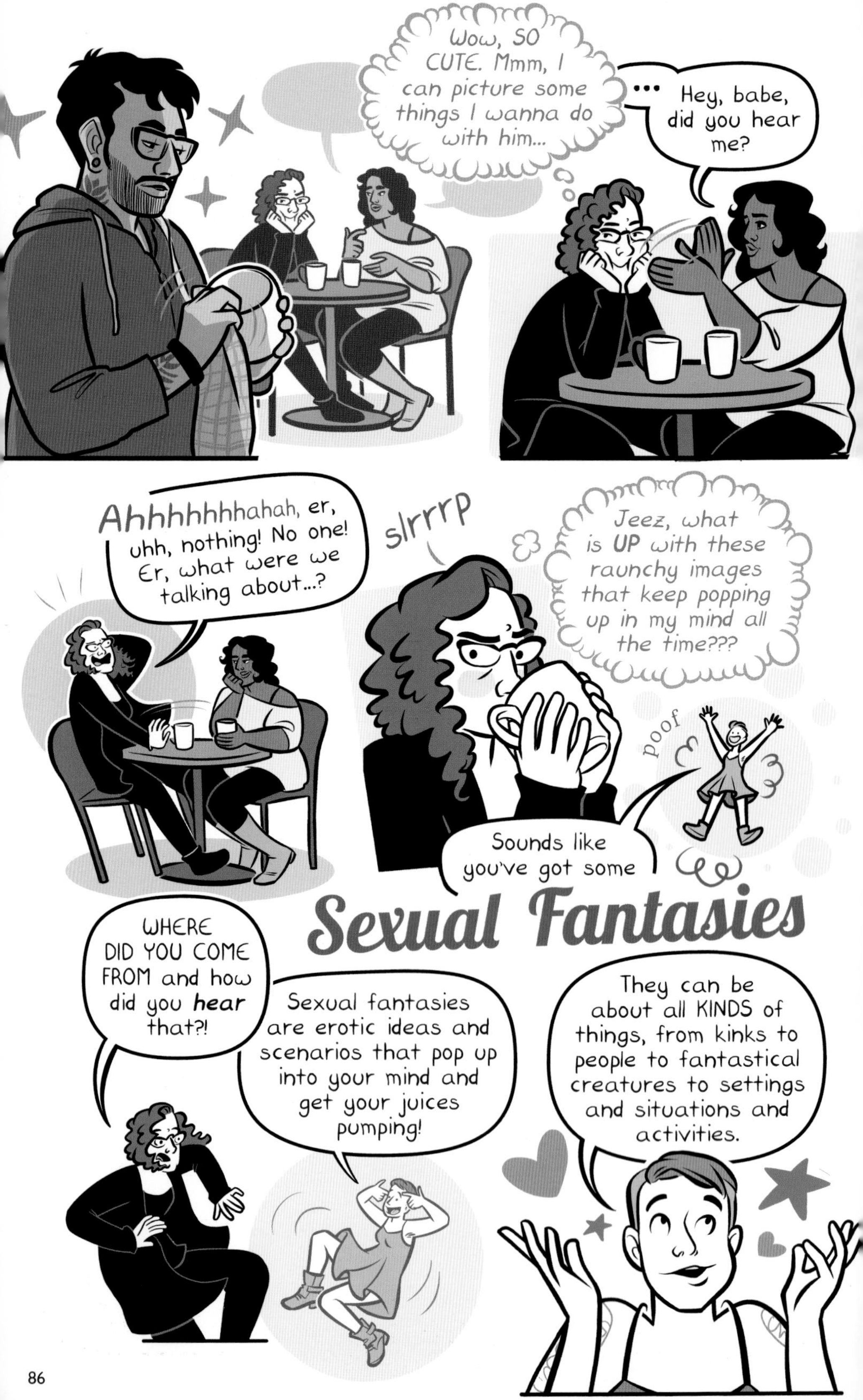
Wow, SO CUTE. Mmm, I can picture some things I wanna do with him...
...
Hey, babe, did you hear me?
Ahhhhhhhahah, er, uhh, nothing! No one! Er, what were we talking about...?
slrrrp
Jeez, what is UP with these raunchy images that keep popping up in my mind all the time???
poof
Sounds like you've got some
Sexual Fantasies
WHERE DID YOU COME FROM and how did you hear that?!
Sexual fantasies are erotic ideas and scenarios that pop up into your mind and get your juices pumping!
They can be about all KINDS of things, from kinks to people to fantastical creatures to settings and situations and activities.

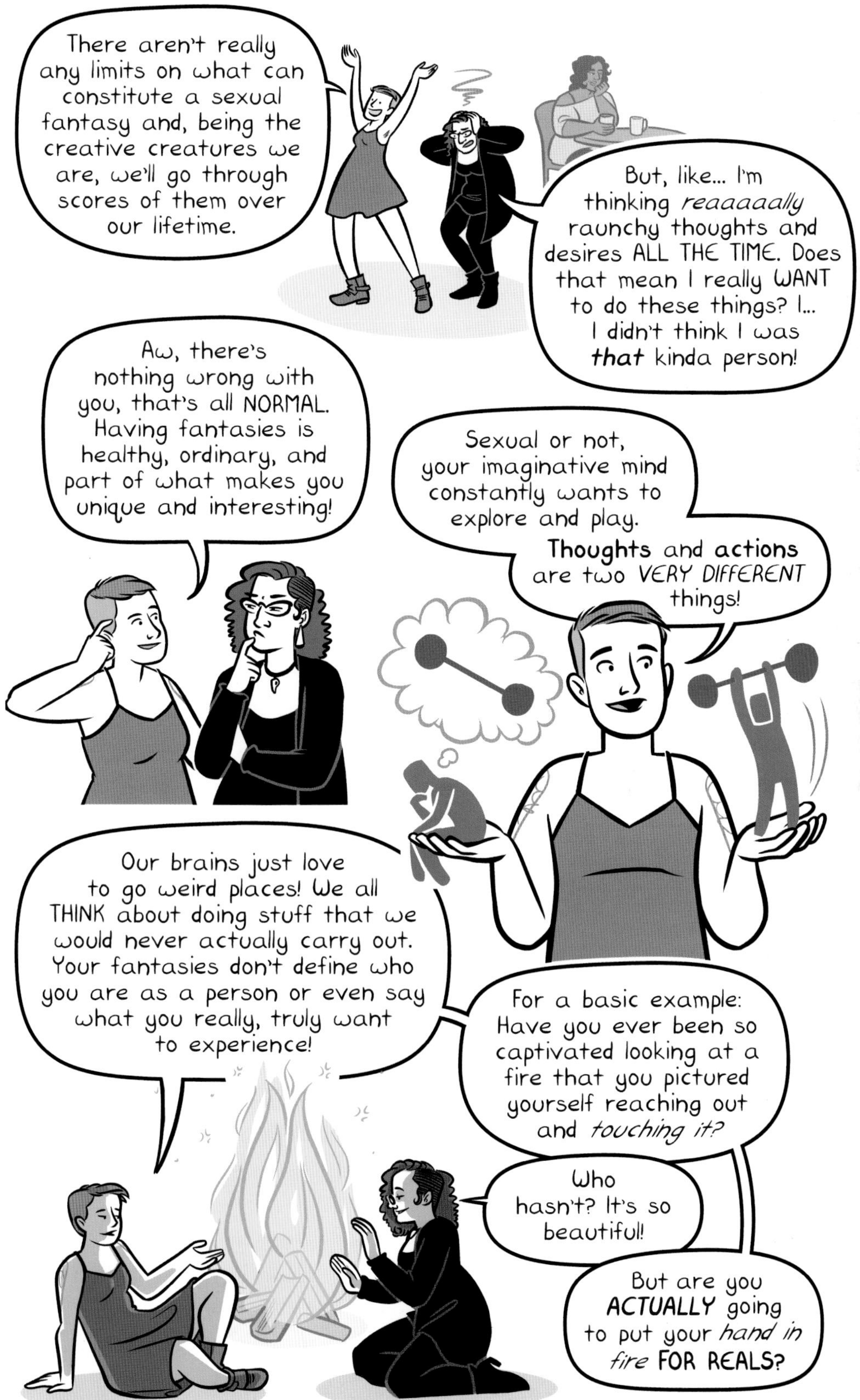
There aren't really any limits on what can constitute a sexual fantasy and, being the creative creatures we are, we'll go through scores of them over our lifetime.
But, like... I'm thinking *reaaaaally* raunchy thoughts and desires ALL THE TIME. Does that mean I really WANT to do these things? I... I didn't think I was **that** kinda person!
Aw, there's nothing wrong with you, that's all NORMAL. Having fantasies is healthy, ordinary, and part of what makes you unique and interesting!
Sexual or not, your imaginative mind constantly wants to explore and play.
Thoughts and **actions** are two *VERY DIFFERENT* things!
Our brains just love to go weird places! We all THINK about doing stuff that we would never actually carry out. Your fantasies don't define who you are as a person or even say what you really, truly want to experience!
For a basic example: Have you ever been so captivated looking at a fire that you pictured yourself reaching out and *touching it?*
Who hasn't? It's so beautiful!
But are you **ACTUALLY** going to put your *hand in fire* **FOR REALS?**

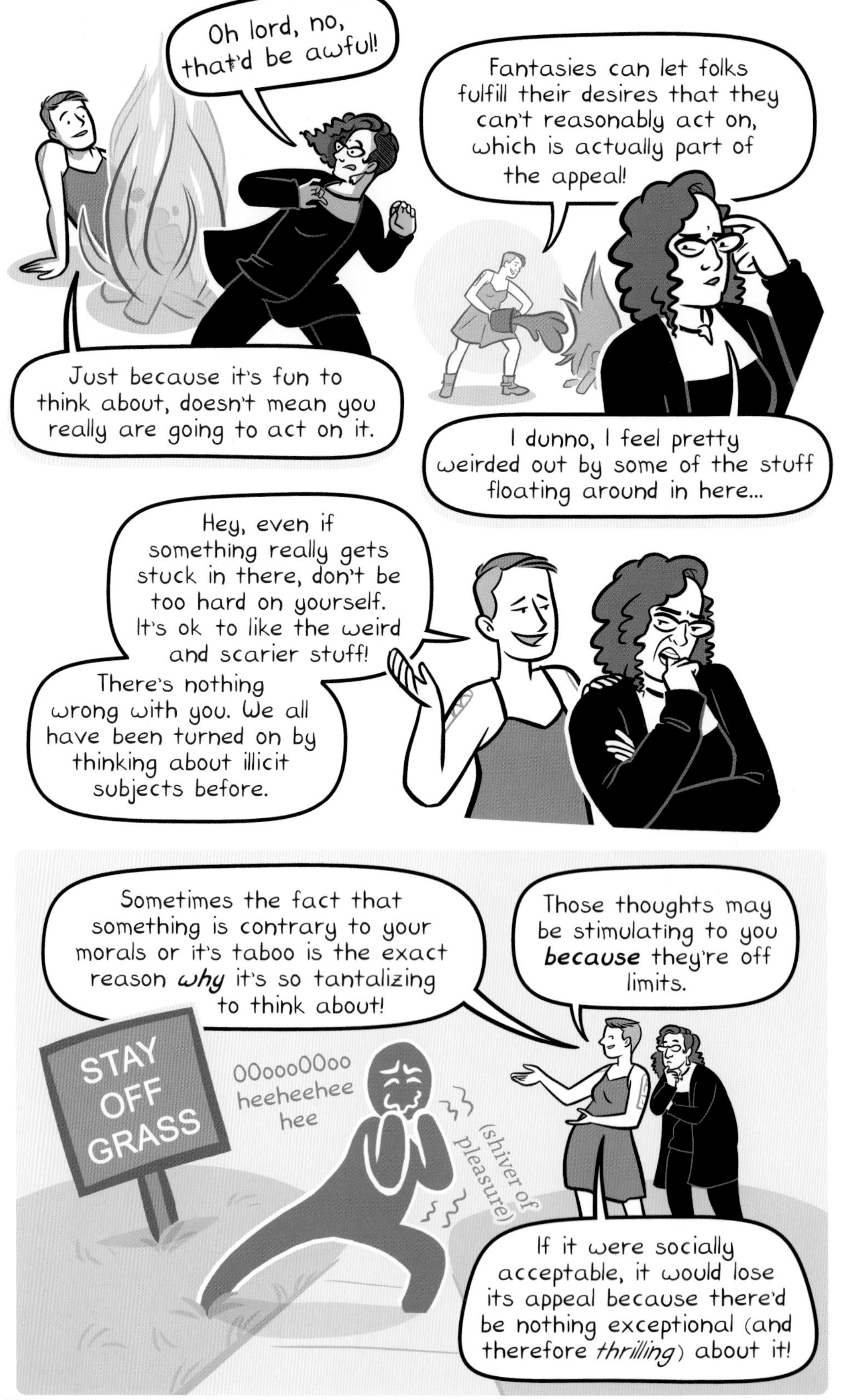
Oh lord, no, that'd be awful!
Just because it's fun to think about, doesn't mean you really are going to act on it.
Fantasies can let folks fulfill their desires that they can't reasonably act on, which is actually part of the appeal!
I dunno, I feel pretty weirded out by some of the stuff floating around in here...
Hey, even if something really gets stuck in there, don't be too hard on yourself. It's ok to like the weird and scarier stuff!
There's nothing wrong with you. We all have been turned on by thinking about illicit subjects before.
Sometimes the fact that something is contrary to your morals or it's taboo is the exact reason *why* it's so tantalizing to think about!
Those thoughts may be stimulating to you ***because*** they're off limits.
STAY OFF GRASS
OOoooOOoo heeheehee hee
(shiver of pleasure)
If it were socially acceptable, it would lose its appeal because there'd be nothing exceptional (and therefore *thrilling*) about it!

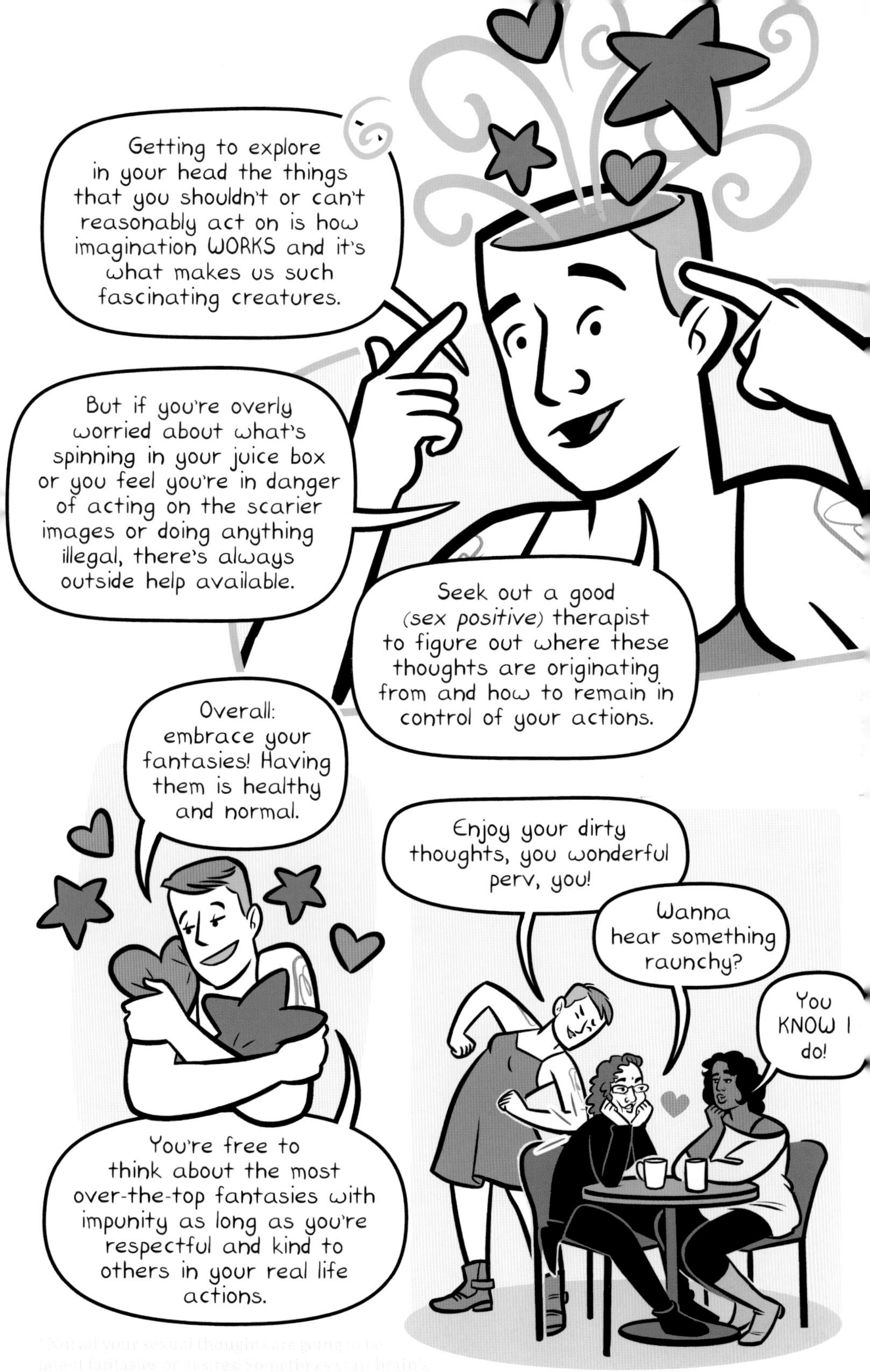
Getting to explore in your head the things that you shouldn't or can't reasonably act on is how imagination WORKS and it's what makes us such fascinating creatures.
But if you're overly worried about what's spinning in your juice box or you feel you're in danger of acting on the scarier images or doing anything illegal, there's always outside help available.
Seek out a good (*sex positive*) therapist to figure out where these thoughts are originating from and how to remain in control of your actions.
Overall: embrace your fantasies! Having them is healthy and normal.
You're free to think about the most over-the-top fantasies with impunity as long as you're respectful and kind to others in your real life actions.
Enjoy your dirty thoughts, you wonderful perv, you!
Wanna hear something raunchy?
You KNOW I do!

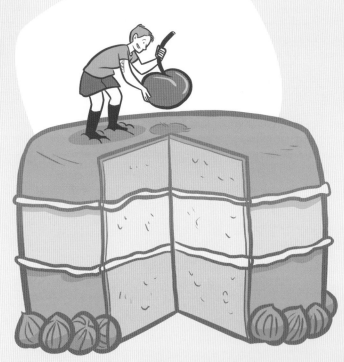

Sexual Response
Cycle

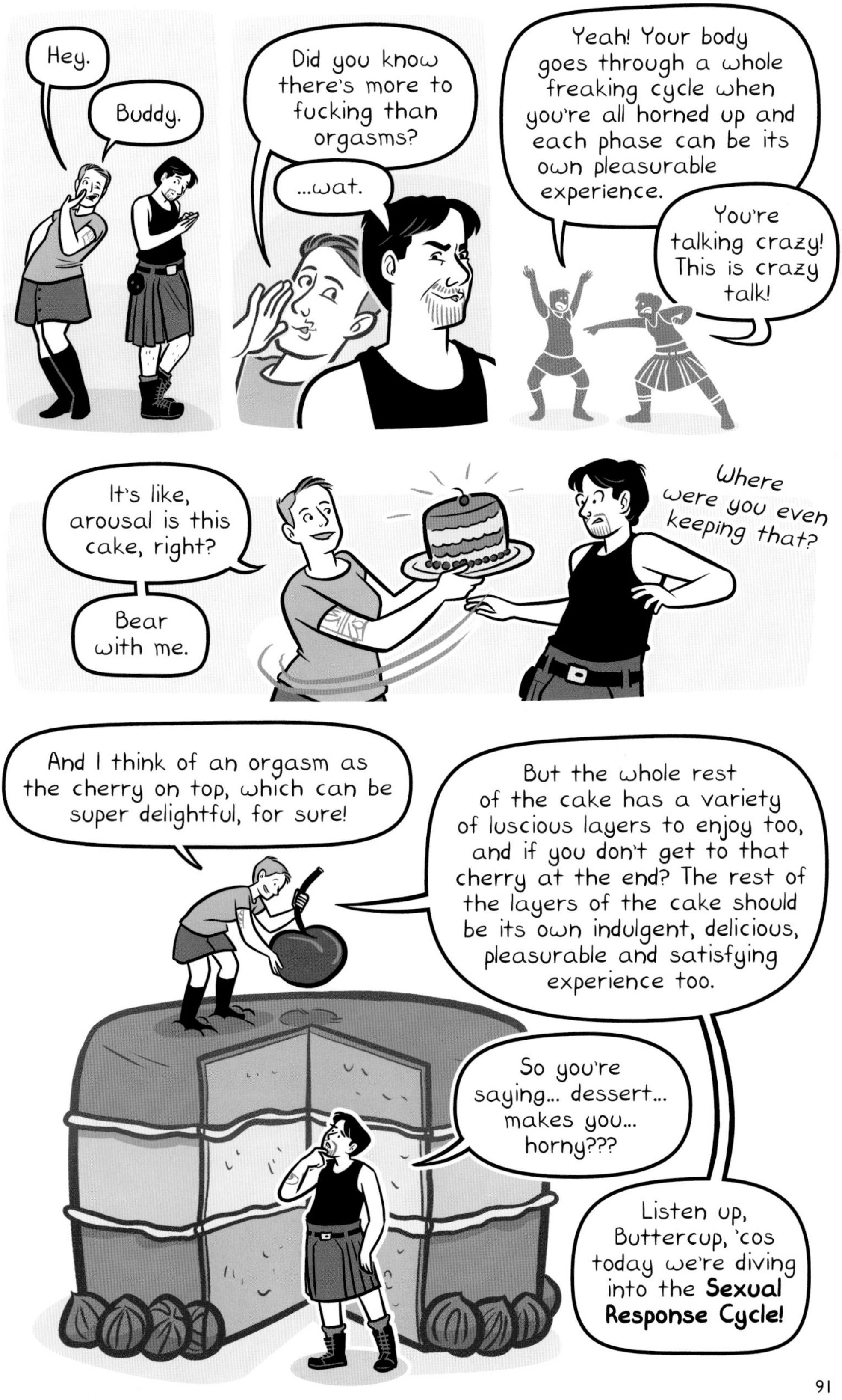
Hey.
Buddy.
Did you know there's more to fucking than orgasms?
...wat.
Yeah! Your body goes through a whole freaking cycle when you're all horned up and each phase can be its own pleasurable experience.
You're talking crazy! This is crazy talk!
It's like, arousal is this cake, right?
Bear with me.
Where were you even keeping that?
And I think of an orgasm as the cherry on top, which can be super delightful, for sure!
But the whole rest of the cake has a variety of luscious layers to enjoy too, and if you don't get to that cherry at the end? The rest of the layers of the cake should be its own indulgent, delicious, pleasurable and satisfying experience too.
So you're saying... dessert... makes you... horny???
Listen up, Buttercup, 'cos today we're diving into the **Sexual Response Cycle!**

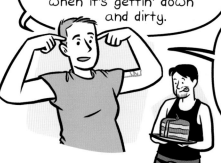

Let's take a look at the different stages your mind and body may go through when it's gettin' down and dirty.

(A Version of)
The Sexual Response Cycle*

*I mashed the classic **Masters & Johnson 4 Phase Cycle** together with **Kaplan's Triphasic Model**, just to kinda cover all the bases. I'm sure researchers will continue to evolve the SRC stages over time, but for now it *generally* looks like this.

Desire

This is your **mind getting excited and interested**, the brain getting switched on! It can be over anything, a sight, a smell, a memory. Something that gets you hungry for sexy times. It's easy to focus on the genital response, but really the brain is your most important sexual organ.

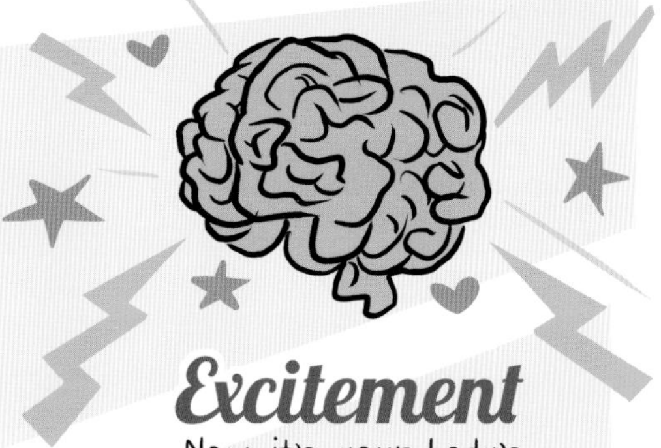

Excitement

Now it's your body's turn to get turned on! This stage begins the **physical changes** your body may go through in response to stimulation, like an increase in blood pressure, heart rate, and breathing. Blood will flow to your genitals, possibly making penises and clitorises swell and harden, vaginas may produce some lubrication and lengthen, dicks may squeeze out a drop or two of pre-ejaculate, and nips may get perky.

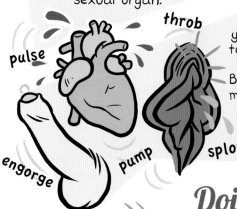

throb

pulse

engorge

pump

splort

Doin' It
(The Plateau phase)

This is when you're **making the action happen**, when your body's switched on, thrumming along and doing its business! Fantasies, feelings, and all sorts will flow through your head while your body will respond more and more to touch, genitals will continue to swell, vaginas will tent around their cervix, faces and chests might get redder (called the Sex Flush! How cute!), a moan or two might escape, muscle spasms around the body might be had, and breathing may modify, from panting to holding your breath.

Orgasm

The explosive phase! The accumulation of all those other processes hit their peak. Your body will tighten up its orgasmic muscles. Your breathing, heartbeat and blood pressure might all jump up. And your body might move or rock as you release all that built-up muscular sexual tension!

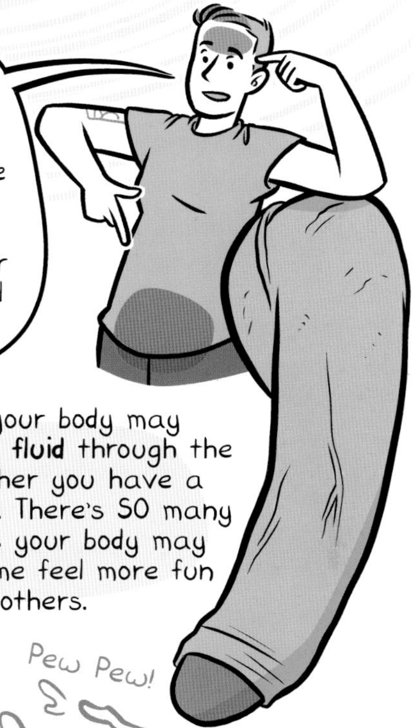

No two orgasms are exactly alike. Some of them feel hard and intense, some soft and tingly, others can be so unremarkable you're not even sure you really had one! Sometimes it can happen more in your head rather than in your genitals, other times it'll feel like a purely physical contraction without much pleasure!

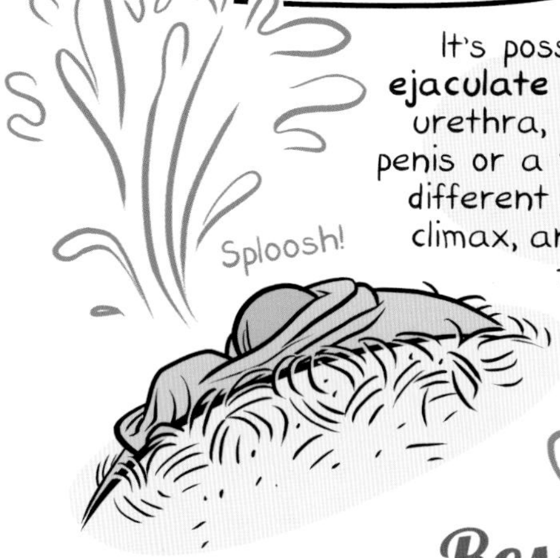

It's possible your body may **ejaculate some fluid** through the urethra, whether you have a penis or a vulva. There's SO many different ways your body may climax, and some feel more fun than others.

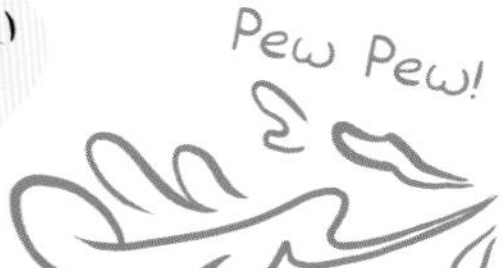

Sploosh!

Pew Pew!

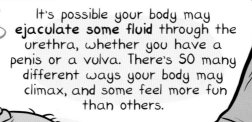

Resolution

The slow come down! Your brain will get its chemical fix, endorphins and all sorts. It can be like waking up back into reality — but really it can be super different for everyone! Your body will settle back to its baseline. Breathing, body parts, heart rate, blood pressure, everything slows back down or deflates back to normal.

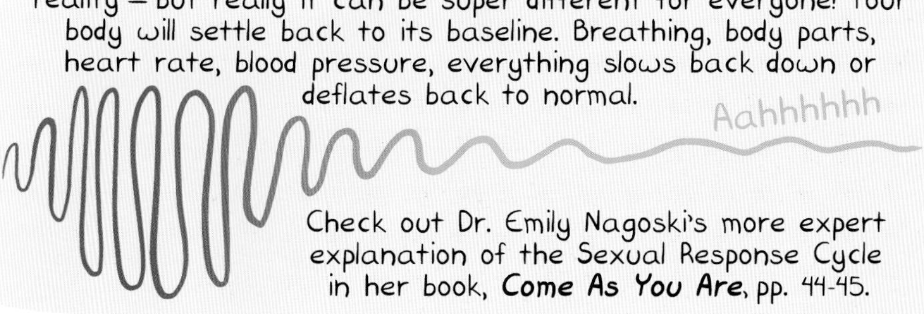

Aahhhhhh

Check out Dr. Emily Nagoski's more expert explanation of the Sexual Response Cycle in her book, **Come As You Are**, pp. 44-45.

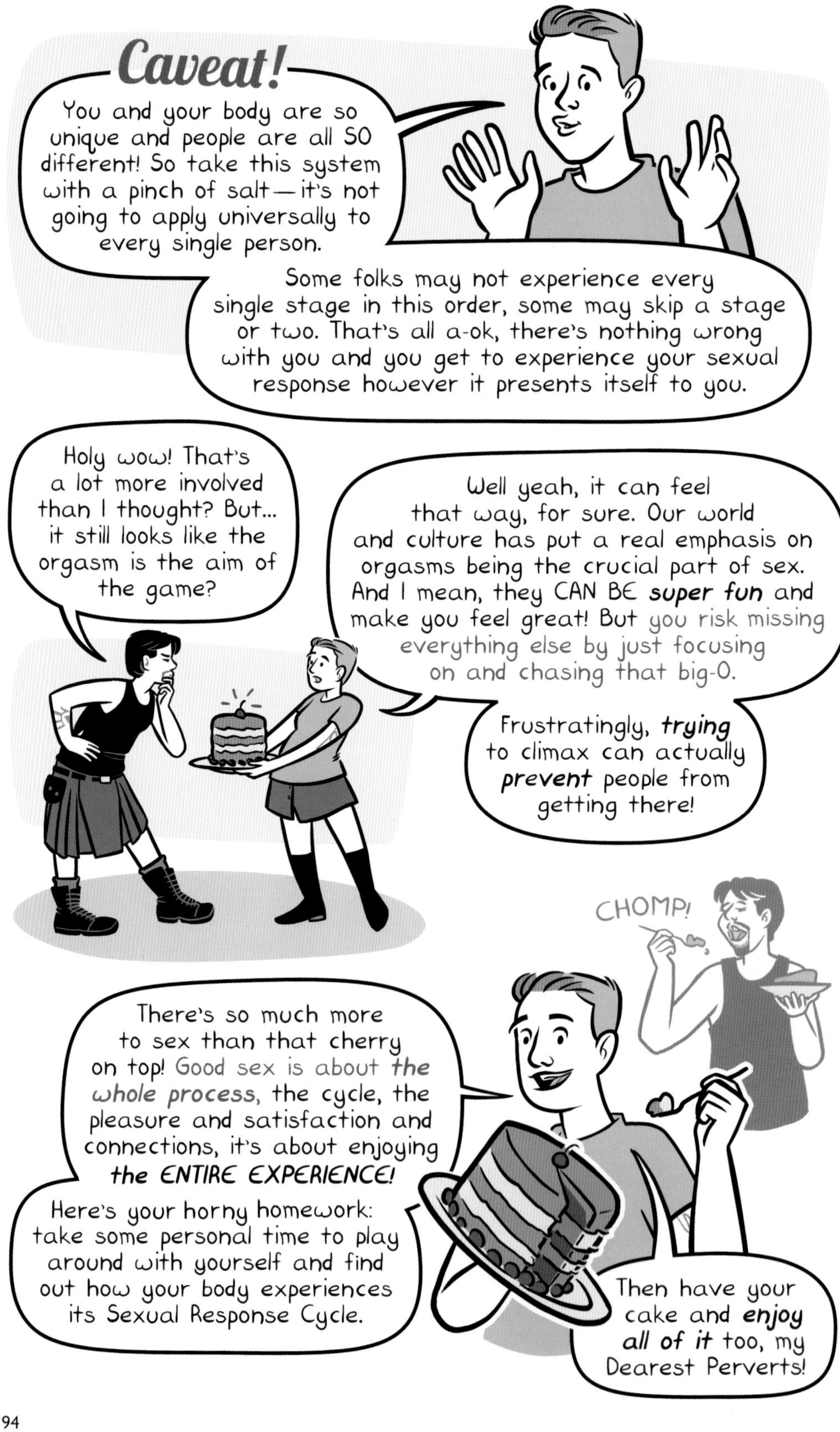
Caveat!
You and your body are so unique and people are all SO different! So take this system with a pinch of salt—it's not going to apply universally to every single person.
Some folks may not experience every single stage in this order, some may skip a stage or two. That's all a-ok, there's nothing wrong with you and you get to experience your sexual response however it presents itself to you.
Holy wow! That's a lot more involved than I thought? But... it still looks like the orgasm is the aim of the game?
Well yeah, it can feel that way, for sure. Our world and culture has put a real emphasis on orgasms being the crucial part of sex. And I mean, they CAN BE super fun and make you feel great! But you risk missing everything else by just focusing on and chasing that big-O.
Frustratingly, trying to climax can actually prevent people from getting there!
CHOMP!
There's so much more to sex than that cherry on top! Good sex is about the whole process, the cycle, the pleasure and satisfaction and connections, it's about enjoying the ENTIRE EXPERIENCE!
Here's your horny homework: take some personal time to play around with yourself and find out how your body experiences its Sexual Response Cycle.
Then have your cake and enjoy all of it too, my Dearest Perverts!

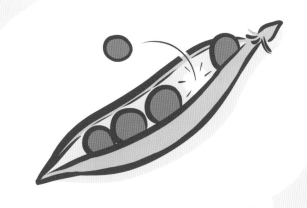

Masturbating
– Vulva –

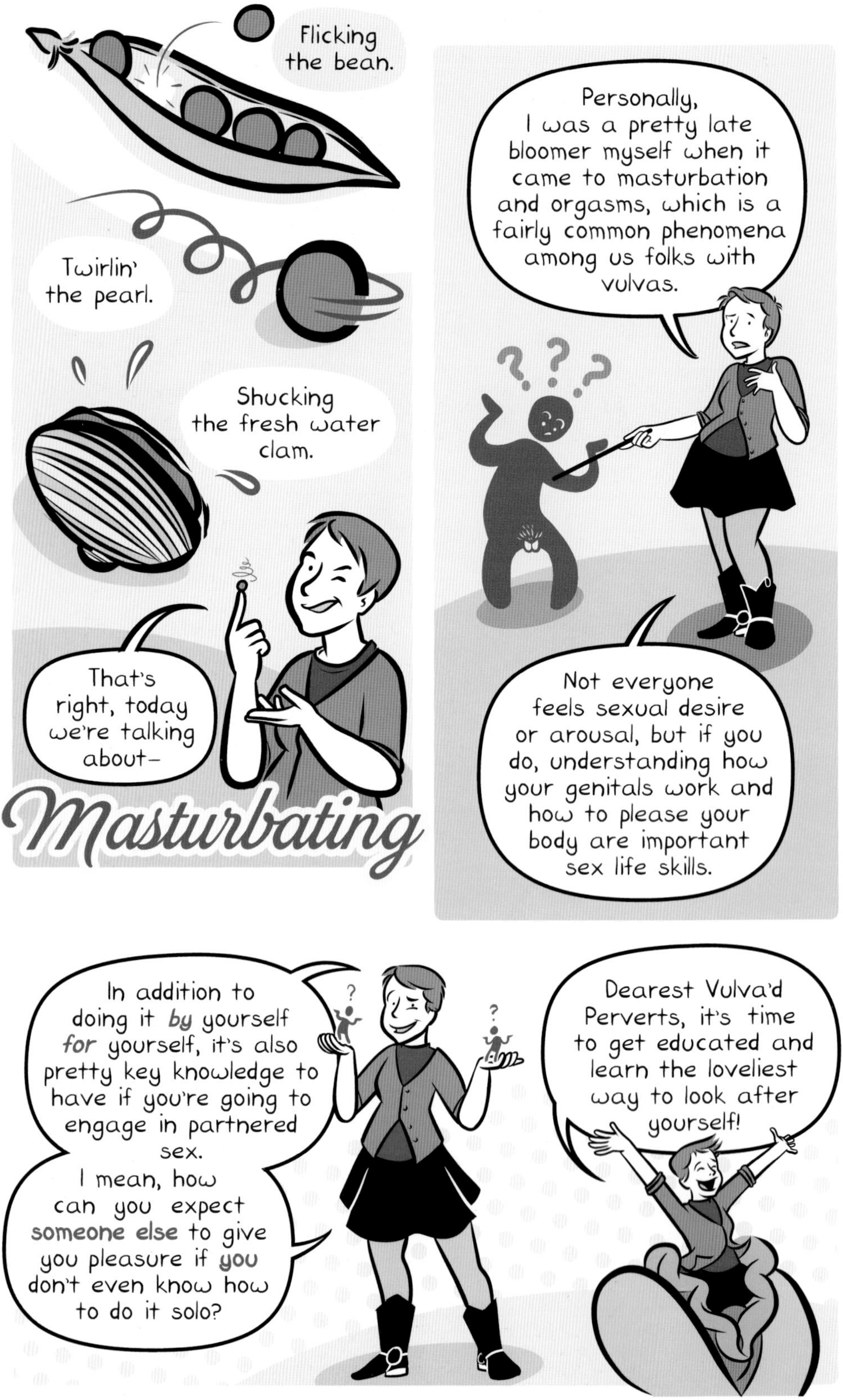

Flicking the bean.
Twirlin' the pearl.
Shucking the fresh water clam.
That's right, today we're talking about–
Masturbating
Personally, I was a pretty late bloomer myself when it came to masturbation and orgasms, which is a fairly common phenomena among us folks with vulvas.
Not everyone feels sexual desire or arousal, but if you do, understanding how your genitals work and how to please your body are important sex life skills.
In addition to doing it *by* yourself *for* yourself, it's also pretty key knowledge to have if you're going to engage in partnered sex.
I mean, how can you expect **someone else** to give you pleasure if **you** don't even know how to do it solo?
Dearest Vulva'd Perverts, it's time to get educated and learn the loveliest way to look after yourself!

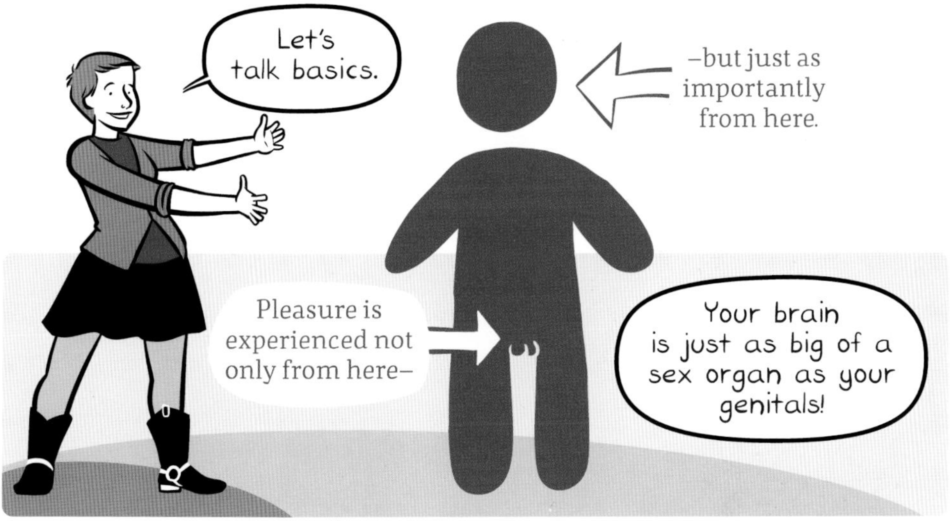
Let's talk basics.
–but just as importantly from here.
Pleasure is experienced not only from here–
Your brain is just as big of a sex organ as your genitals!

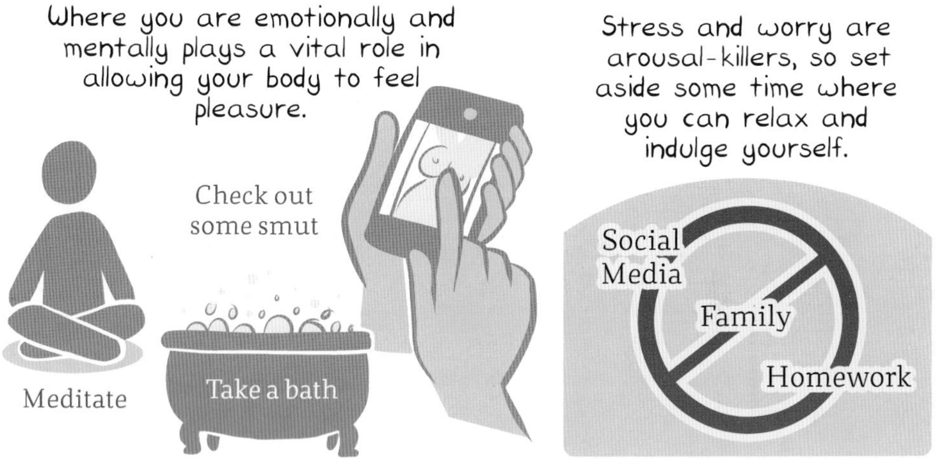
Where you are emotionally and mentally plays a vital role in allowing your body to feel pleasure.
Stress and worry are arousal-killers, so set aside some time where you can relax and indulge yourself.
Check out some smut
Meditate
Take a bath
Social Media
Family
Homework

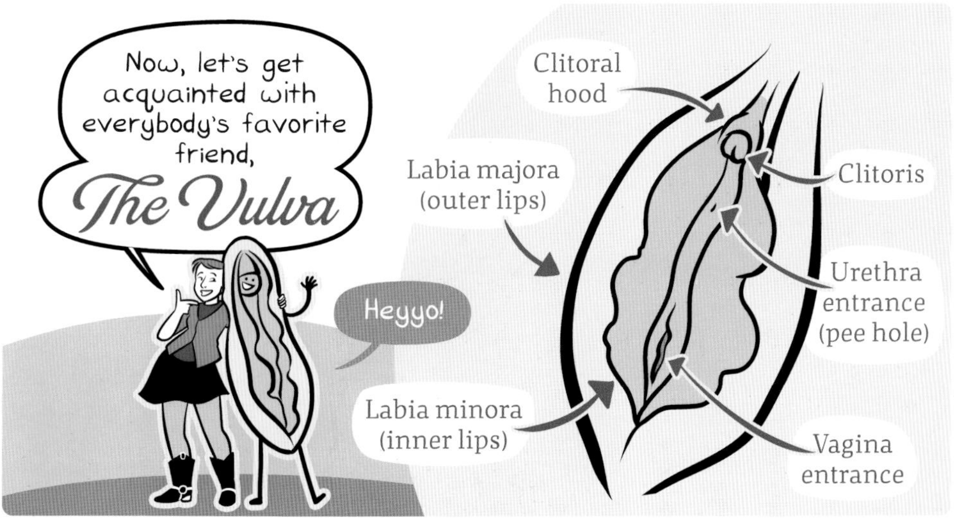
Now, let's get acquainted with everybody's favorite friend, The Vulva
Heyyo!
Clitoral hood
Labia majora (outer lips)
Clitoris
Urethra entrance (pee hole)
Labia minora (inner lips)
Vagina entrance

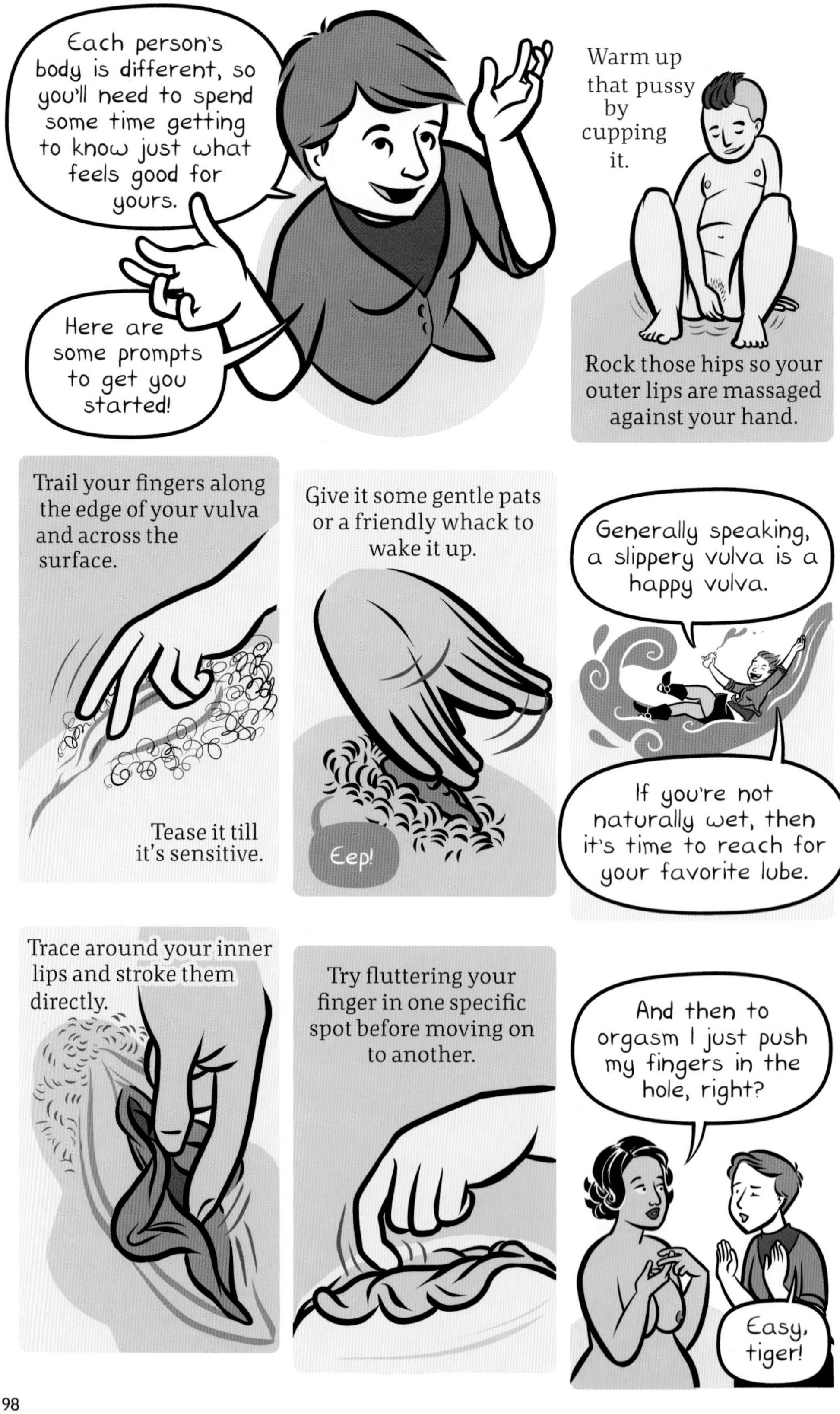
Each person's body is different, so you'll need to spend some time getting to know just what feels good for yours.
Here are some prompts to get you started!
Warm up that pussy by cupping it.
Rock those hips so your outer lips are massaged against your hand.
Trail your fingers along the edge of your vulva and across the surface.
Tease it till it's sensitive.
Give it some gentle pats or a friendly whack to wake it up.
Eep!
Generally speaking, a slippery vulva is a happy vulva.
If you're not naturally wet, then it's time to reach for your favorite lube.
Trace around your inner lips and stroke them directly.
Try fluttering your finger in one specific spot before moving on to another.
And then to orgasm I just push my fingers in the hole, right?
Easy, tiger!

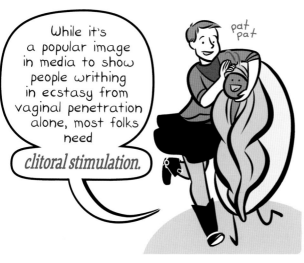

While it's a popular image in media to show people writing in ecstasy from vaginal penetration alone, most folks need *clitoral stimulation.*

pat pat

Circle your finger around the perimeter of the clit.

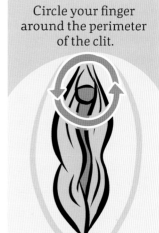

Press broad pressure directly against it and move fingers in a circular motion.

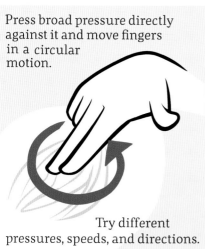

Try different pressures, speeds, and directions.

Take pauses!

A brief break can ramp up your sensitivity, making your cunt ache for more.

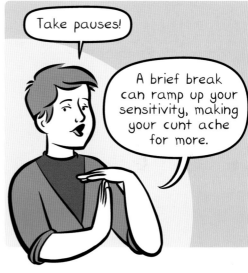

If you want to feel full or penetrated, slip a finger or two inside your vagina.

BZZZZZZZZZZZZ

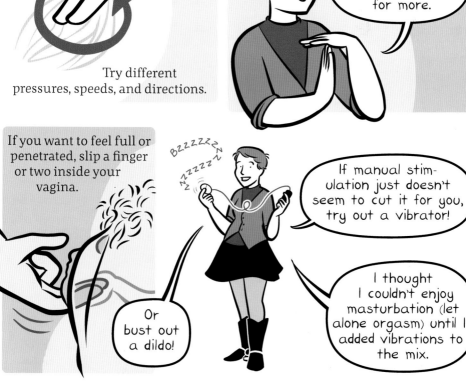

If manual stim-ulation just doesn't seem to cut it for you, try out a vibrator!

Or bust out a dildo!

I thought I couldn't enjoy masturbation (let alone orgasm) until I added vibrations to the mix.

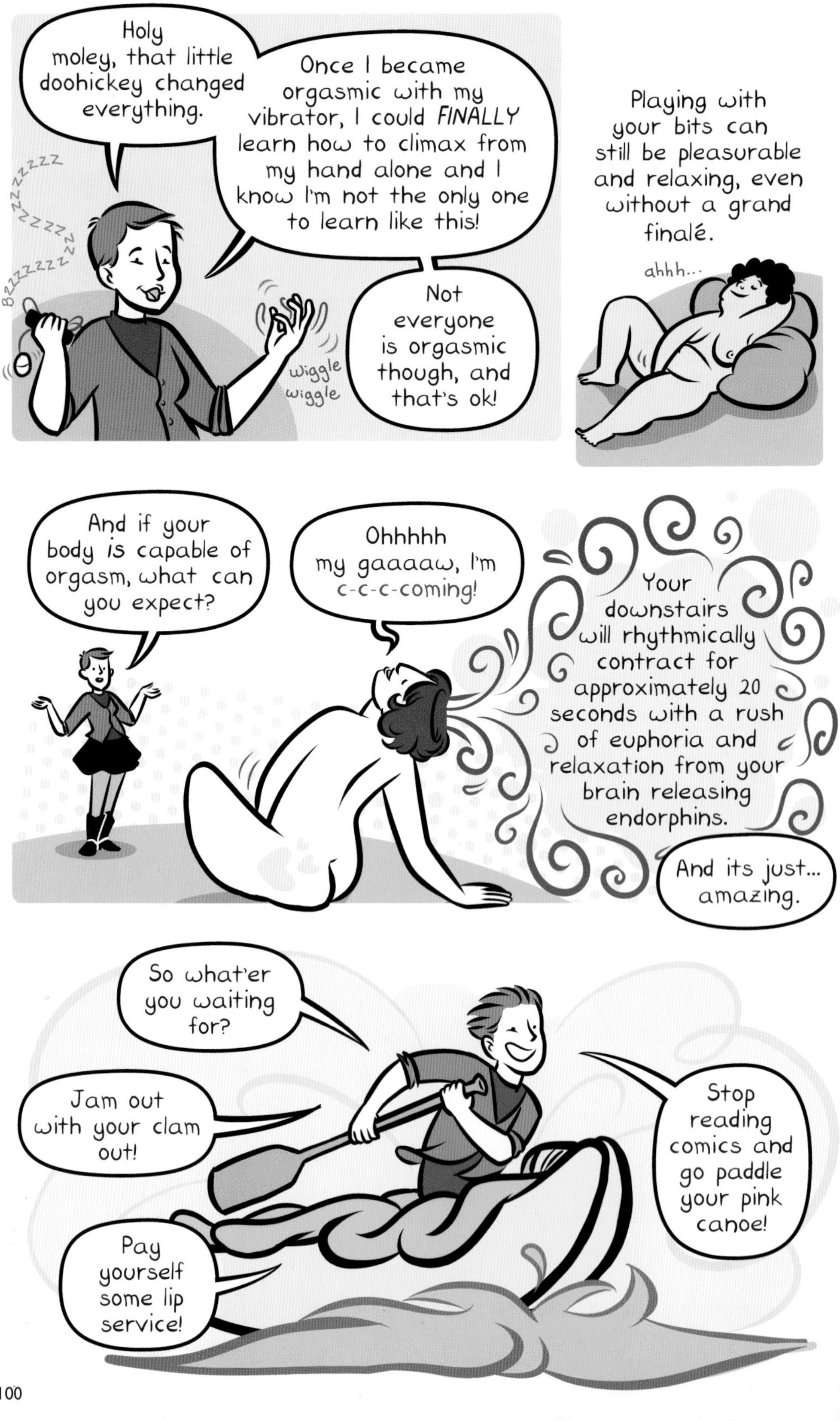
Holy moley, that little doohickey changed everything.
Bzzzzzzzz
Once I became orgasmic with my vibrator, I could *FINALLY* learn how to climax from my hand alone and I know I'm not the only one to learn like this!
wiggle wiggle
Not everyone is orgasmic though, and that's ok!
Playing with your bits can still be pleasurable and relaxing, even without a grand finalé.
ahhh...
And if your body *is* capable of orgasm, what can you expect?
Ohhhhh my gaaaaw, I'm c-c-c-coming!
Your downstairs will rhythmically contract for approximately 20 seconds with a rush of euphoria and relaxation from your brain releasing endorphins.
And its just... amazing.
So what'er you waiting for?
Jam out with your clam out!
Stop reading comics and go paddle your pink canoe!
Pay yourself some lip service!

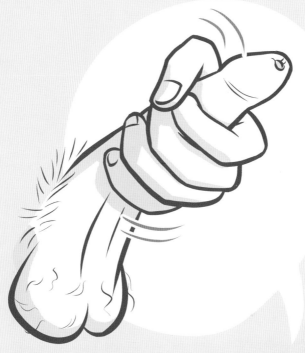

Masturbating
– Penis –

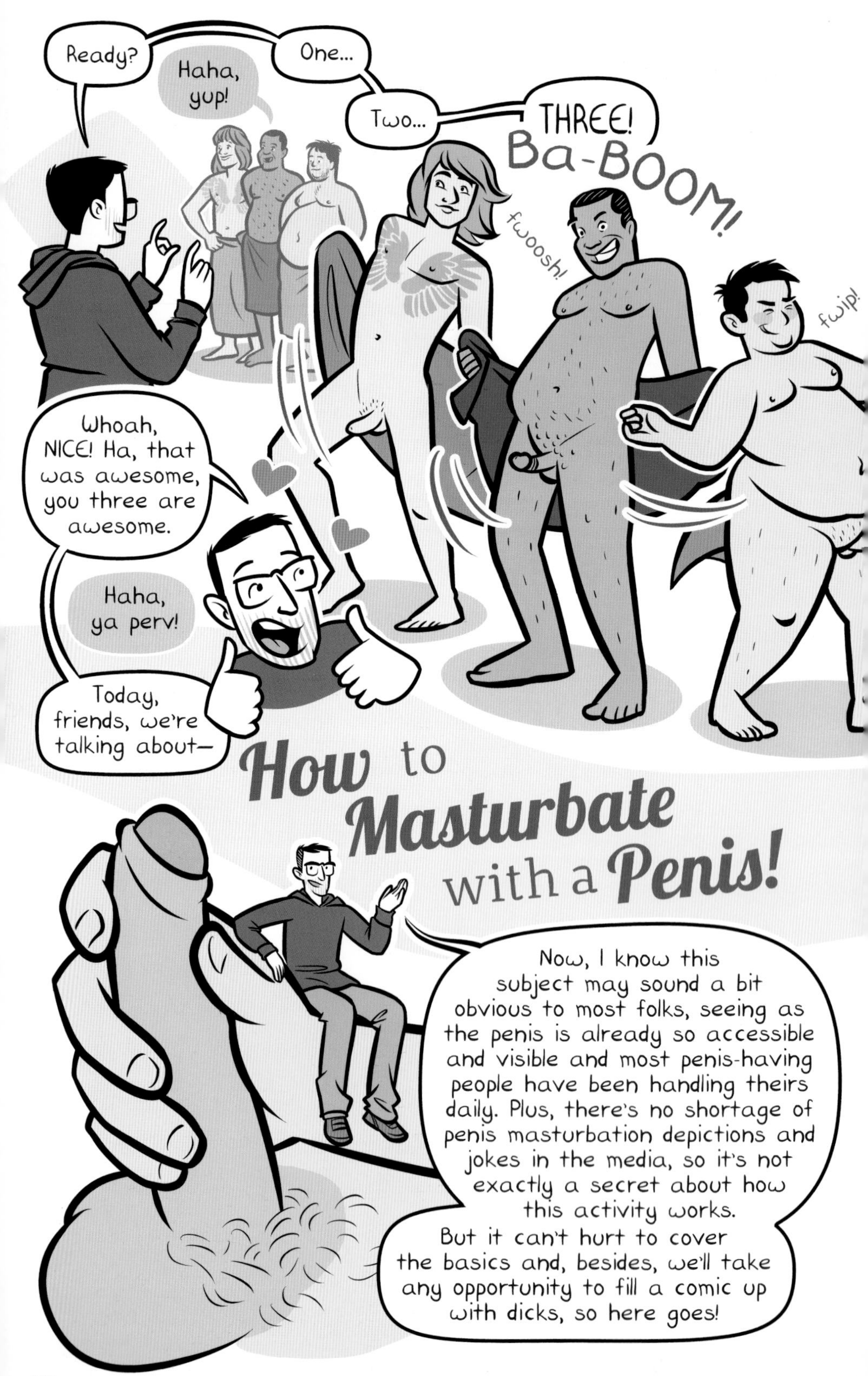
Ready?
Haha, yup!
One...
Two...
THREE!
Ba-BOOM!
fwooosh!
fwip!
Whoah, NICE! Ha, that was awesome, you three are awesome.
Haha, ya perv!
Today, friends, we're talking about—
How to Masturbate with a Penis!
Now, I know this subject may sound a bit obvious to most folks, seeing as the penis is already so accessible and visible and most penis-having people have been handling theirs daily. Plus, there's no shortage of penis masturbation depictions and jokes in the media, so it's not exactly a secret about how this activity works.
But it can't hurt to cover the basics and, besides, we'll take any opportunity to fill a comic up with dicks, so here goes!

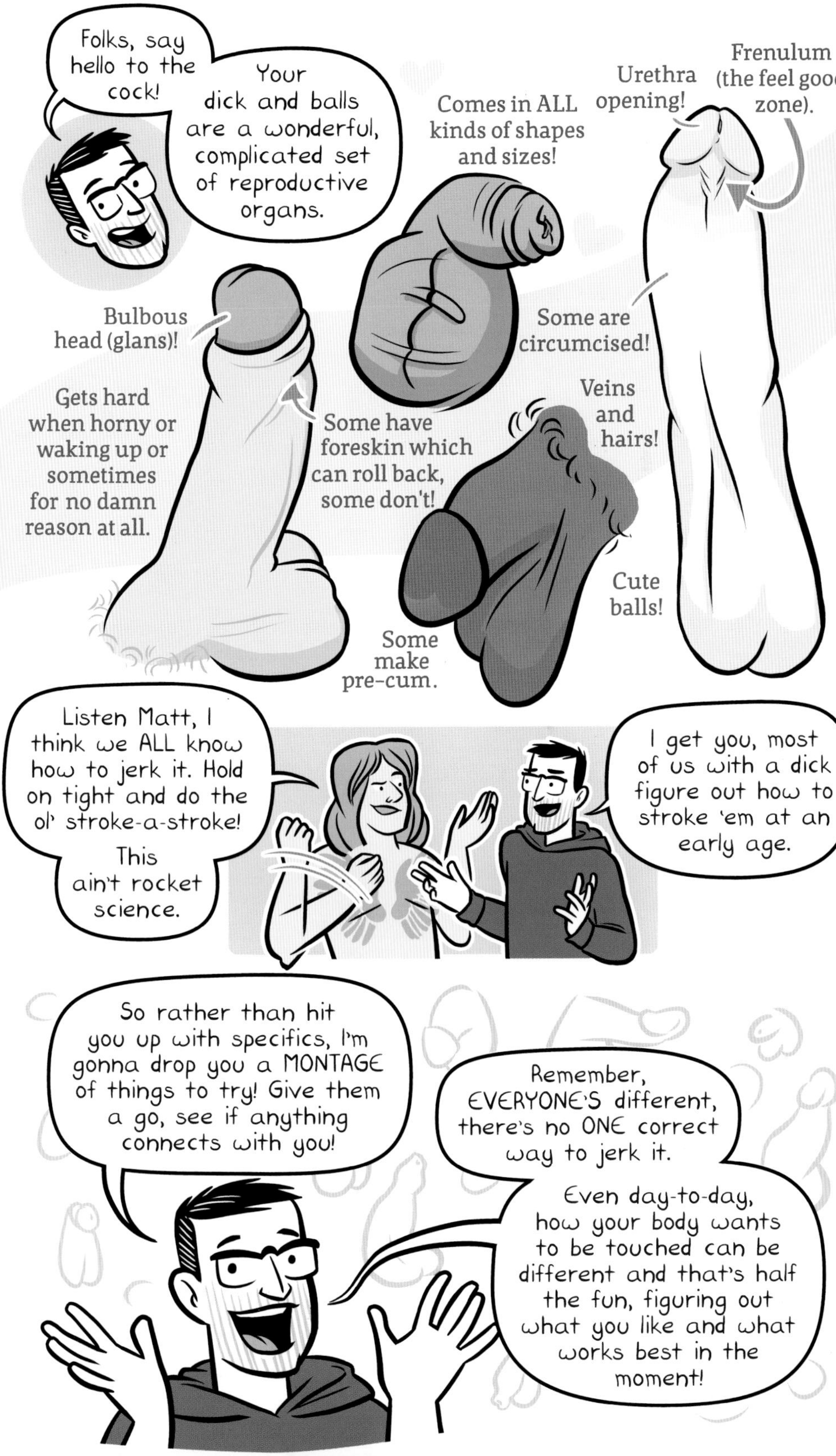

Folks, say hello to the cock!
Your dick and balls are a wonderful, complicated set of reproductive organs.
Comes in ALL kinds of shapes and sizes!
Urethra opening!
Frenulum (the feel good zone).
Bulbous head (glans)!
Some are circumcised!
Gets hard when horny or waking up or sometimes for no damn reason at all.
Some have foreskin which can roll back, some don't!
Veins and hairs!
Cute balls!
Some make pre-cum.
Listen Matt, I think we ALL know how to jerk it. Hold on tight and do the ol' stroke-a-stroke!
This ain't rocket science.
I get you, most of us with a dick figure out how to stroke 'em at an early age.
So rather than hit you up with specifics, I'm gonna drop you a MONTAGE of things to try! Give them a go, see if anything connects with you!
Remember, EVERYONE'S different, there's no ONE correct way to jerk it.
Even day-to-day, how your body wants to be touched can be different and that's half the fun, figuring out what you like and what works best in the moment!

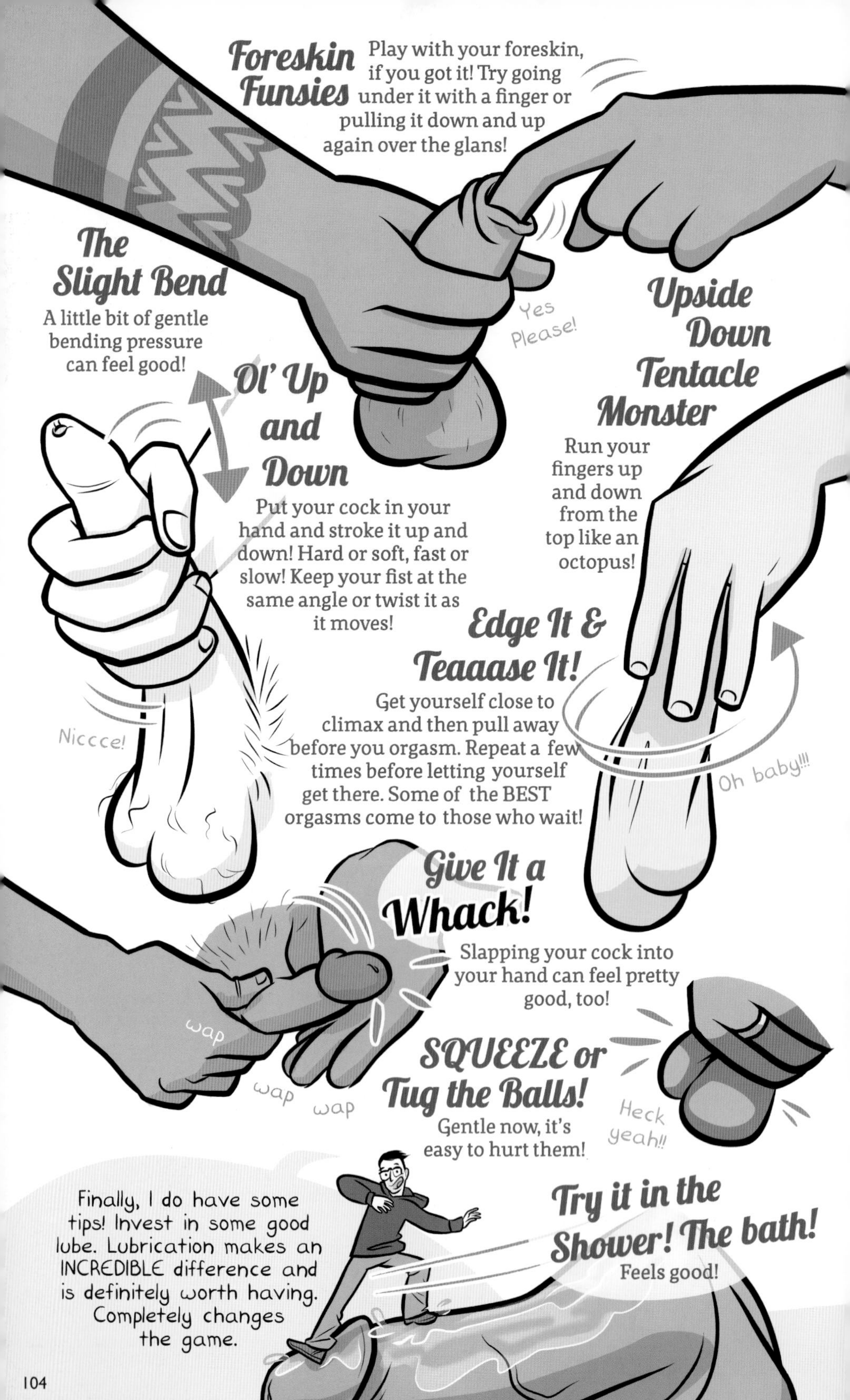
Foreskin Funsies
Play with your foreskin, if you got it! Try going under it with a finger or pulling it down and up again over the glans!
Yes Please!
The Slight Bend
A little bit of gentle bending pressure can feel good!
Ol' Up and Down
Put your cock in your hand and stroke it up and down! Hard or soft, fast or slow! Keep your fist at the same angle or twist it as it moves!
Niccce!
Upside Down Tentacle Monster
Run your fingers up and down from the top like an octopus!
Edge It & Teaaase It!
Get yourself close to climax and then pull away before you orgasm. Repeat a few times before letting yourself get there. Some of the BEST orgasms come to those who wait!
Oh baby!!!
Give It a Whack!
Slapping your cock into your hand can feel pretty good, too!
wap
wap
wap
SQUEEZE or Tug the Balls!
Gentle now, it's easy to hurt them!
Heck yeah!!
Finally, I do have some tips! Invest in some good lube. Lubrication makes an INCREDIBLE difference and is definitely worth having. Completely changes the game.
Try it in the Shower! The bath!
Feels good!

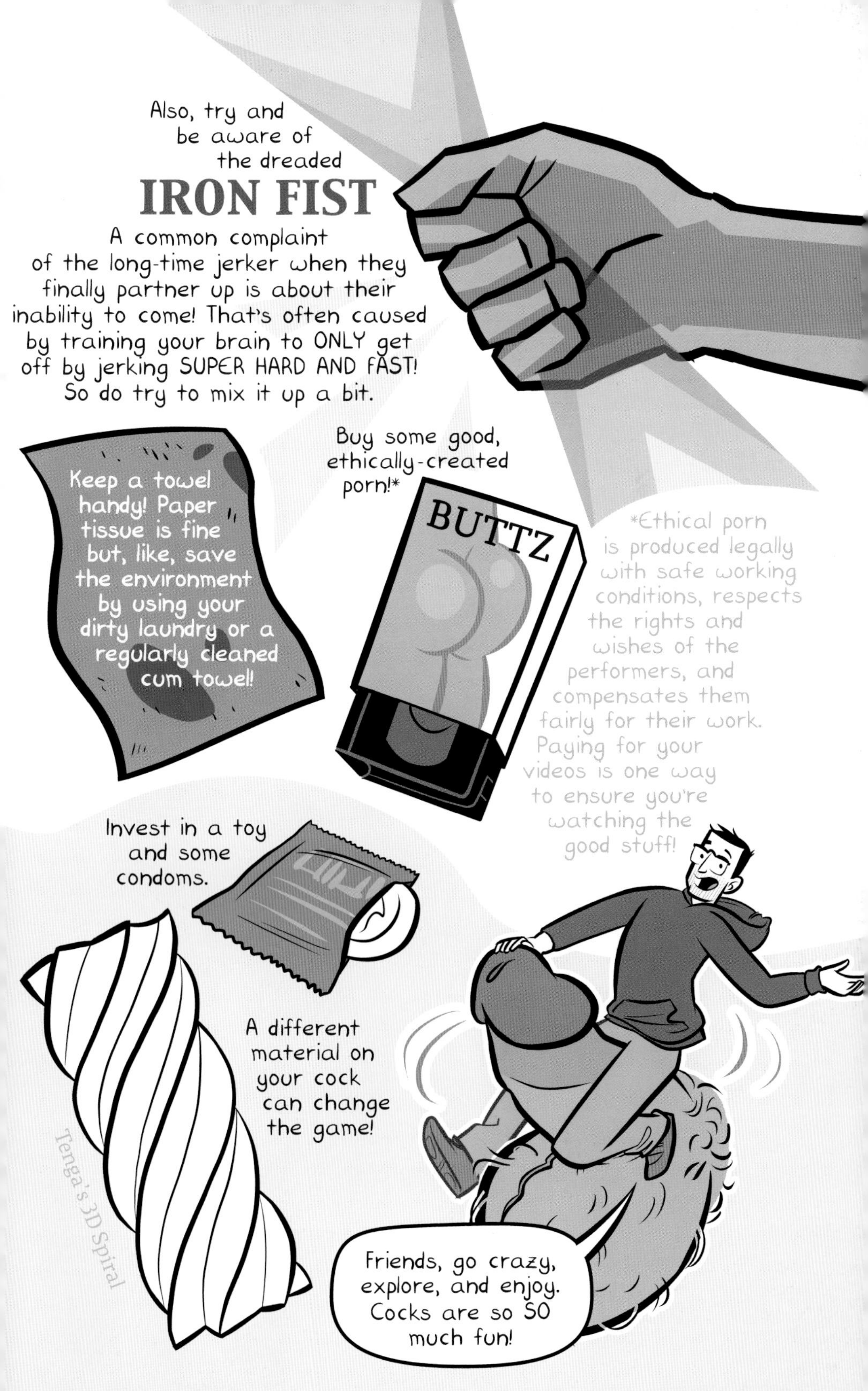

Also, try and be aware of the dreaded

IRON FIST

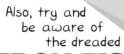

A common complaint of the long-time jerker when they finally partner up is about their inability to come! That's often caused by training your brain to ONLY get off by jerking SUPER HARD AND FAST! So do try to mix it up a bit.

Keep a towel handy! Paper tissue is fine but, like, save the environment by using your dirty laundry or a regularly cleaned cum towel!

Buy some good, ethically-created porn!*

BUTTZ

*Ethical porn is produced legally with safe working conditions, respects the rights and wishes of the performers, and compensates them fairly for their work. Paying for your videos is one way to ensure you're watching the good stuff!

Invest in a toy and some condoms.

A different material on your cock can change the game!

Tenga's 3D Spiral

Friends, go crazy, explore, and enjoy. Cocks are so SO much fun!

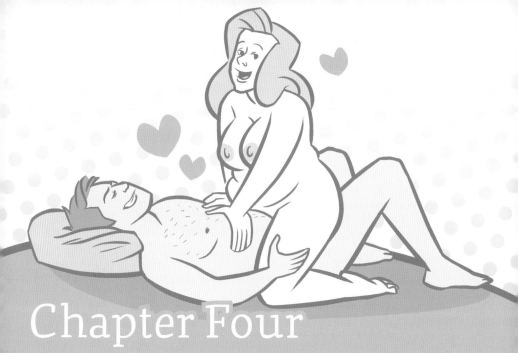

Chapter Four

Doin' It With Others

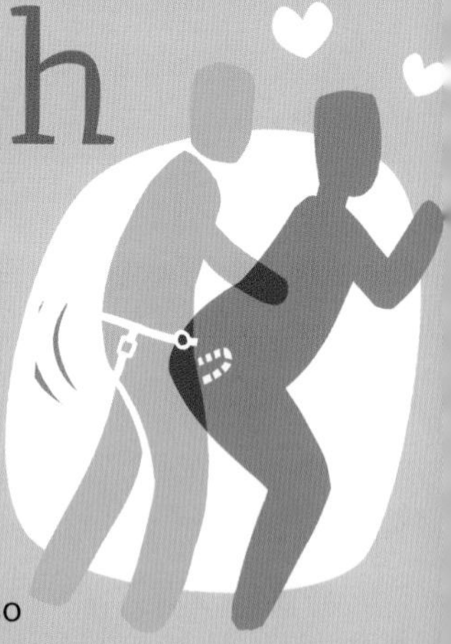

It's the part of the book where we talk about having sex... with OTHERS! Man, how does that even WORK? Read on, chums, and find out some of the ways people can smoosh their bodies together. You know by now that I love my cheesy analogies, so here is another one: having sex is a lot like dancing. There's so many different ways to move your body with another person, different rhythms and speeds and styles to try out together. It's a skill that you can develop with practice and communication! And just like dancing, it might not appeal to everyone! Some people don't especially crave it and some don't enjoy it and both of those things are A-OK. You don't have to dance if you don't feel like it and you don't gotta fuck either, that is totally normal and healthy.

There is no One Right Way to have sex. What you've seen in movies, watched in porn, or read about in dirty fanfiction is good for entertainment and arousal, but it's not necessarily a recipe for having The Good Sex. Good Sex means having sex in the way that feels best for you and your partner, whether you're together for one night or one lifetime. Talk about it together and try different activities!

Ok, ok, it's all well and good to talk about sex, but how do you actually DO it? Time to read on and get some instructional comics!

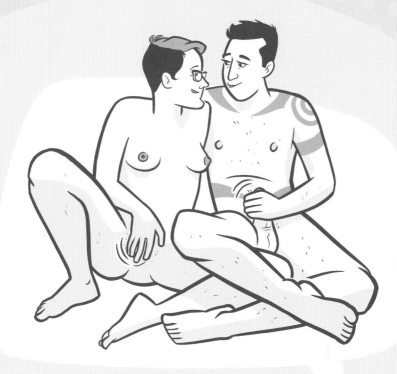

Mutual
Masturbation

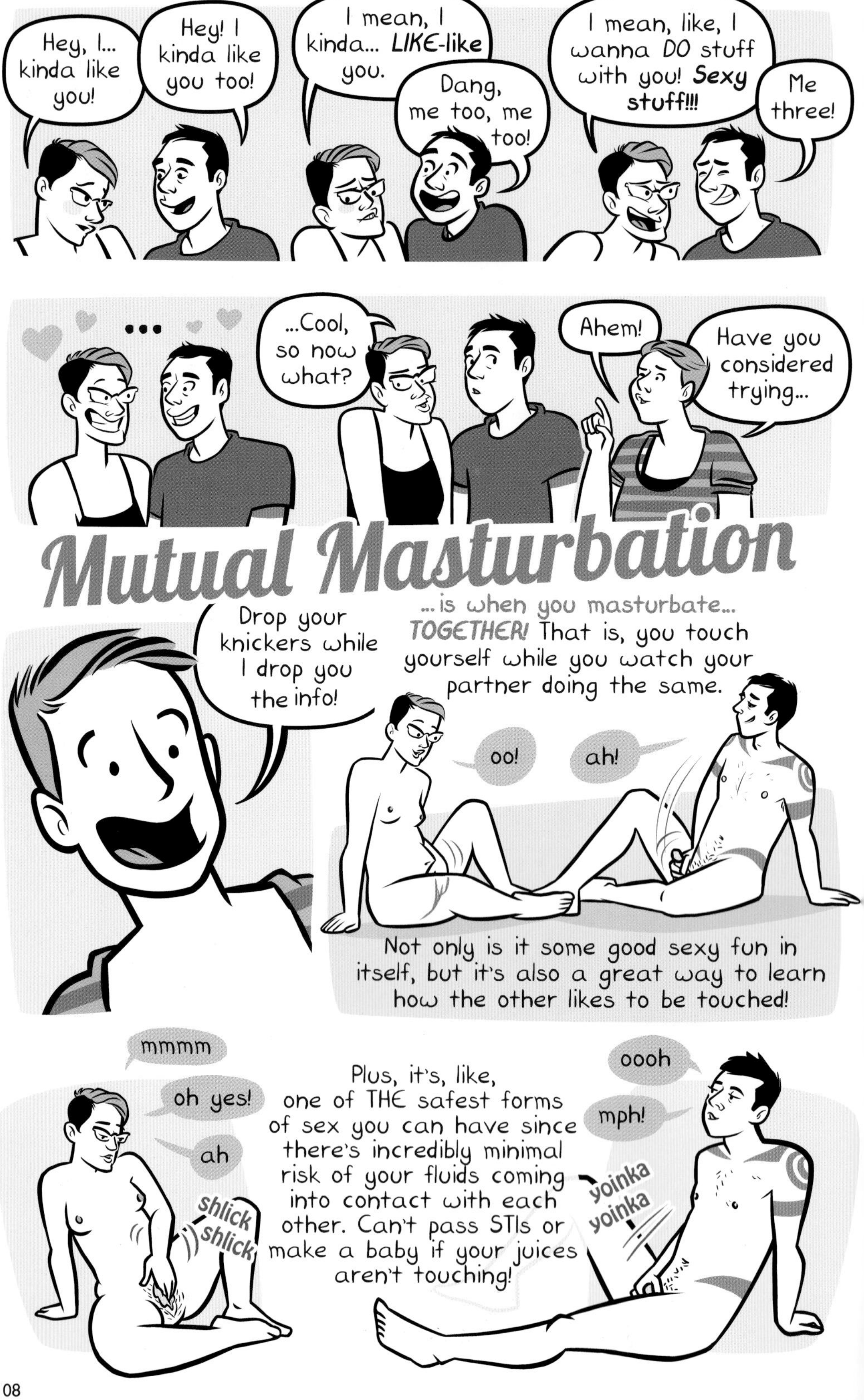
Hey, I... kinda like you!
Hey! I kinda like you too!
I mean, I kinda... LIKE-like you.
Dang, me too, me too!
I mean, like, I wanna DO stuff with you! Sexy stuff!!!
Me three!
...Cool, so now what?
Ahem!
Have you considered trying...
Mutual Masturbation
Drop your knickers while I drop you the info!
...is when you masturbate... TOGETHER! That is, you touch yourself while you watch your partner doing the same.
oo!
ah!
Not only is it some good sexy fun in itself, but it's also a great way to learn how the other likes to be touched!
mmmm
oh yes!
ah
shlick shlick
Plus, it's, like, one of THE safest forms of sex you can have since there's incredibly minimal risk of your fluids coming into contact with each other. Can't pass STIs or make a baby if your juices aren't touching!
oooh
mph!
yoinka yoinka

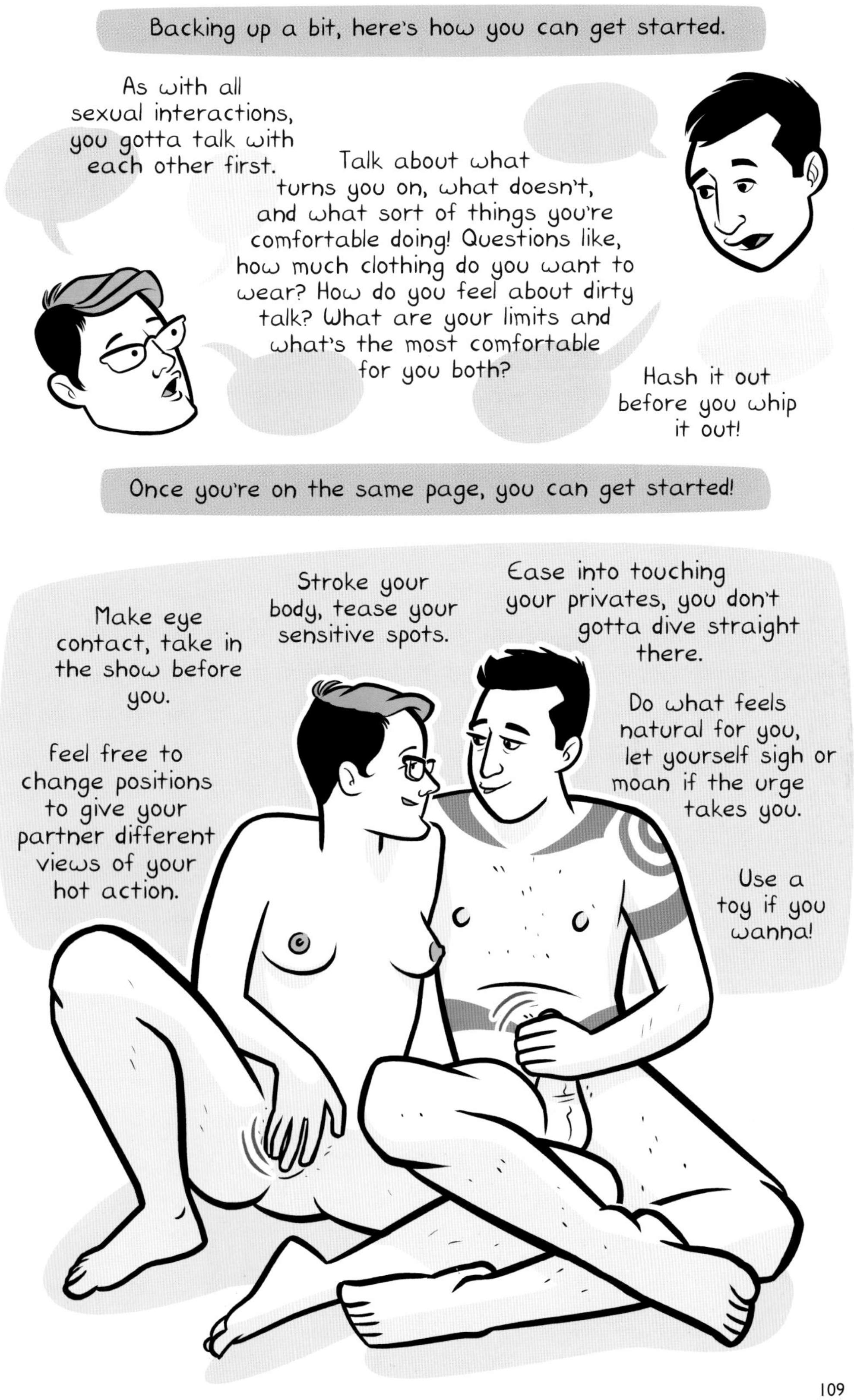
Backing up a bit, here's how you can get started.
As with all sexual interactions, you gotta talk with each other first.
Talk about what turns you on, what doesn't, and what sort of things you're comfortable doing! Questions like, how much clothing do you want to wear? How do you feel about dirty talk? What are your limits and what's the most comfortable for you both?
Hash it out before you whip it out!
Once you're on the same page, you can get started!
Make eye contact, take in the show before you.
Stroke your body, tease your sensitive spots.
Ease into touching your privates, you don't gotta dive straight there.
Feel free to change positions to give your partner different views of your hot action.
Do what feels natural for you, let yourself sigh or moan if the urge takes you.
Use a toy if you wanna!

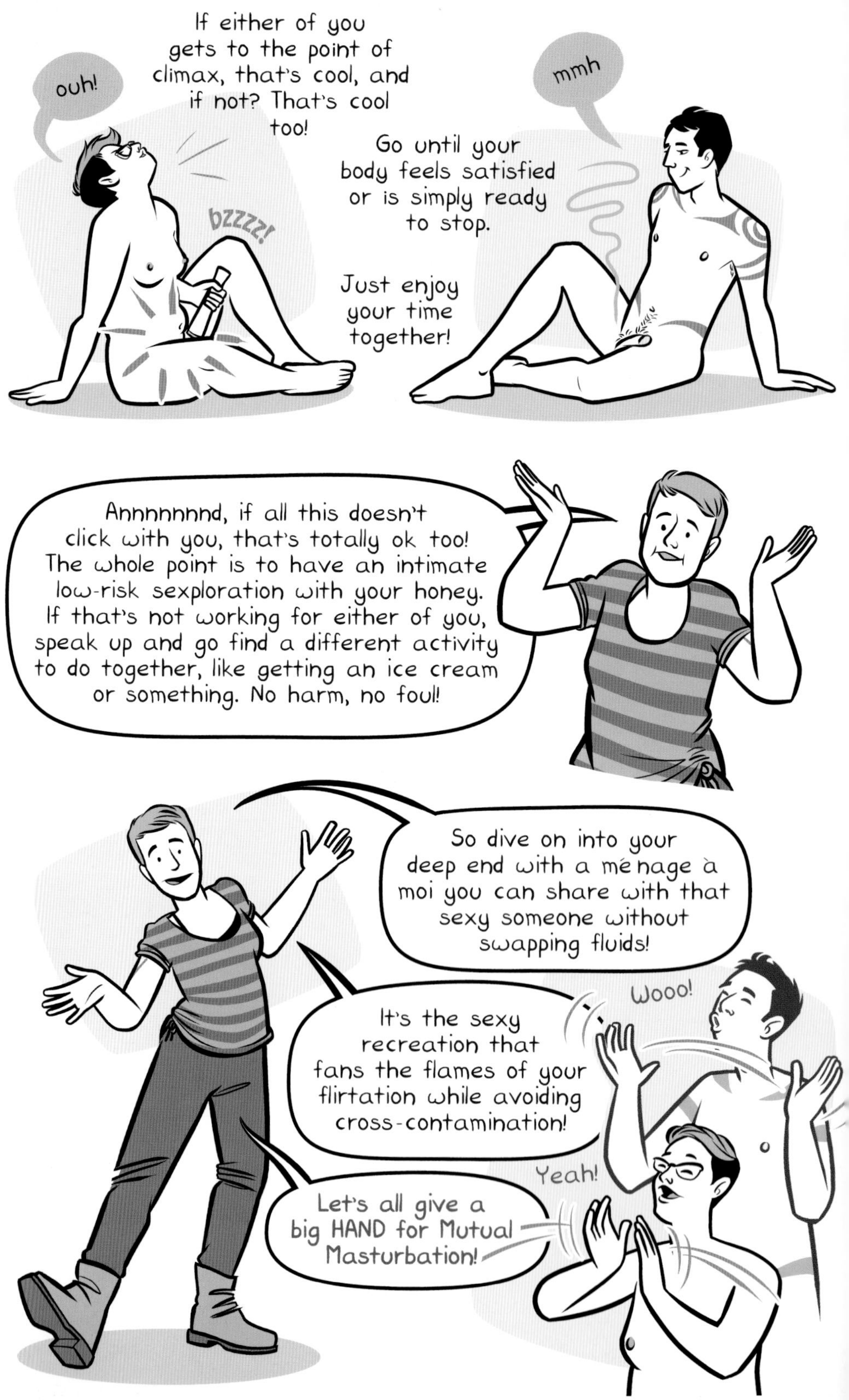
ouh!
If either of you gets to the point of climax, that's cool, and if not? That's cool too!
bzzzz!
mmh
Go until your body feels satisfied or is simply ready to stop.
Just enjoy your time together!
Annnnnnnd, if all this doesn't click with you, that's totally ok too! The whole point is to have an intimate low-risk sexploration with your honey. If that's not working for either of you, speak up and go find a different activity to do together, like getting an ice cream or something. No harm, no foul!
So dive on into your deep end with a ménage à moi you can share with that sexy someone without swapping fluids!
Wooo!
It's the sexy recreation that fans the flames of your flirtation while avoiding cross-contamination!
Yeah!
Let's all give a big HAND for Mutual Masturbation!

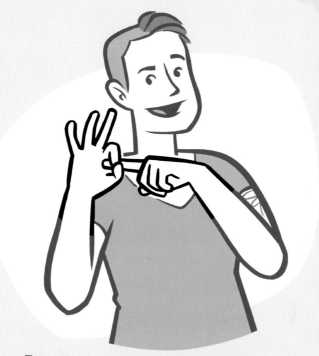

Manual Sex

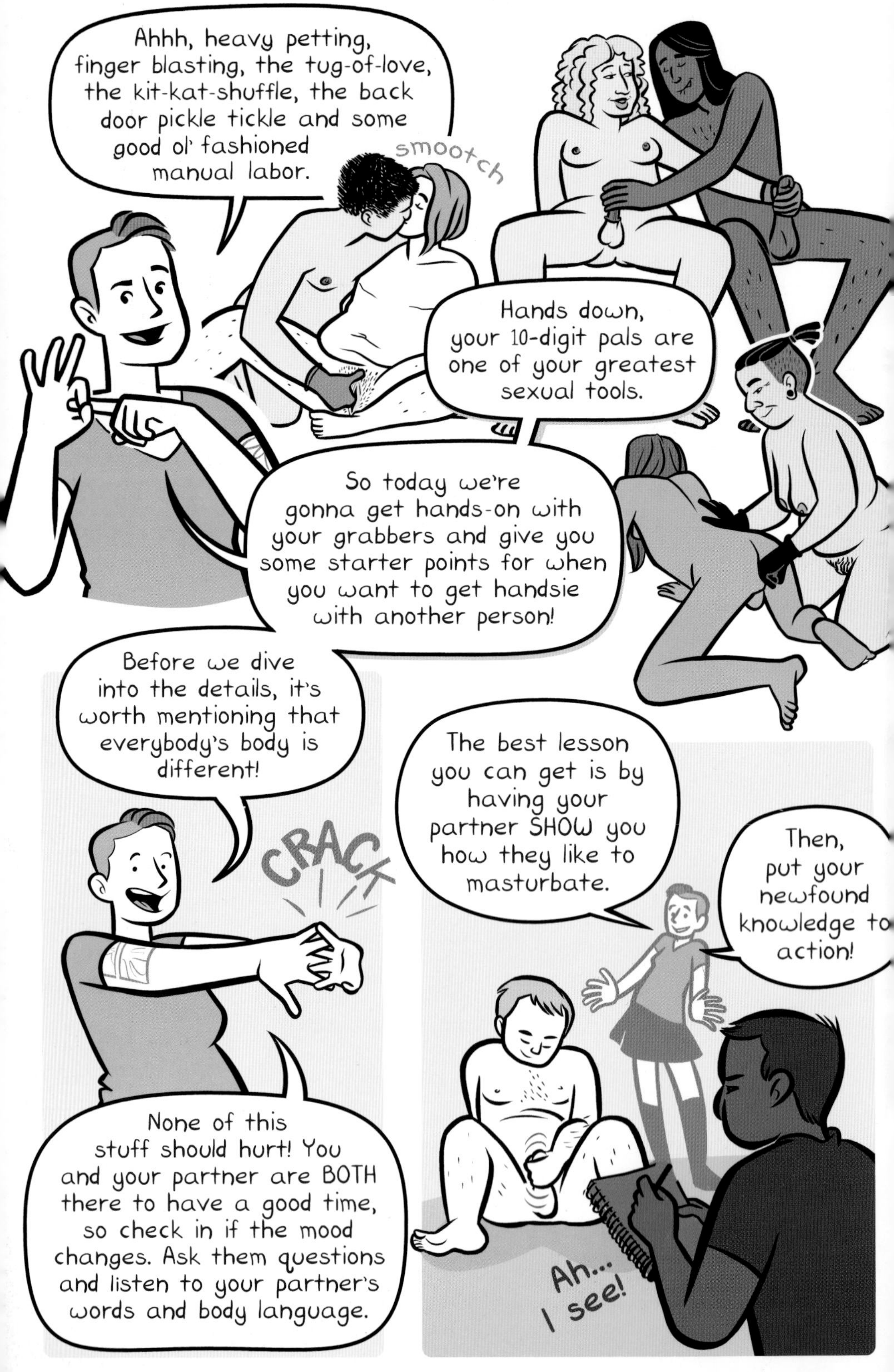
Ahhh, heavy petting, finger blasting, the tug-of-love, the kit-kat-shuffle, the back door pickle tickle and some good ol' fashioned manual labor.
smootch
Hands down, your 10-digit pals are one of your greatest sexual tools.
So today we're gonna get hands-on with your grabbers and give you some starter points for when you want to get handsie with another person!
Before we dive into the details, it's worth mentioning that everybody's body is different!
CRACK
None of this stuff should hurt! You and your partner are BOTH there to have a good time, so check in if the mood changes. Ask them questions and listen to your partner's words and body language.
The best lesson you can get is by having your partner SHOW you how they like to masturbate.
Then, put your newfound knowledge to action!
Ah... I see!

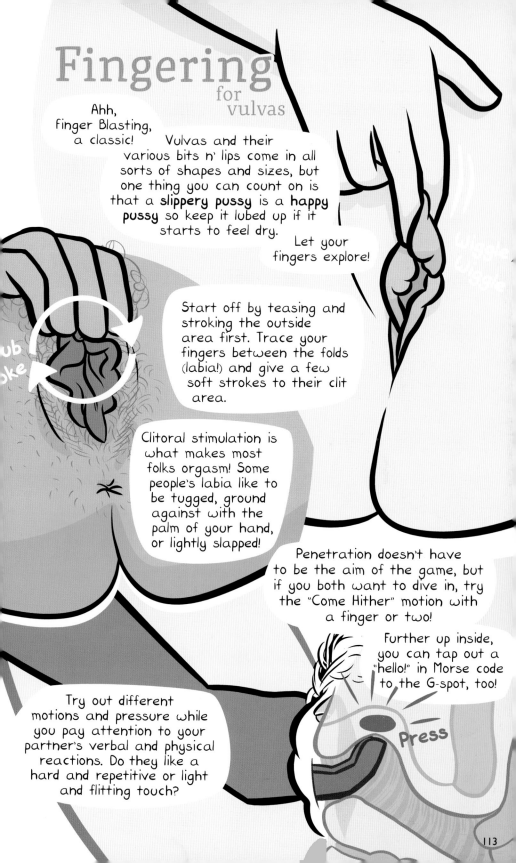

Fingering
for vulvas

Ahh, finger Blasting, a classic! Vulvas and their various bits n' lips come in all sorts of shapes and sizes, but one thing you can count on is that a **slippery pussy** is a **happy pussy** so keep it lubed up if it starts to feel dry.

Let your fingers explore!

wiggle wiggle

rub stroke

Start off by teasing and stroking the outside area first. Trace your fingers between the folds (labia!) and give a few soft strokes to their clit area.

Clitoral stimulation is what makes most folks orgasm! Some people's labia like to be tugged, ground against with the palm of your hand, or lightly slapped!

Penetration doesn't have to be the aim of the game, but if you both want to dive in, try the "Come Hither" motion with a finger or two!

Further up inside, you can tap out a "hello!" in Morse code to the G-spot, too!

Try out different motions and pressure while you pay attention to your partner's verbal and physical reactions. Do they like a hard and repetitive or light and flitting touch?

Press

Handjobs
for penises

The Ol' Rub 'n' Tug!

Some folks like drier contact, others prefer to keep things slippery with some lube!

Test out different grip pressures and listen to the cock in your hand. It'll tell you how it feels about what you're doing by the way it surges, pulses, hardens, or softens.

You can use both hands to cover more ground!

The head can be very sensitive, try running your thumb over the frenulum periodically.

Jerk Twist

Try twisting your hand around the cock shaft and head every now and then, if they still have it, sliding the foreskin up and over the top and then back down again.

Don't forget to give a little love to the balls! Give 'em a gentle tug, cup them in your hand, or roll them in your palm.

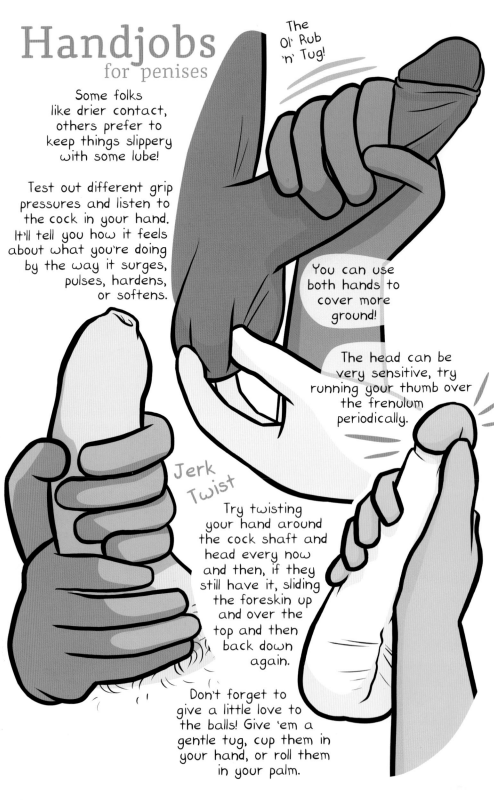

Get'cher pinky all stinky with some...

Butt Fingering
for anuses

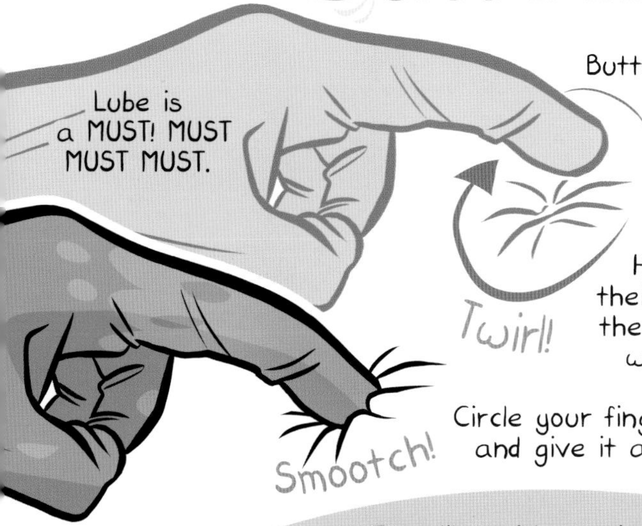
Twirl!
Smootch!

Lube is a MUST! MUST MUST MUST.

Butts can be very fickle, so this is ALL about listening to your partner, reading their body, and starting SLOW.

Help your partner relax their rectum by entertaining their other sensitives areas with your opposite hand.

Circle your finger against the rim and give it a little tap or two.

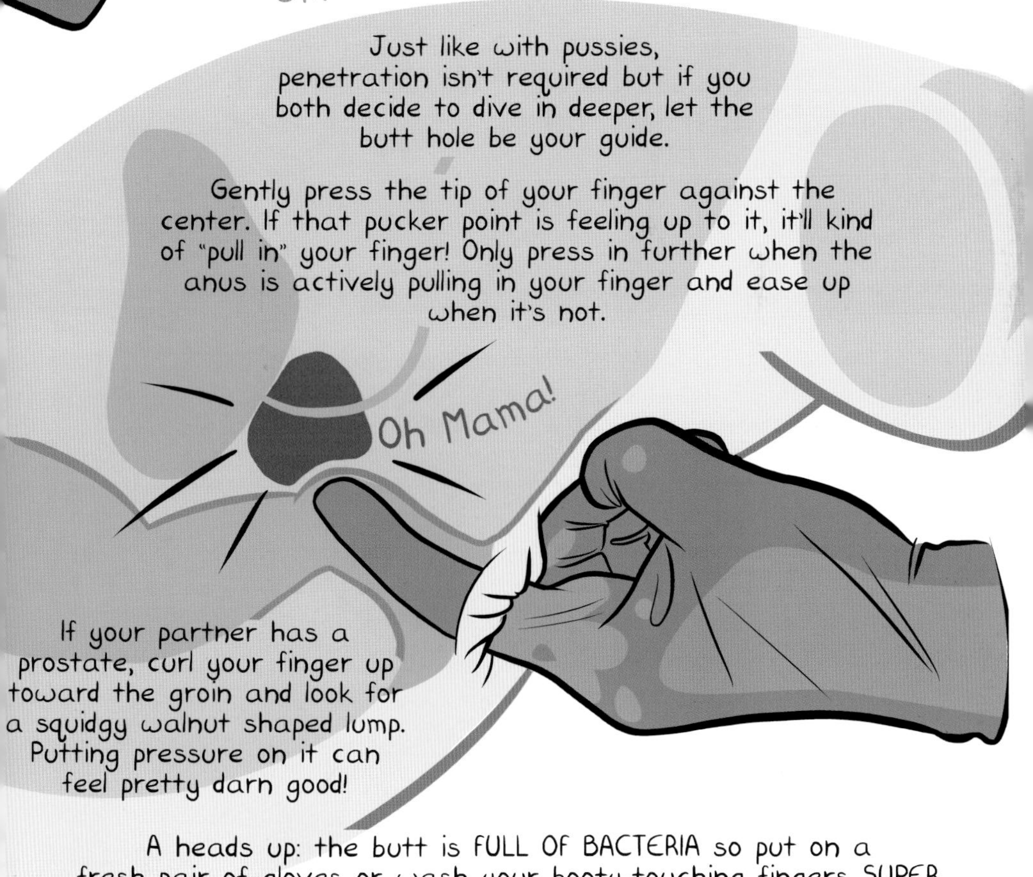
Oh Mama!

Just like with pussies, penetration isn't required but if you both decide to dive in deeper, let the butt hole be your guide.

Gently press the tip of your finger against the center. If that pucker point is feeling up to it, it'll kind of "pull in" your finger! Only press in further when the anus is actively pulling in your finger and ease up when it's not.

If your partner has a prostate, curl your finger up toward the groin and look for a squidgy walnut shaped lump. Putting pressure on it can feel pretty darn good!

A heads up: the butt is FULL OF BACTERIA so put on a fresh pair of gloves or wash your booty-touching fingers SUPER well with soap before touching other parts of the body, ESPECIALLY the vulva!

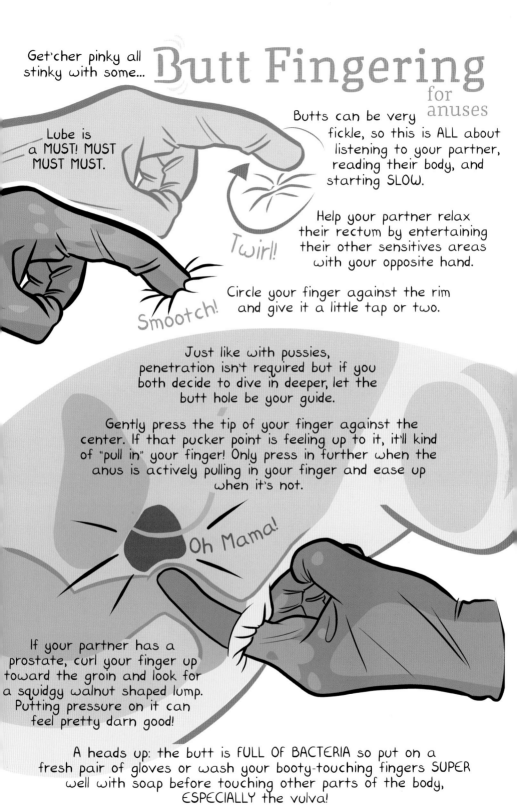

Fisting

for vaginas & anuses

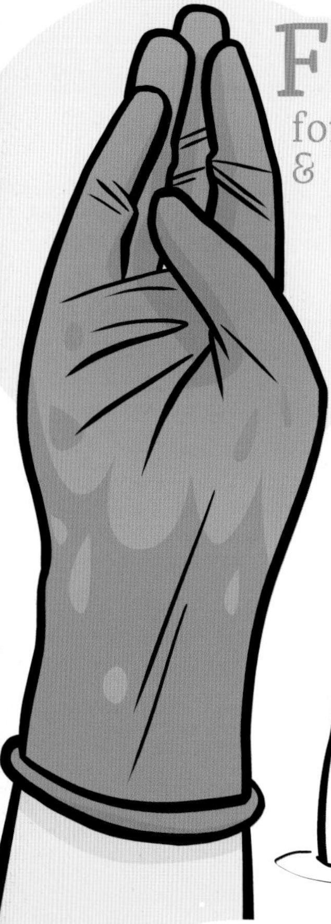

This is **varsity level** hand sex and NOT for beginners or the impatient! This is also something that not everyone is physically capable of having done to them.

COMMUNICATE CONSTANTLY.

Use SO much lube. And then use even more. The vagina or anus needs to be ULTRA warmed up and already spacious from lots of fingers or toys going in to prepare it to be fisted.

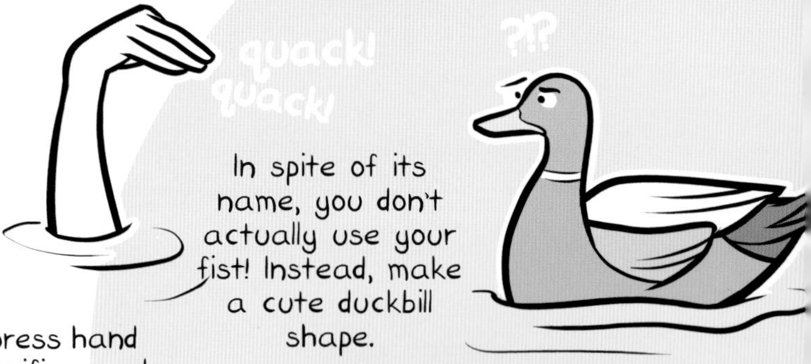
quack!
quack!
?!?

In spite of its name, you don't actually use your fist! Instead, make a cute duckbill shape.

GENTLY press hand into the orifice, and let the opening pull in the hand. Do not push against resistance! Stop if it hurts!!!!

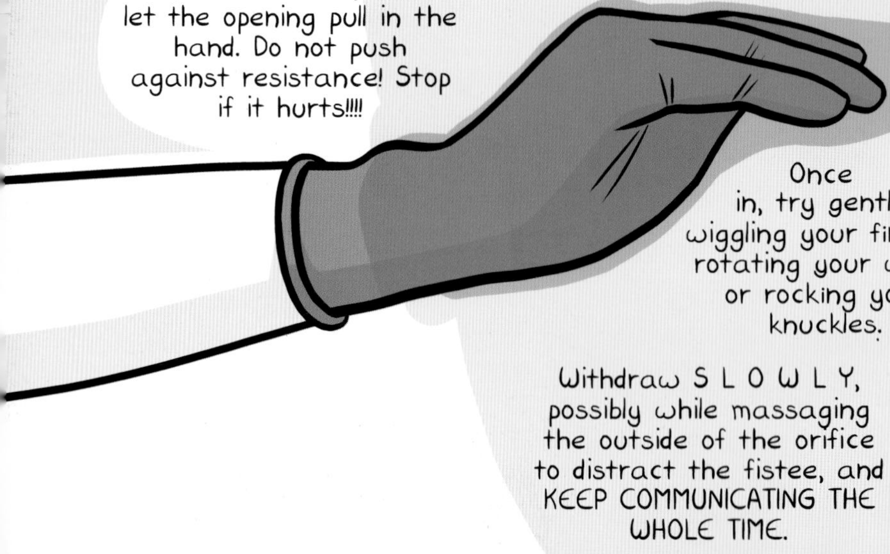

Once in, try gently wiggling your fingers, rotating your wrist, or rocking your knuckles.

Withdraw S L O W L Y, possibly while massaging the outside of the orifice to distract the fistee, and KEEP COMMUNICATING THE WHOLE TIME.

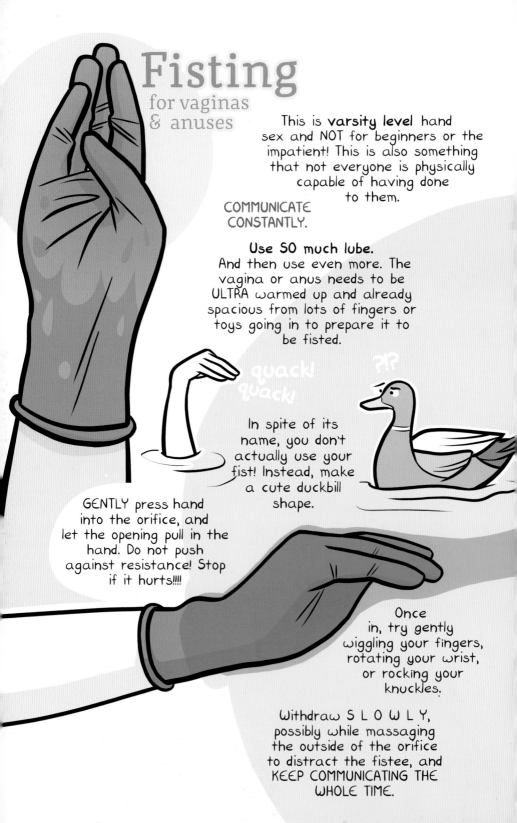

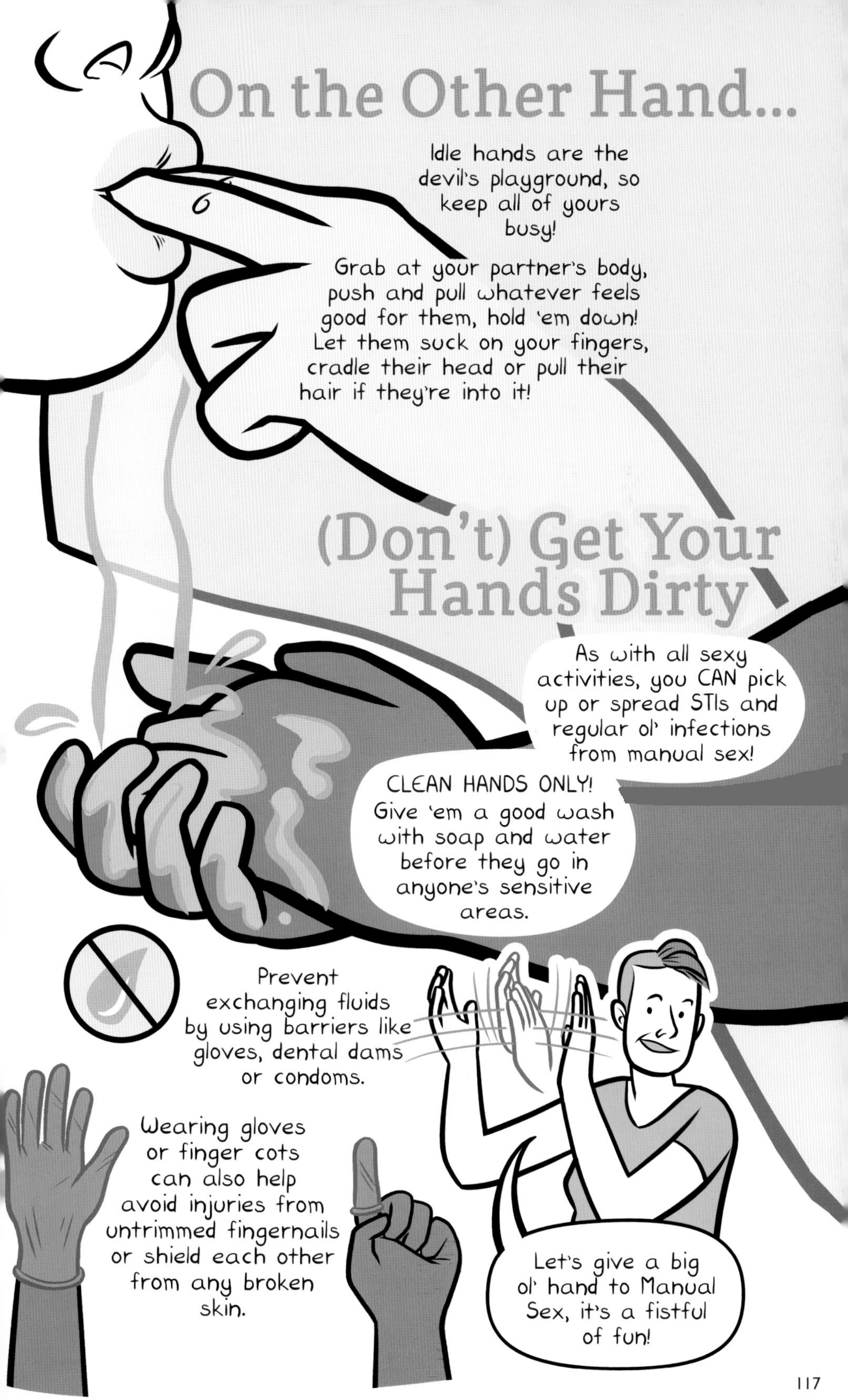
On the Other Hand...
Idle hands are the devil's playground, so keep all of yours busy!
Grab at your partner's body, push and pull whatever feels good for them, hold 'em down! Let them suck on your fingers, cradle their head or pull their hair if they're into it!
(Don't) Get Your Hands Dirty
As with all sexy activities, you CAN pick up or spread STIs and regular ol' infections from manual sex!
CLEAN HANDS ONLY! Give 'em a good wash with soap and water before they go in anyone's sensitive areas.
Prevent exchanging fluids by using barriers like gloves, dental dams or condoms.
Wearing gloves or finger cots can also help avoid injuries from untrimmed fingernails or shield each other from any broken skin.
Let's give a big ol' hand to Manual Sex, it's a fistful of fun!

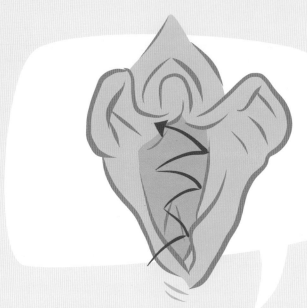

Oral Sex
for a Vulva

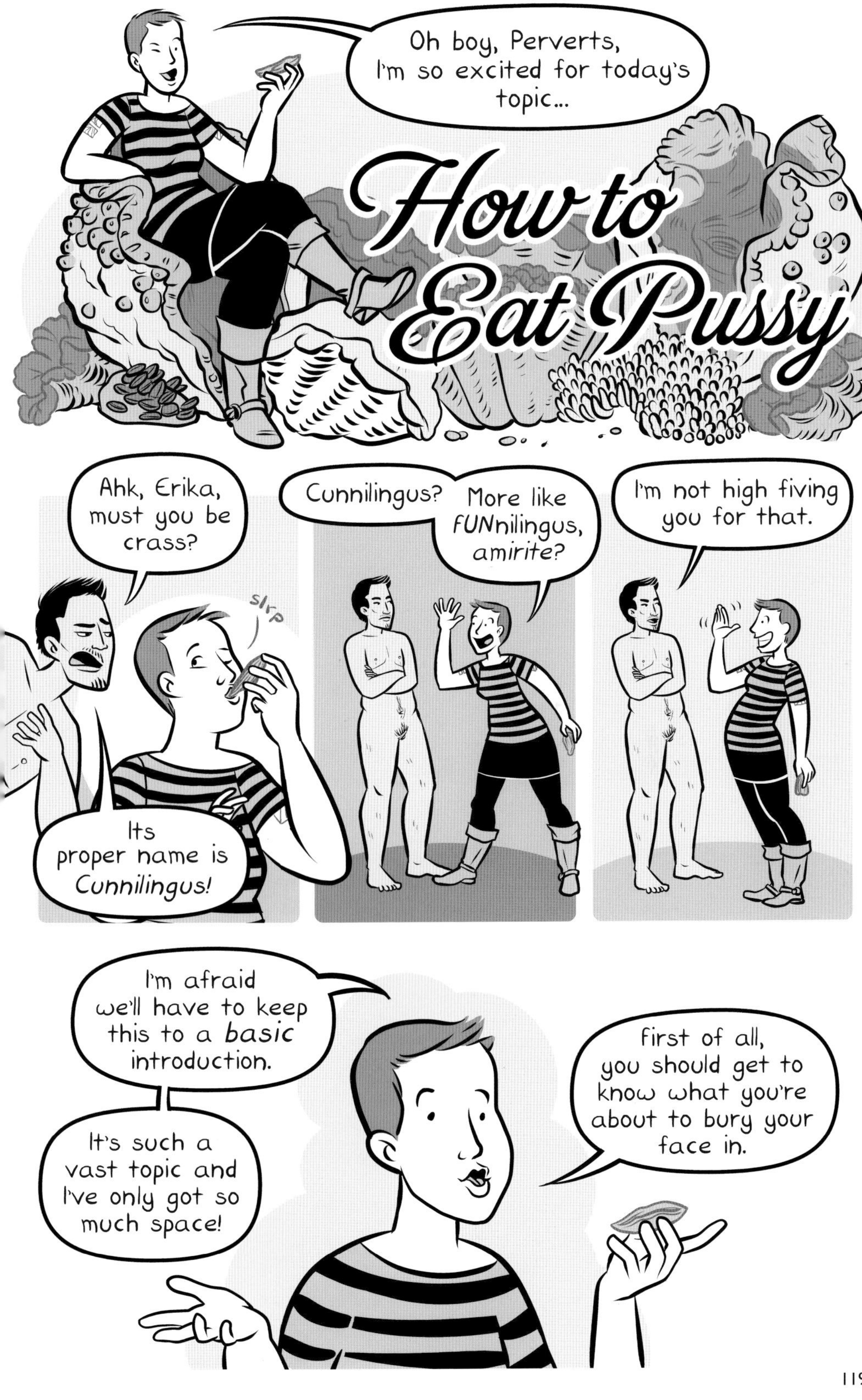
Oh boy, Perverts, I'm so excited for today's topic...
How to Eat Pussy
Ahk, Erika, must you be crass?
slrp
Its proper name is Cunnilingus!
Cunnilingus?
More like FUNnilingus, amirite?
I'm not high fiving you for that.
I'm afraid we'll have to keep this to a basic introduction.
It's such a vast topic and I've only got so much space!
first of all, you should get to know what you're about to bury your face in.

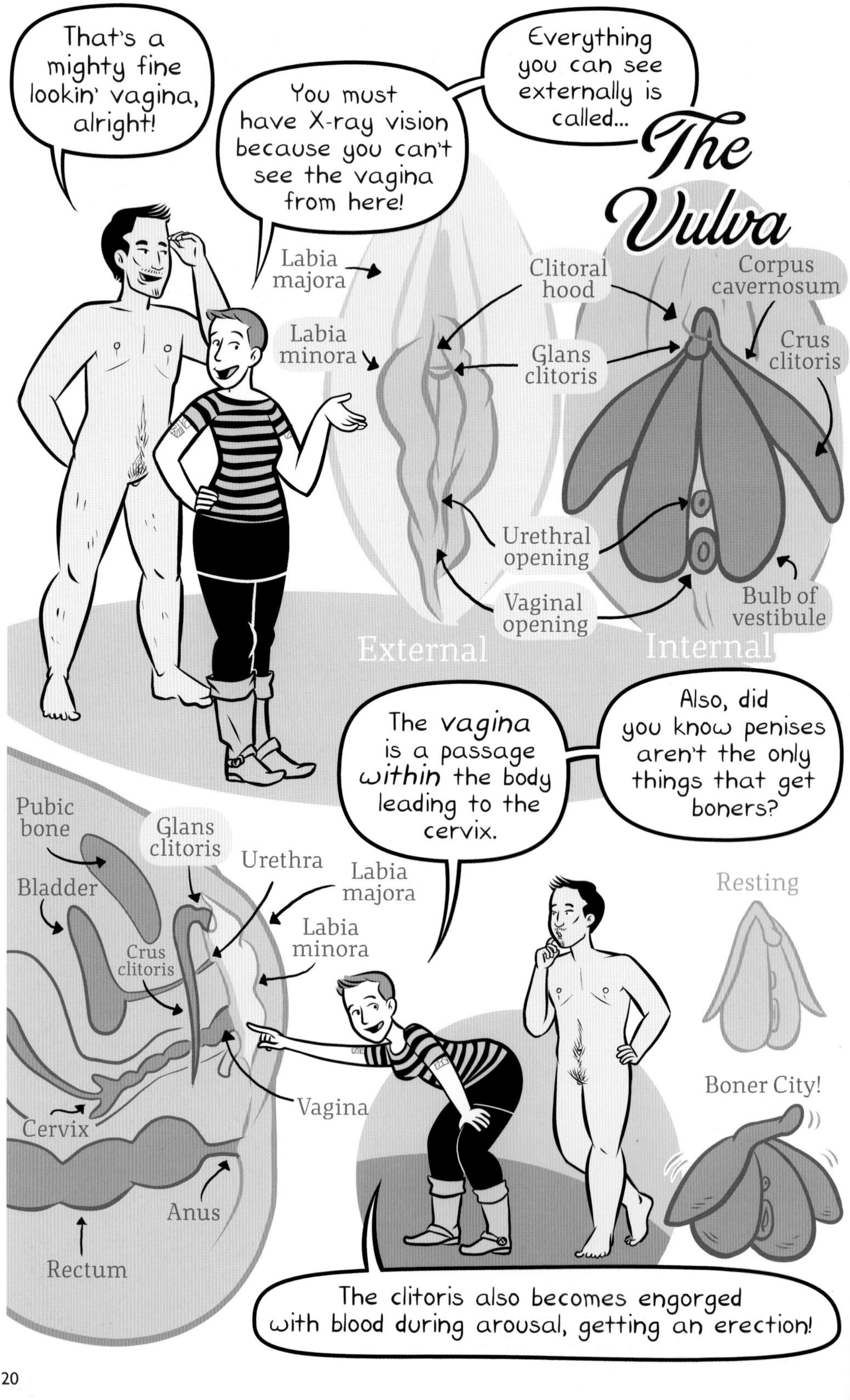

That's a mighty fine lookin' vagina, alright!
You must have X-ray vision because you can't see the vagina from here!
Everything you can see externally is called...
The Vulva
Labia majora
Labia minora
Clitoral hood
Glans clitoris
Corpus cavernosum
Crus clitoris
Urethral opening
Vaginal opening
Bulb of vestibule
External
Internal
The vagina is a passage within the body leading to the cervix.
Also, did you know penises aren't the only things that get boners?
Pubic bone
Bladder
Glans clitoris
Urethra
Labia majora
Labia minora
Crus clitoris
Vagina
Cervix
Anus
Rectum
Resting
Boner City!
The clitoris also becomes engorged with blood during arousal, getting an erection!

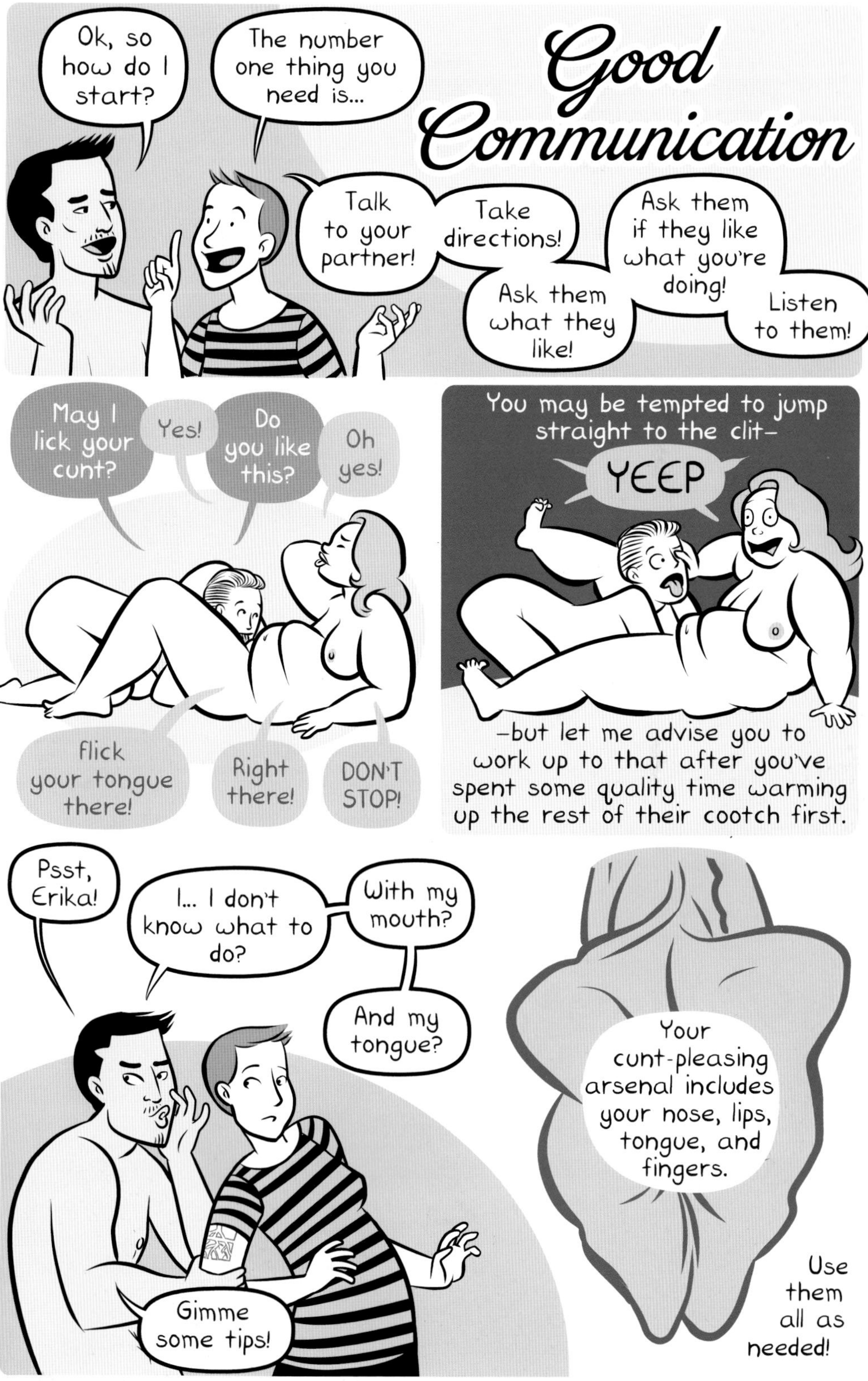
Ok, so how do I start?
The number one thing you need is...
Good Communication
Talk to your partner!
Take directions!
Ask them what they like!
Ask them if they like what you're doing!
Listen to them!
May I lick your cunt?
Yes!
Do you like this?
Oh yes!
Flick your tongue there!
Right there!
DON'T STOP!
You may be tempted to jump straight to the clit–
YEEP
–but let me advise you to work up to that after you've spent some quality time warming up the rest of their cootch first.
Psst, Erika!
I... I don't know what to do?
With my mouth?
And my tongue?
Gimme some tips!
Your cunt-pleasing arsenal includes your nose, lips, tongue, and fingers.
Use them all as needed!

Take Your Tongue Cross Cuntry

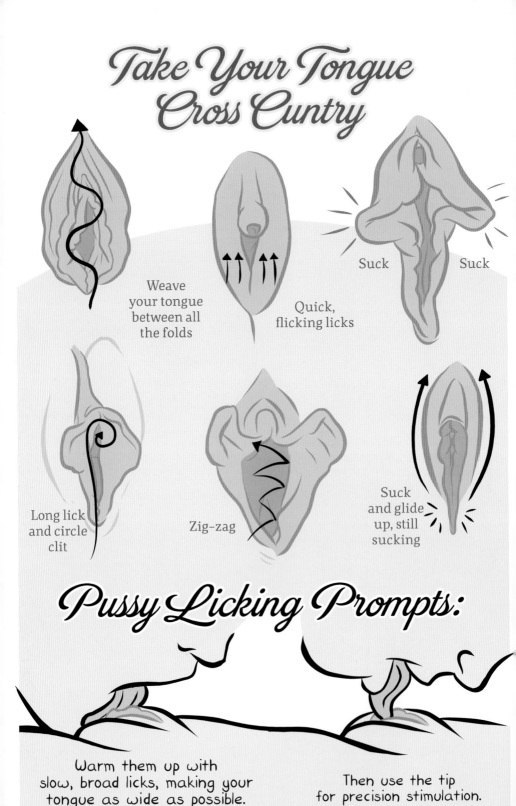

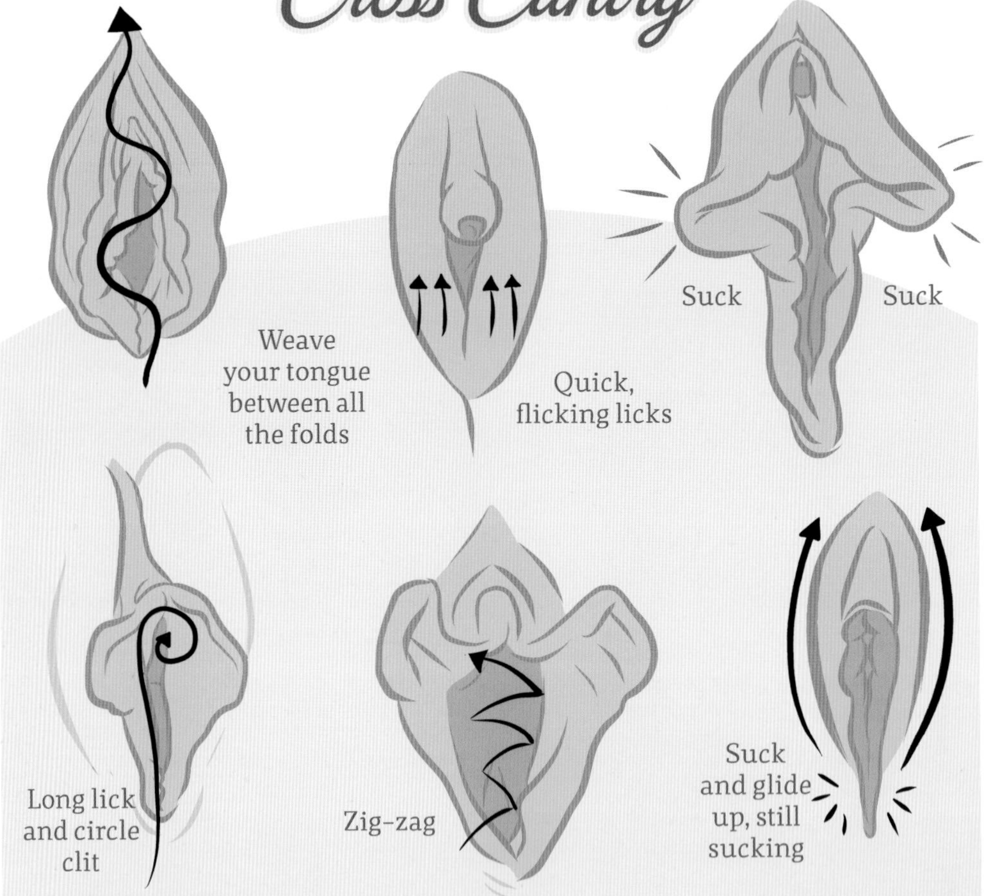
Weave your tongue between all the folds
Quick, flicking licks
Suck
Suck
Long lick and circle clit
Zig-zag
Suck and glide up, still sucking

Pussy Licking Prompts:

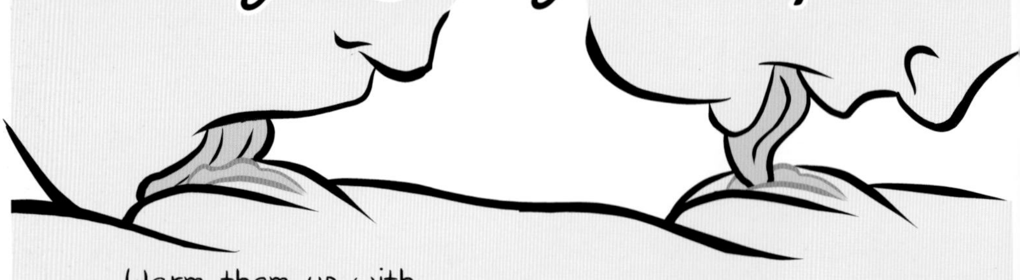

Warm them up with slow, broad licks, making your tongue as wide as possible.

Then use the tip for precision stimulation.

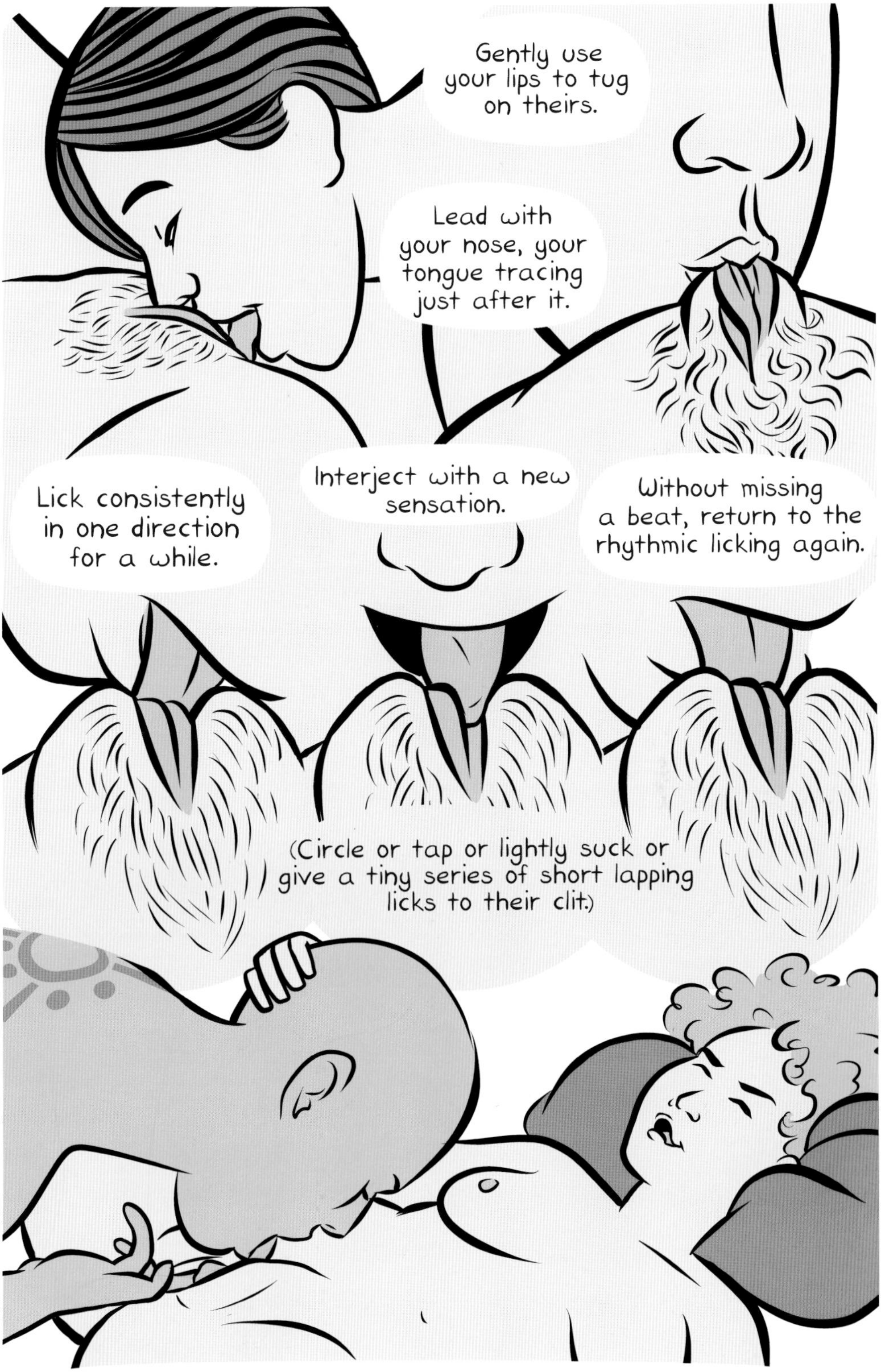
Gently use your lips to tug on theirs.
Lead with your nose, your tongue tracing just after it.
Lick consistently in one direction for a while.
Interject with a new sensation.
Without missing a beat, return to the rhythmic licking again.
(Circle or tap or lightly suck or give a tiny series of short lapping licks to their clit.)

Slip a finger or two inside their vagina while you keep licking.

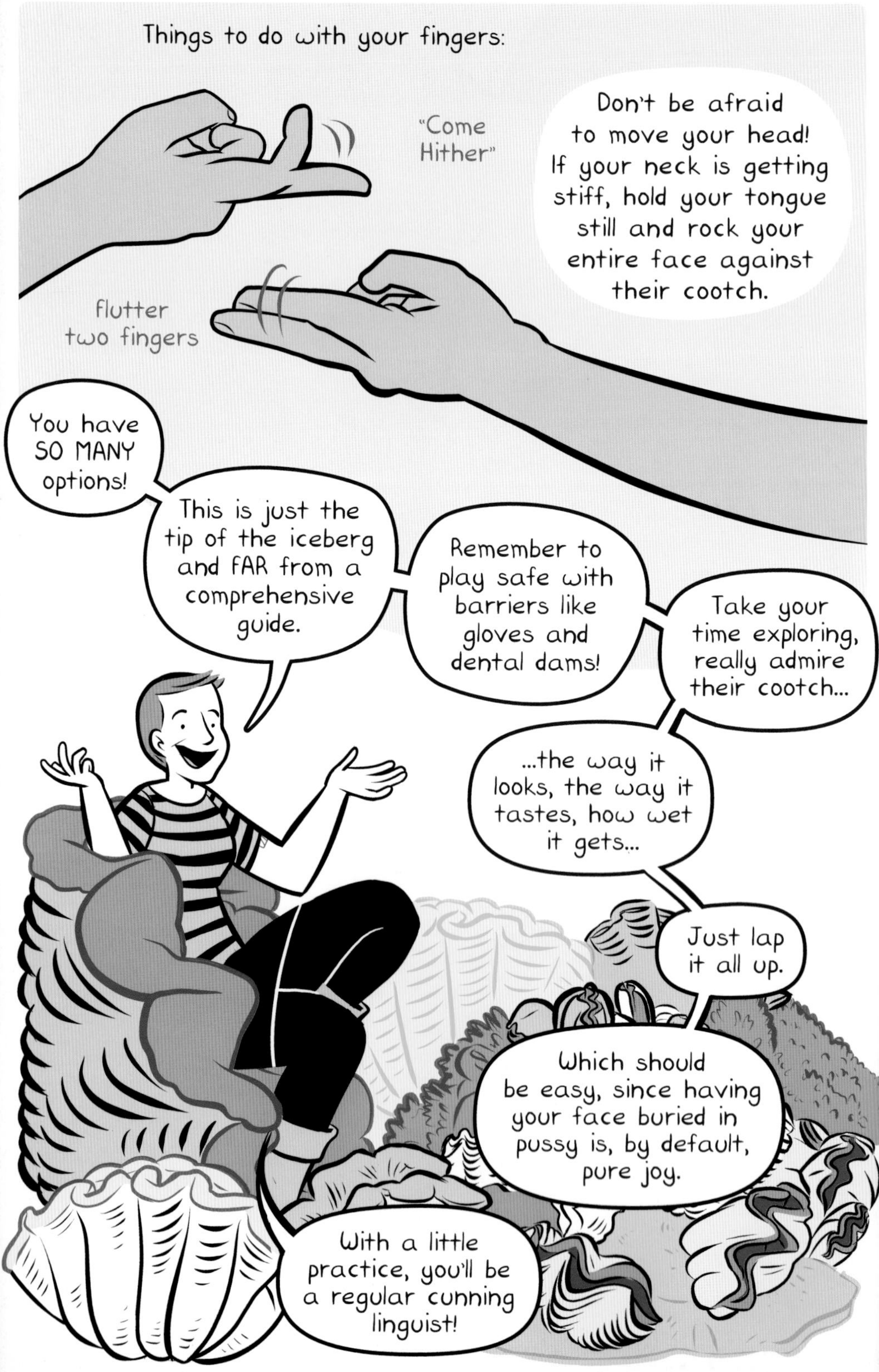

Things to do with your fingers:
"Come Hither"
flutter two fingers
Don't be afraid to move your head! If your neck is getting stiff, hold your tongue still and rock your entire face against their cootch.
You have SO MANY options!
This is just the tip of the iceberg and FAR from a comprehensive guide.
Remember to play safe with barriers like gloves and dental dams!
Take your time exploring, really admire their cootch...
...the way it looks, the way it tastes, how wet it gets...
Just lap it all up.
Which should be easy, since having your face buried in pussy is, by default, pure joy.
With a little practice, you'll be a regular cunning linguist!

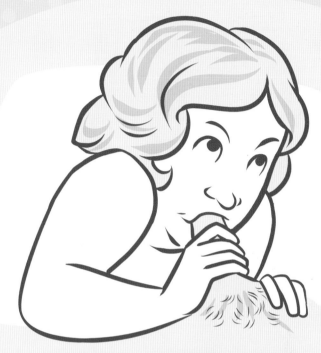

Oral Sex
for a Penis

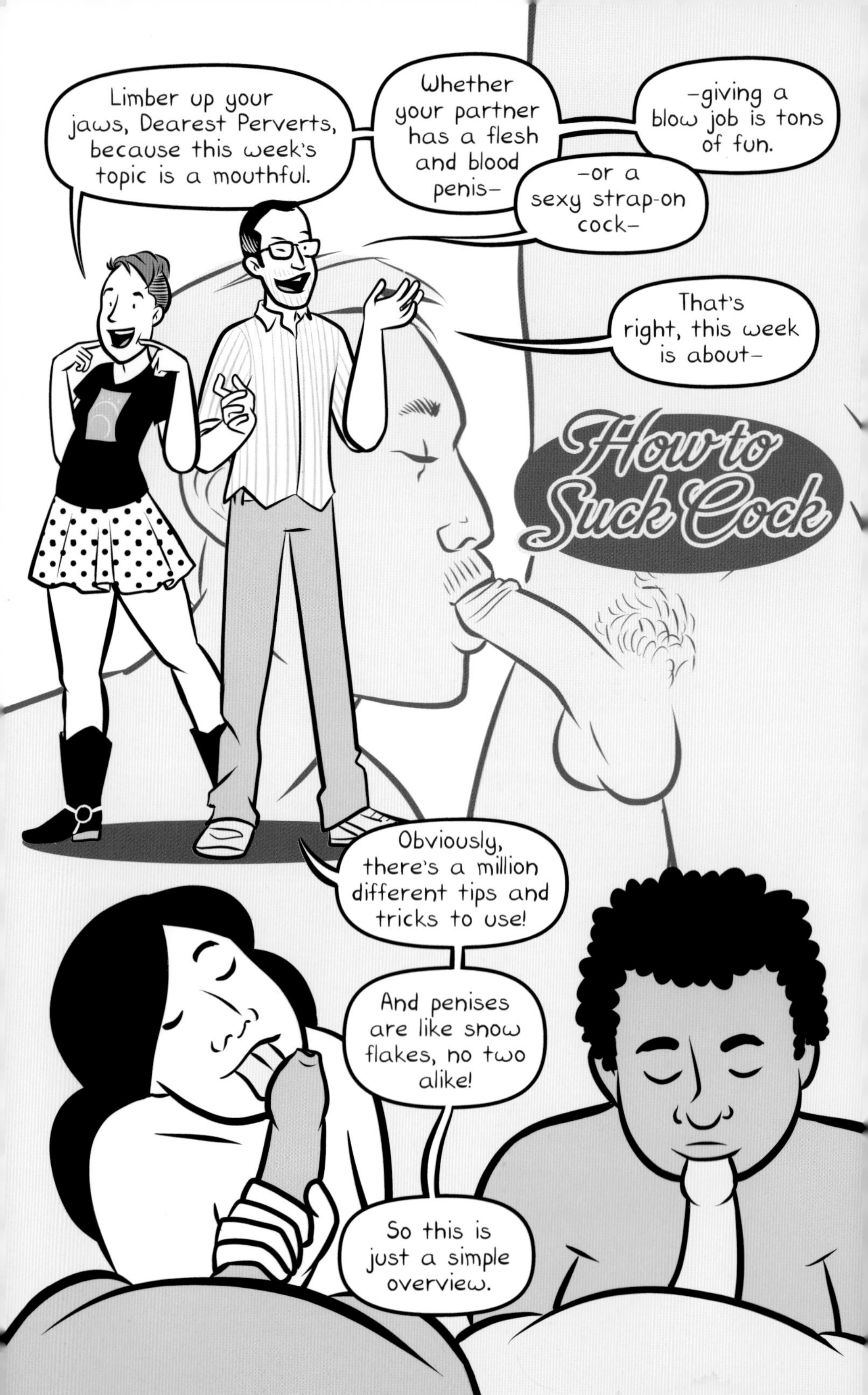
Limber up your jaws, Dearest Perverts, because this week's topic is a mouthful.
Whether your partner has a flesh and blood penis–
–or a sexy strap-on cock–
–giving a blow job is tons of fun.
That's right, this week is about–
How to Suck Cock
Obviously, there's a million different tips and tricks to use!
And penises are like snow flakes, no two alike!
So this is just a simple overview.

Meet the Penis

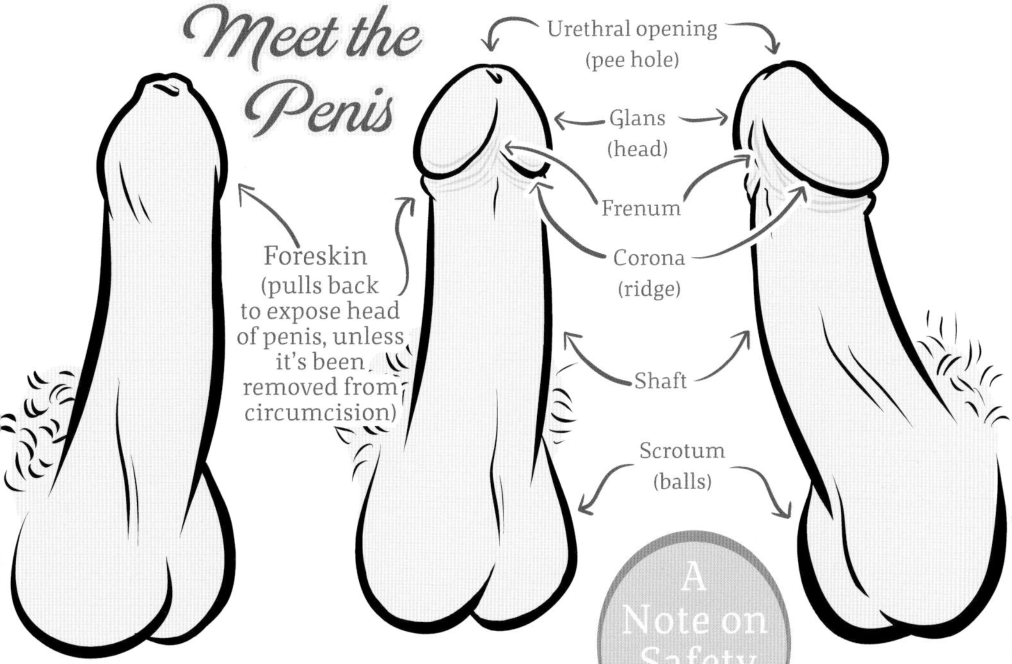

Urethral opening
(pee hole)
Glans
(head)
Frenum
Corona
(ridge)
Foreskin
(pulls back
to expose head
of penis, unless
it's been
removed from
circumcision)
Shaft
Scrotum
(balls)

A Note on Safety

STIs can be transmitted between saliva and semen, so to prevent spreading anything infectious between partners, put a condom on the penis before it goes in anyone's mouth.

Communicate

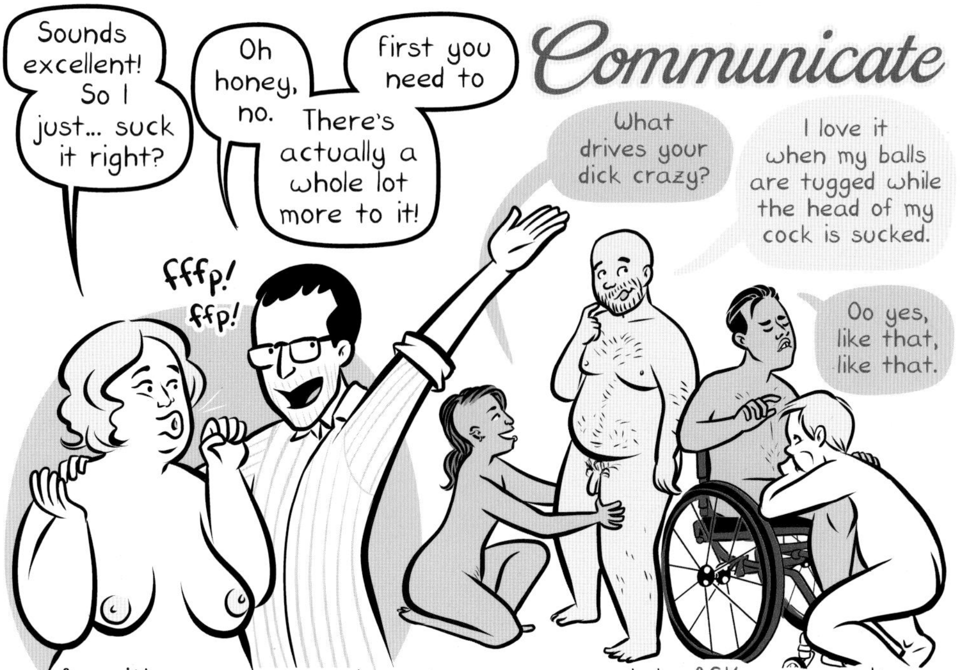

Sounds excellent! So I just... suck it right?
Oh honey, no.
first you need to
There's actually a whole lot more to it!
fffp! ffp!
What drives your dick crazy?
I love it when my balls are tugged while the head of my cock is sucked.
Oo yes, like that, like that.

As with every sex act, you're gonna want to ASK your partner what they like, TELL your partner what you want, give the giver positive reinforcement when they're doing something you do like.

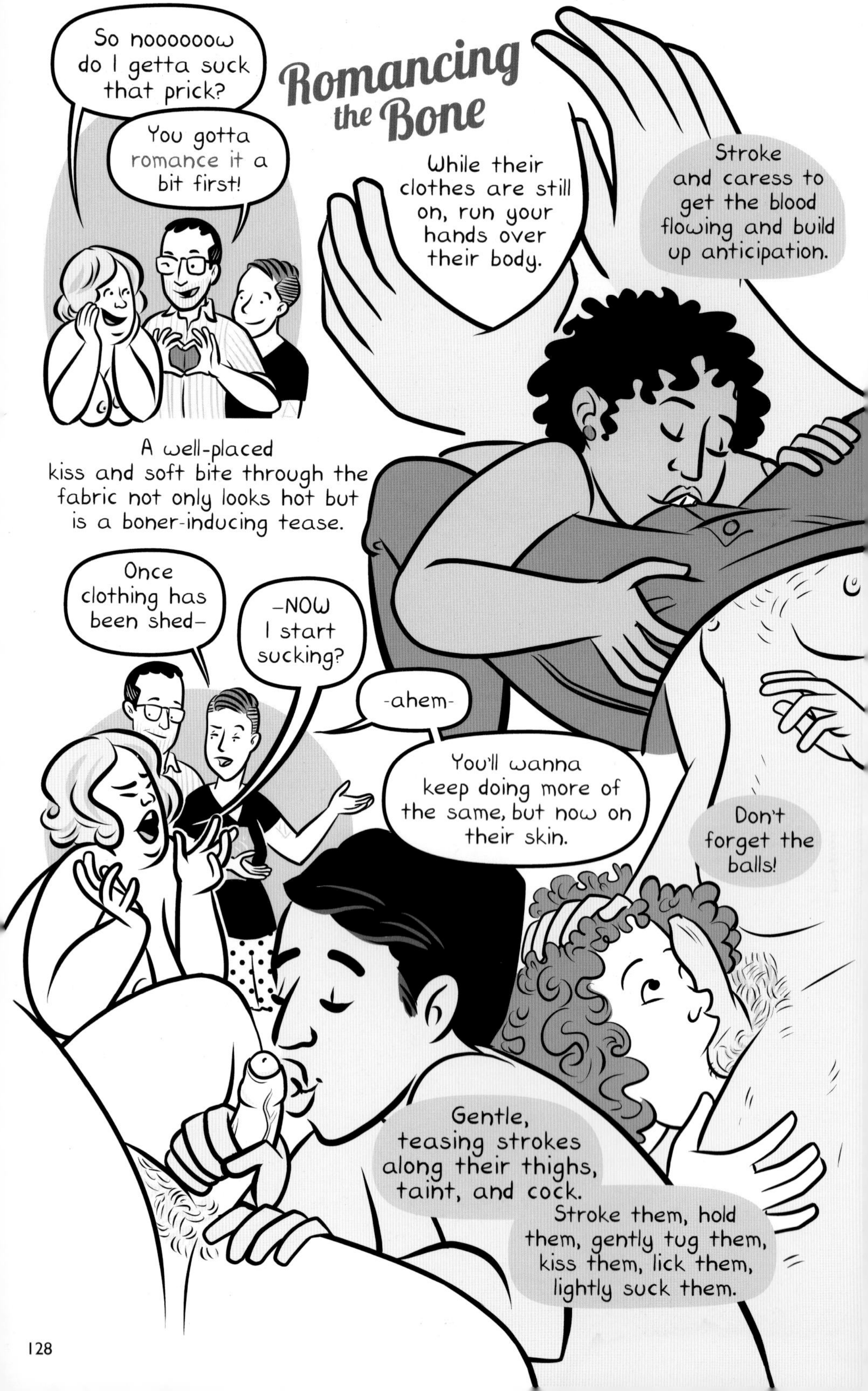
So noooooow do I getta suck that prick?
You gotta romance it a bit first!
Romancing the Bone
While their clothes are still on, run your hands over their body.
Stroke and caress to get the blood flowing and build up anticipation.
A well-placed kiss and soft bite through the fabric not only looks hot but is a boner-inducing tease.
Once clothing has been shed–
–NOW I start sucking?
-ahem-
You'll wanna keep doing more of the same, but now on their skin.
Don't forget the balls!
Gentle, teasing strokes along their thighs, taint, and cock.
Stroke them, hold them, gently tug them, kiss them, lick them, lightly suck them.

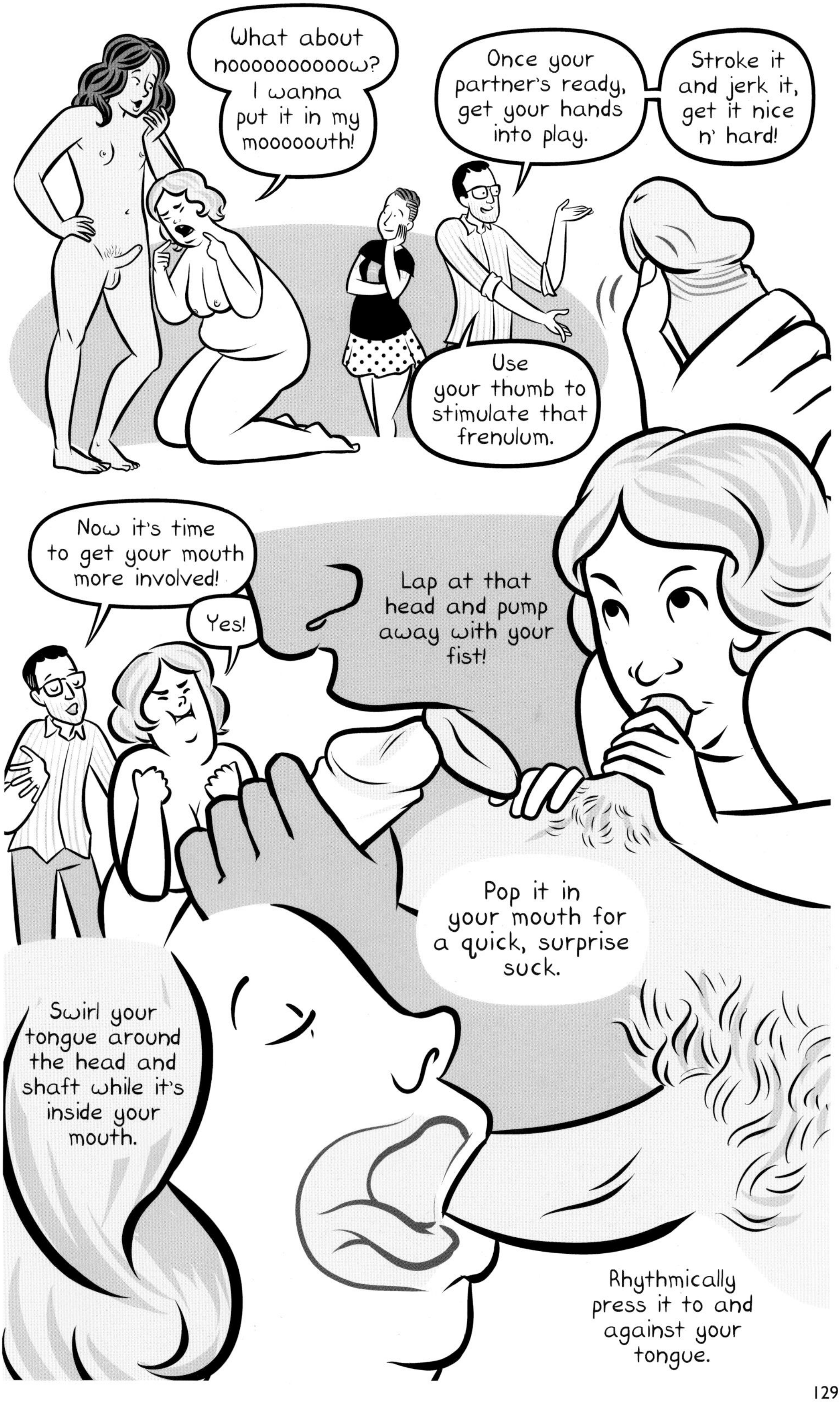
What about nooooooooooow? I wanna put it in my moooooouth!
Once your partner's ready, get your hands into play.
Stroke it and jerk it, get it nice n' hard!
Use your thumb to stimulate that frenulum.
Now it's time to get your mouth more involved!
Yes!
Lap at that head and pump away with your fist!
Pop it in your mouth for a quick, surprise suck.
Swirl your tongue around the head and shaft while it's inside your mouth.
Rhythmically press it to and against your tongue.

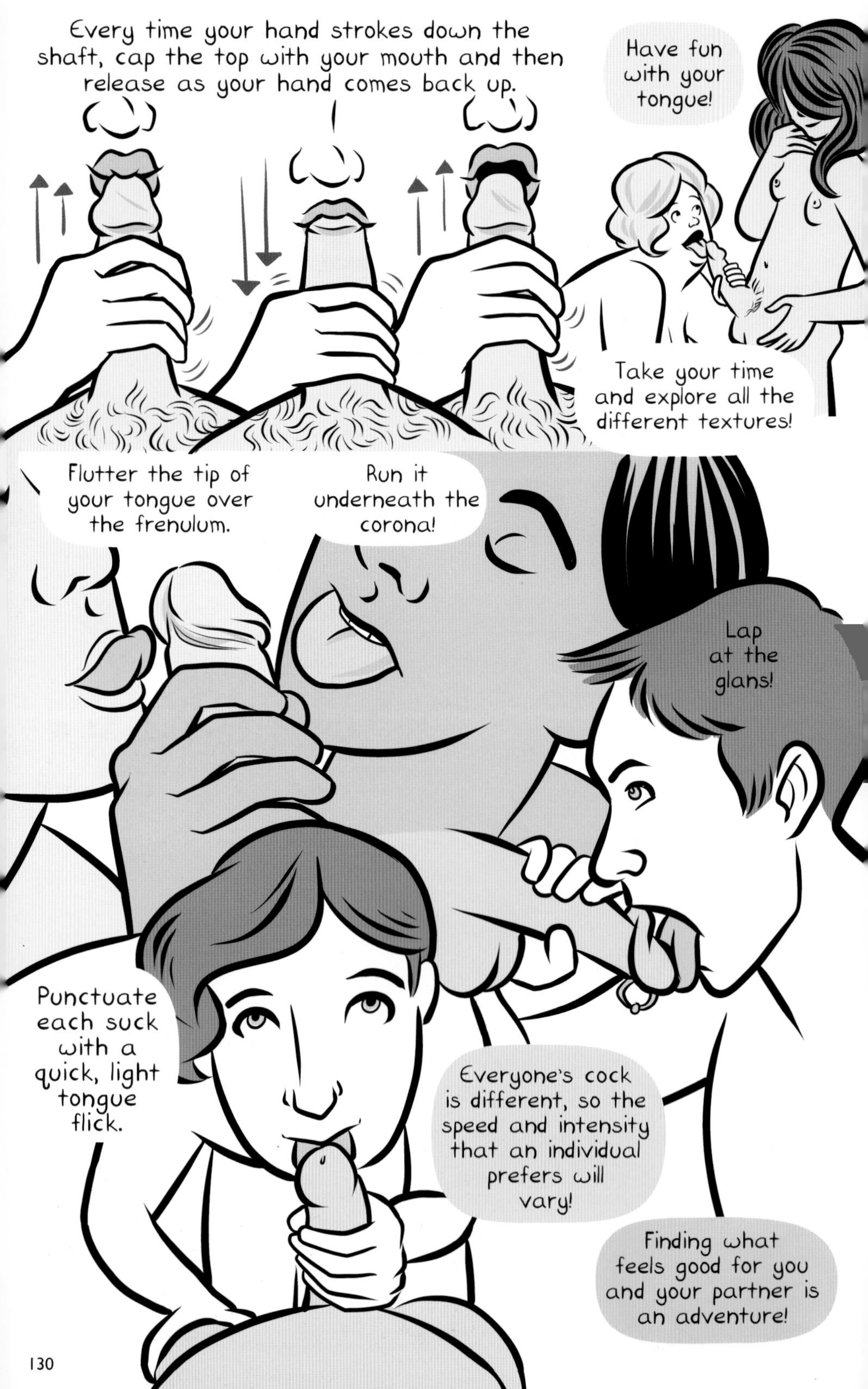

Every time your hand strokes down the shaft, cap the top with your mouth and then release as your hand comes back up.
Have fun with your tongue!
Take your time and explore all the different textures!
Flutter the tip of your tongue over the frenulum.
Run it underneath the corona!
Lap at the glans!
Punctuate each suck with a quick, light tongue flick.
Everyone's cock is different, so the speed and intensity that an individual prefers will vary!
Finding what feels good for you and your partner is an adventure!

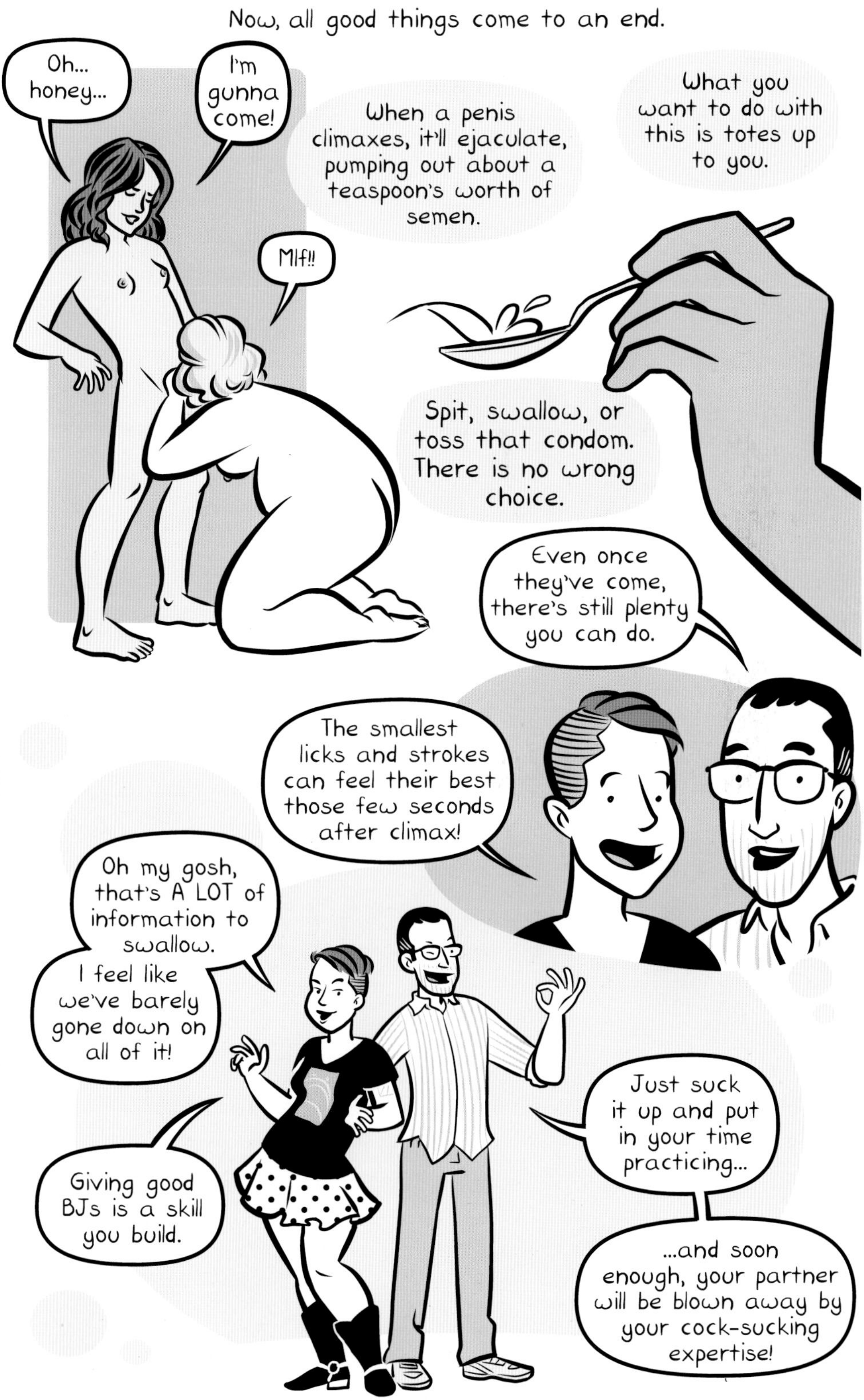
Now, all good things come to an end.
Oh... honey...
I'm gunna come!
When a penis climaxes, it'll ejaculate, pumping out about a teaspoon's worth of semen.
What you want to do with this is totes up to you.
Mlf!!
Spit, swallow, or toss that condom. There is no wrong choice.
Even once they've come, there's still plenty you can do.
The smallest licks and strokes can feel their best those few seconds after climax!
Oh my gosh, that's A LOT of information to swallow.
I feel like we've barely gone down on all of it!
Giving good BJs is a skill you build.
Just suck it up and put in your time practicing...
...and soon enough, your partner will be blown away by your cock-sucking expertise!

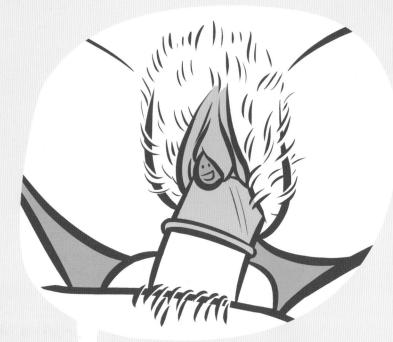

Vaginal
Intercourse

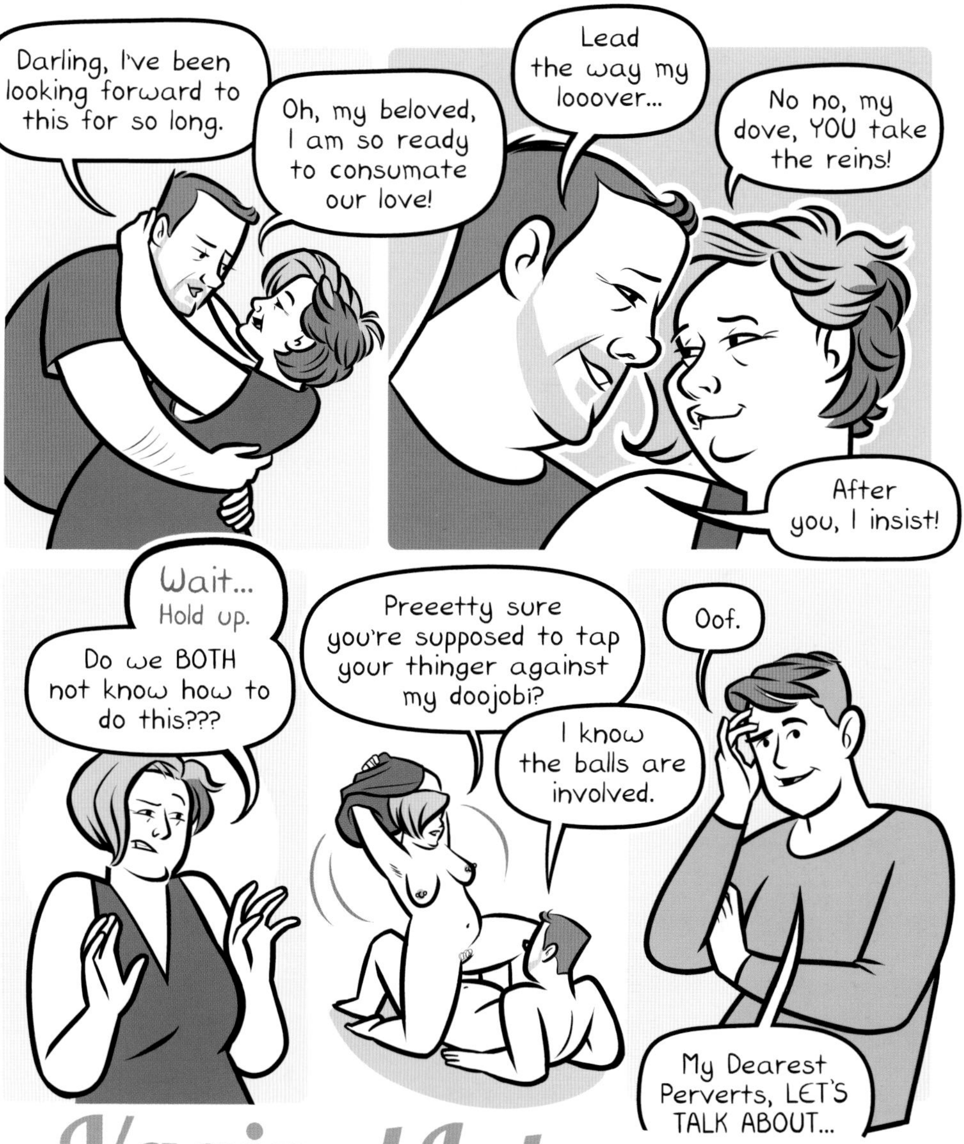
Darling, I've been looking forward to this for so long.
Oh, my beloved, I am so ready to consumate our love!
Lead the way my looover...
No no, my dove, YOU take the reins!
After you, I insist!
Wait... Hold up.
Do we BOTH not know how to do this???
Preeetty sure you're supposed to tap your thinger against my doojobi?
I know the balls are involved.
Oof.
My Dearest Perverts, LET'S TALK ABOUT...

Vaginal Intercourse

What are we talking about here? Well this type of fuckin' is when two people have sex together with their penis and vagina interlocking!

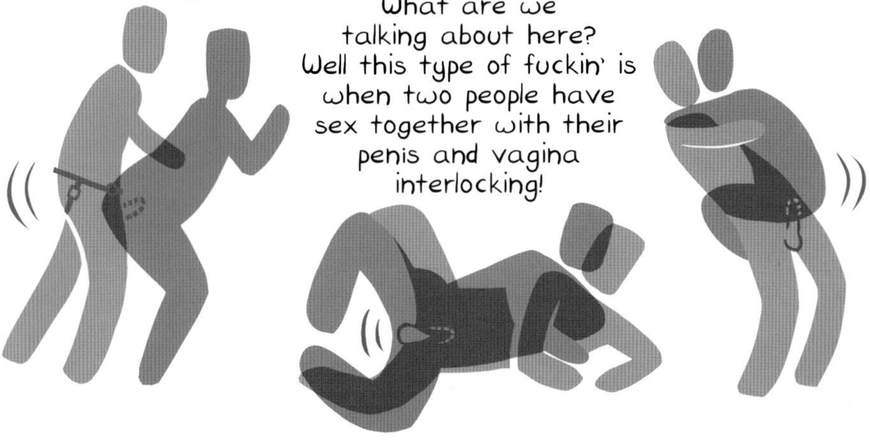

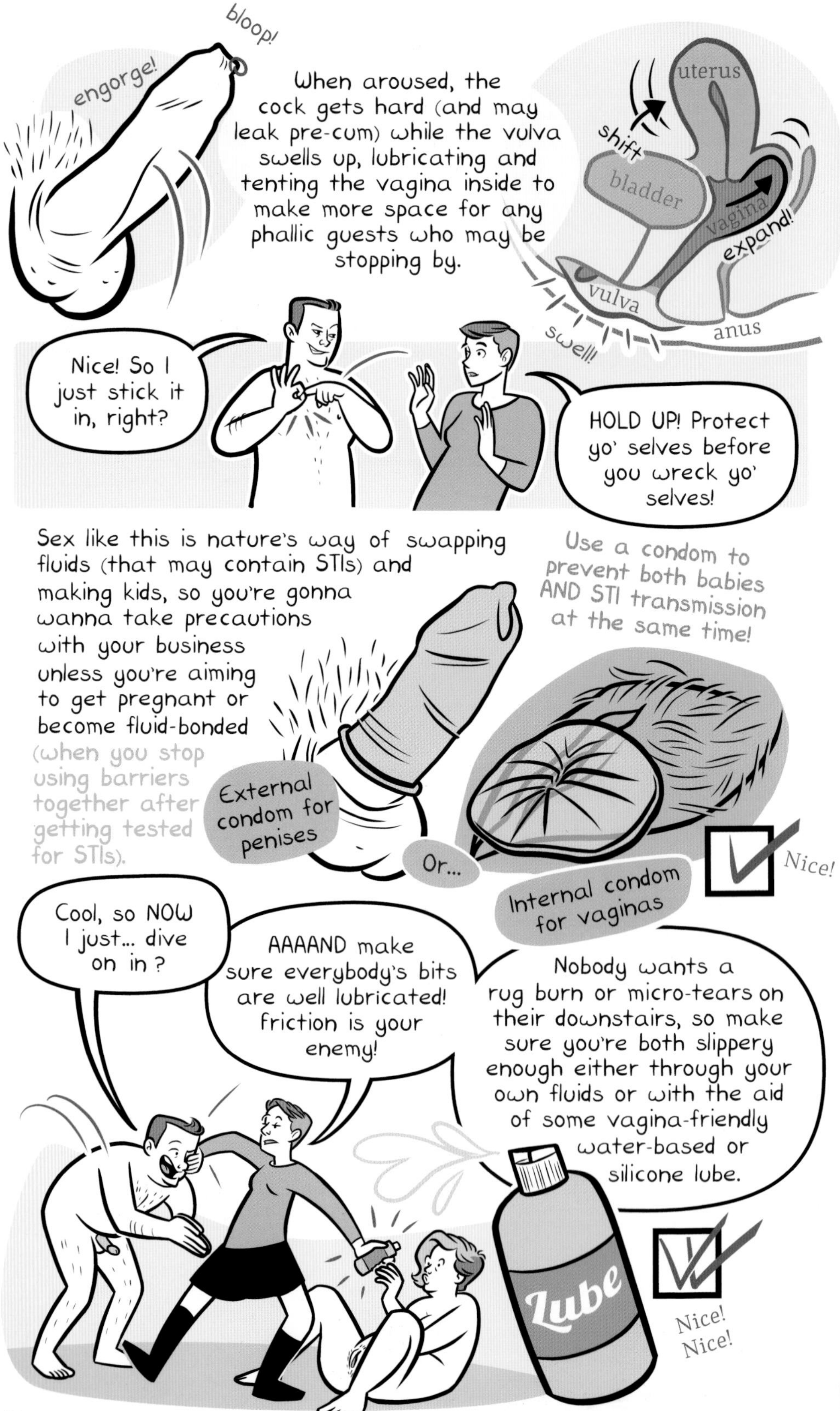
bloop!
engorge!
When aroused, the cock gets hard (and may leak pre-cum) while the vulva swells up, lubricating and tenting the vagina inside to make more space for any phallic guests who may be stopping by.
uterus
shift
bladder
vagina
expand!
vulva
swell!
anus
Nice! So I just stick it in, right?
HOLD UP! Protect yo' selves before you wreck yo' selves!
Sex like this is nature's way of swapping fluids (that may contain STIs) and making kids, so you're gonna wanna take precautions with your business unless you're aiming to get pregnant or become fluid-bonded
(when you stop using barriers together after getting tested for STIs).
Use a condom to prevent both babies AND STI transmission at the same time!
External condom for penises
Or...
Internal condom for vaginas
Nice!
Cool, so NOW I just... dive on in?
AAAAND make sure everybody's bits are well lubricated! Friction is your enemy!
Nobody wants a rug burn or micro-tears on their downstairs, so make sure you're both slippery enough either through your own fluids or with the aid of some vagina-friendly water-based or silicone lube.
Lube
Nice!
Nice!

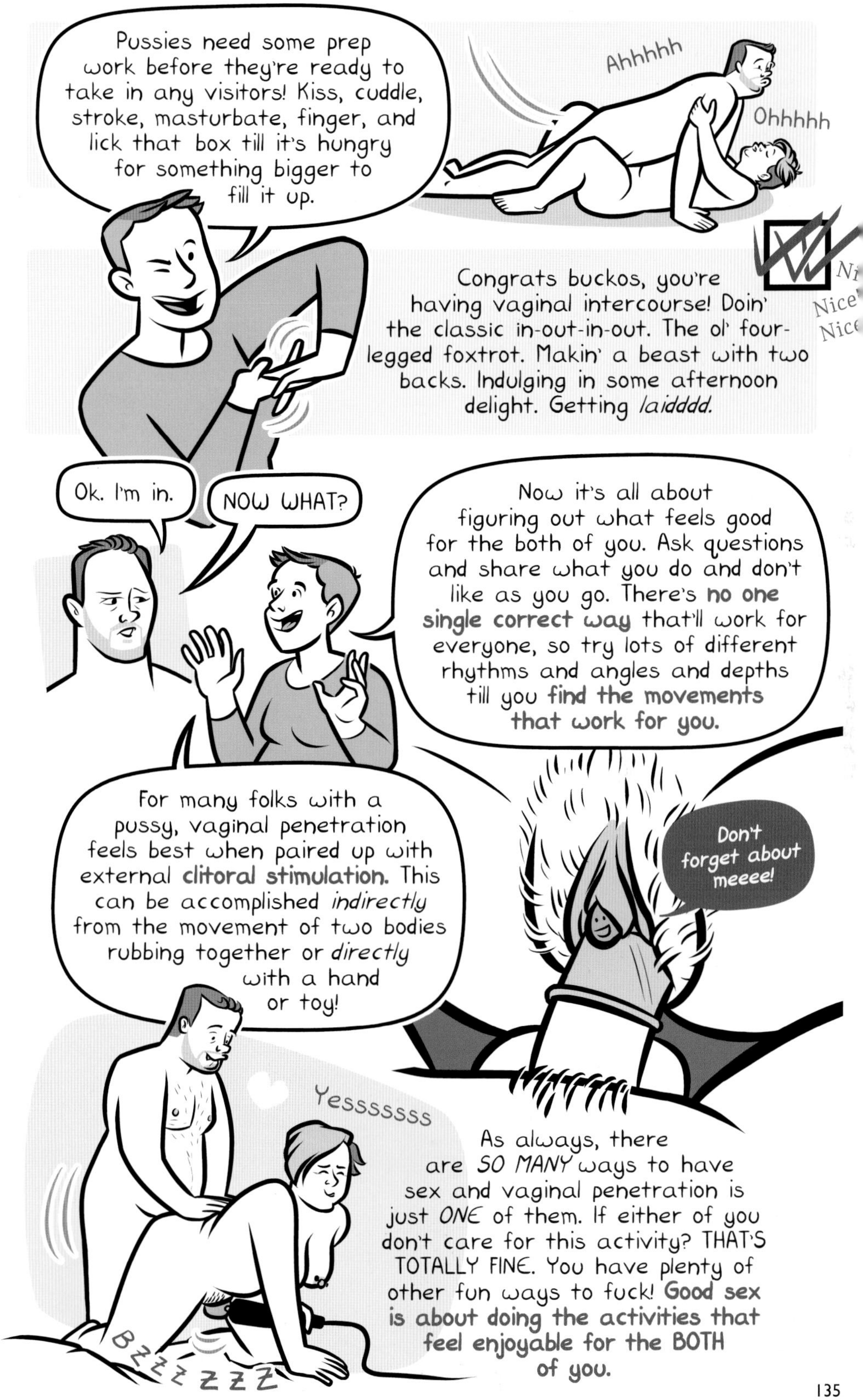

Pussies need some prep work before they're ready to take in any visitors! Kiss, cuddle, stroke, masturbate, finger, and lick that box till it's hungry for something bigger to fill it up.
Ahhhhh
Ohhhhh
Congrats buckos, you're having vaginal intercourse! Doin' the classic in-out-in-out. The ol' four-legged foxtrot. Makin' a beast with two backs. Indulging in some afternoon delight. Getting *laidddd.*
Nice
Ok. I'm in.
NOW WHAT?
Now it's all about figuring out what feels good for the both of you. Ask questions and share what you do and don't like as you go. There's **no one single correct way** that'll work for everyone, so try lots of different rhythms and angles and depths till you **find the movements that work for you.**
For many folks with a pussy, vaginal penetration feels best when paired up with external **clitoral stimulation.** This can be accomplished *indirectly* from the movement of two bodies rubbing together or *directly* with a hand or toy!
Don't forget about meeee!
Yesssssss
BZZZZZZ
As always, there are *SO MANY* ways to have sex and vaginal penetration is just *ONE* of them. If either of you don't care for this activity? THAT'S TOTALLY FINE. You have plenty of other fun ways to fuck! **Good sex is about doing the activities that feel enjoyable for the BOTH of you.**

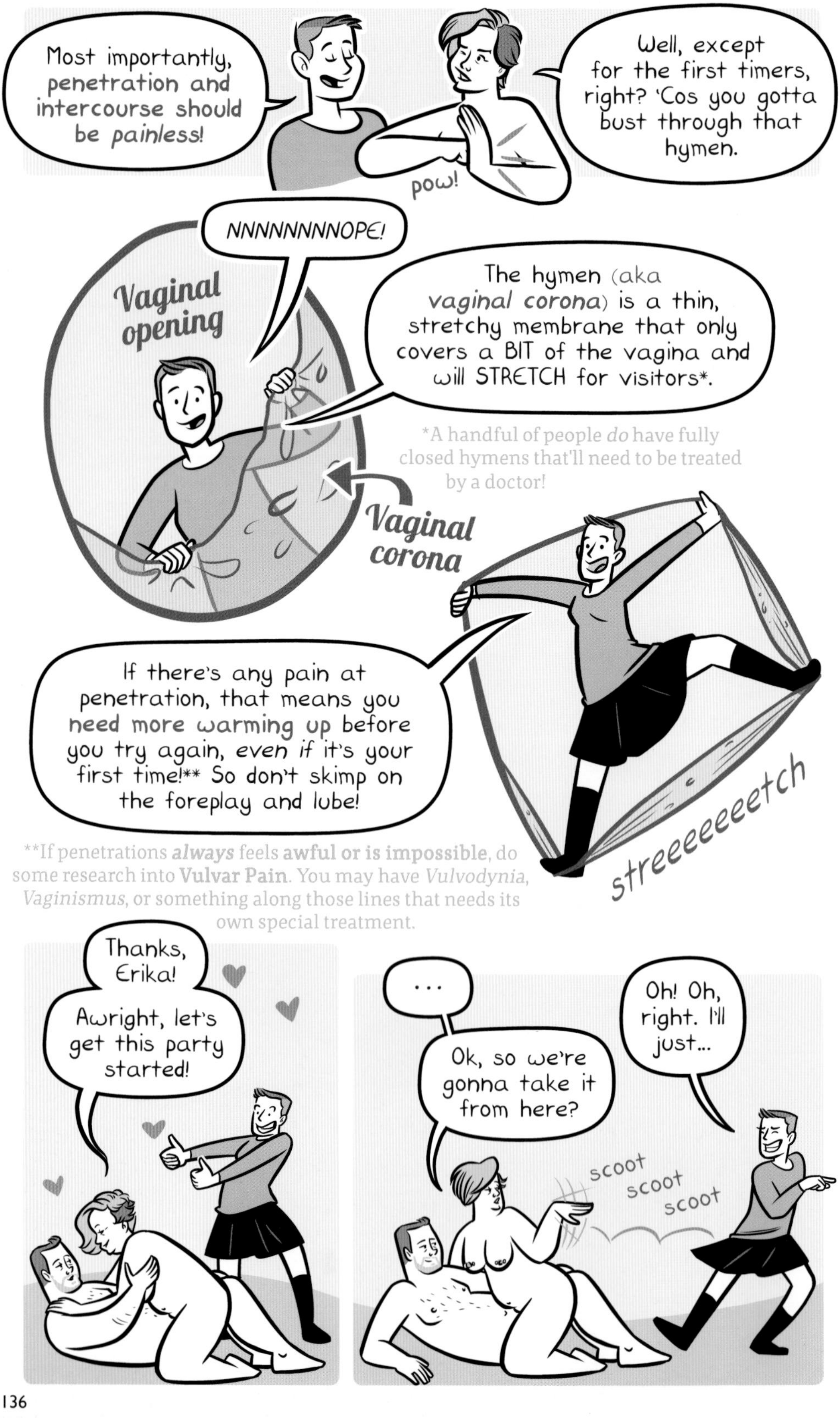

Most importantly, penetration and intercourse should be painless!
Well, except for the first timers, right? 'Cos you gotta bust through that hymen.
pow!
NNNNNNNNOPE!
Vaginal opening
The hymen (aka vaginal corona) is a thin, stretchy membrane that only covers a BIT of the vagina and will STRETCH for visitors*.
*A handful of people do have fully closed hymens that'll need to be treated by a doctor!
Vaginal corona
If there's any pain at penetration, that means you need more warming up before you try again, even if it's your first time!** So don't skimp on the foreplay and lube!
streeeeeeetch
**If penetrations always feels awful or is impossible, do some research into Vulvar Pain. You may have Vulvodynia, Vaginismus, or something along those lines that needs its own special treatment.
Thanks, Erika!
Awright, let's get this party started!
...
Ok, so we're gonna take it from here?
Oh! Oh, right. I'll just...
scoot
scoot
scoot

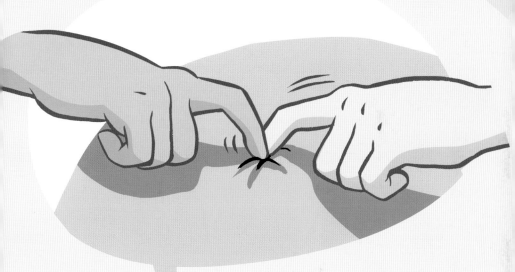

Anal
Introduction

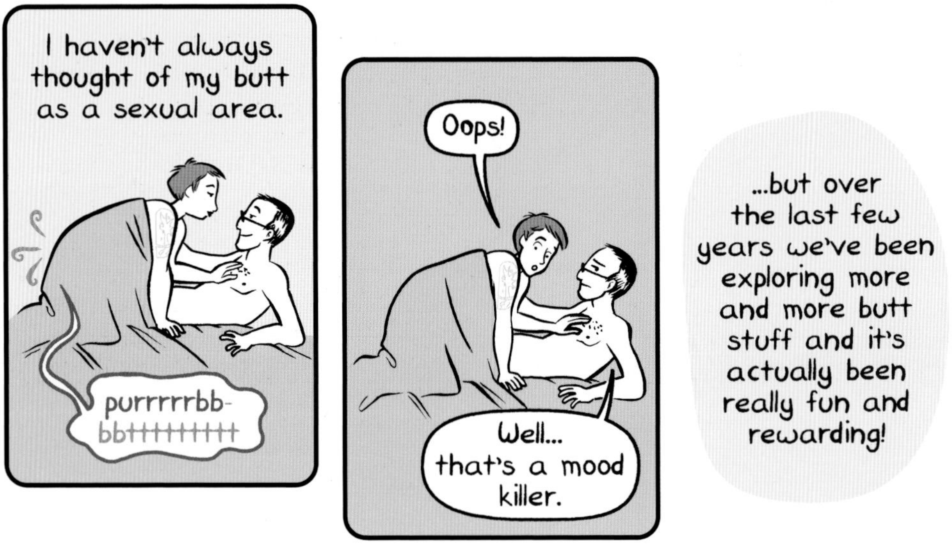
I haven't always thought of my butt as a sexual area.
purrrrrbb-bbttttttttt
Oops!
Well... that's a mood killer.
...but over the last few years we've been exploring more and more butt stuff and it's actually been really fun and rewarding!

So lets dive in together and explore the basics of *Anal Sex*!

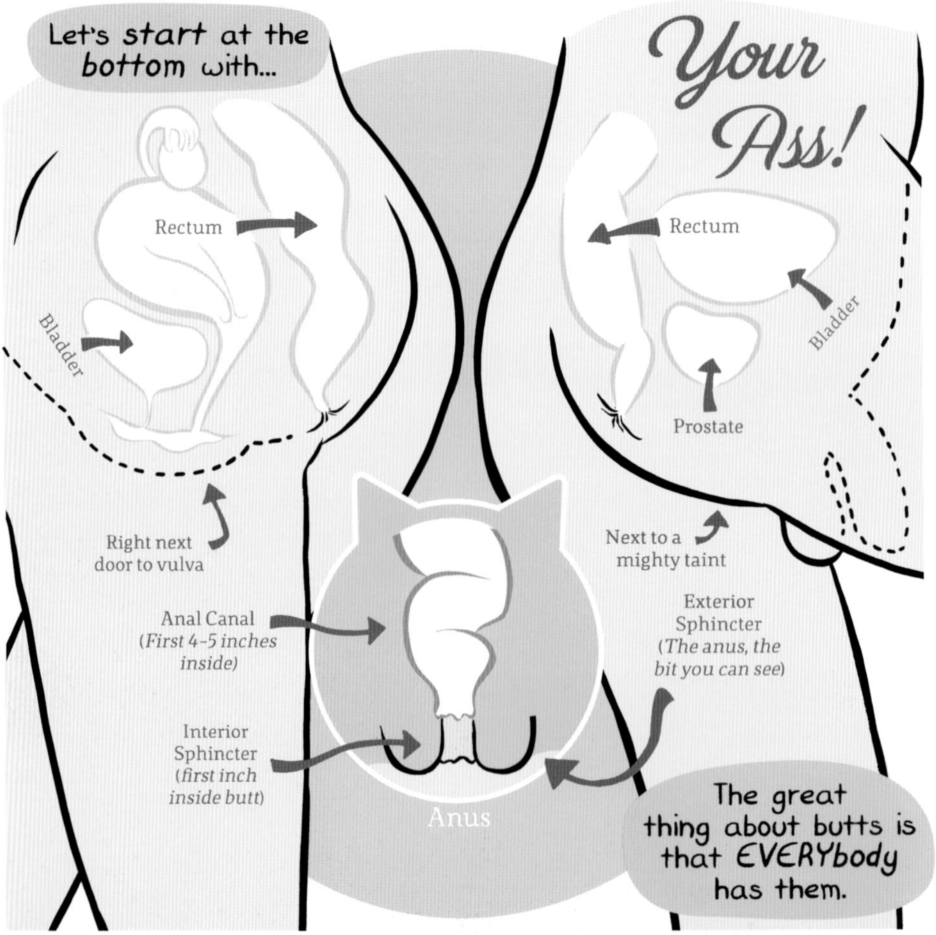
Let's start at the bottom with...
Your Ass!
Rectum
Bladder
Right next door to vulva
Rectum
Bladder
Prostate
Next to a mighty taint
Anal Canal (First 4-5 inches inside)
Interior Sphincter (first inch inside butt)
Anus
Exterior Sphincter (The anus, the bit you can see)
The great thing about butts is that EVERYbody has them.

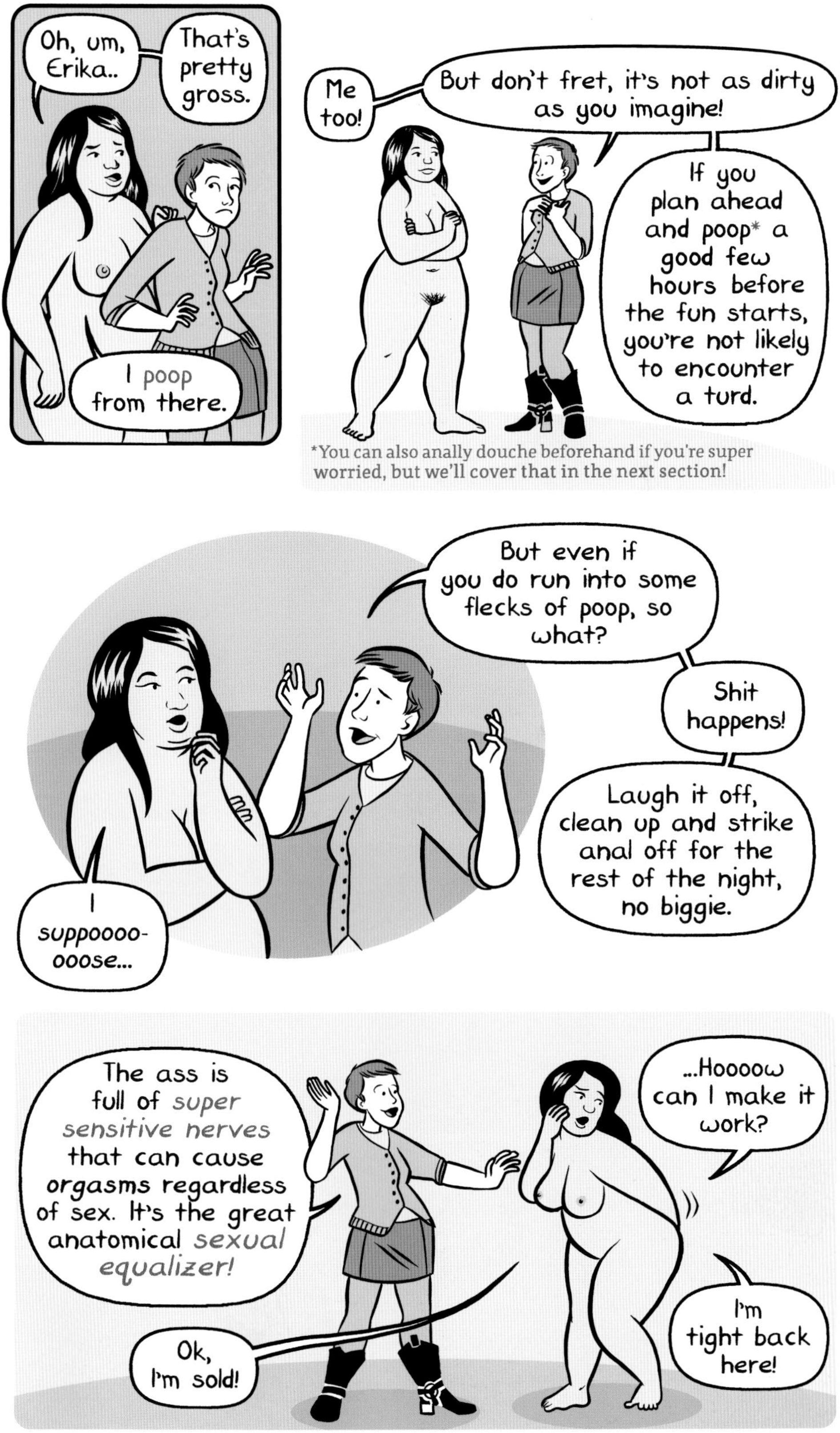
Oh, um, Erika..
That's pretty gross.
I poop from there.
Me too!
But don't fret, it's not as dirty as you imagine!
If you plan ahead and poop* a good few hours before the fun starts, you're not likely to encounter a turd.
*You can also anally douche beforehand if you're super worried, but we'll cover that in the next section!
But even if you do run into some flecks of poop, so what?
Shit happens!
Laugh it off, clean up and strike anal off for the rest of the night, no biggie.
I suppoooo-ooose...
The ass is full of super sensitive nerves that can cause orgasms regardless of sex. It's the great anatomical sexual equalizer!
...Hooooow can I make it work?
I'm tight back here!
Ok, I'm sold!

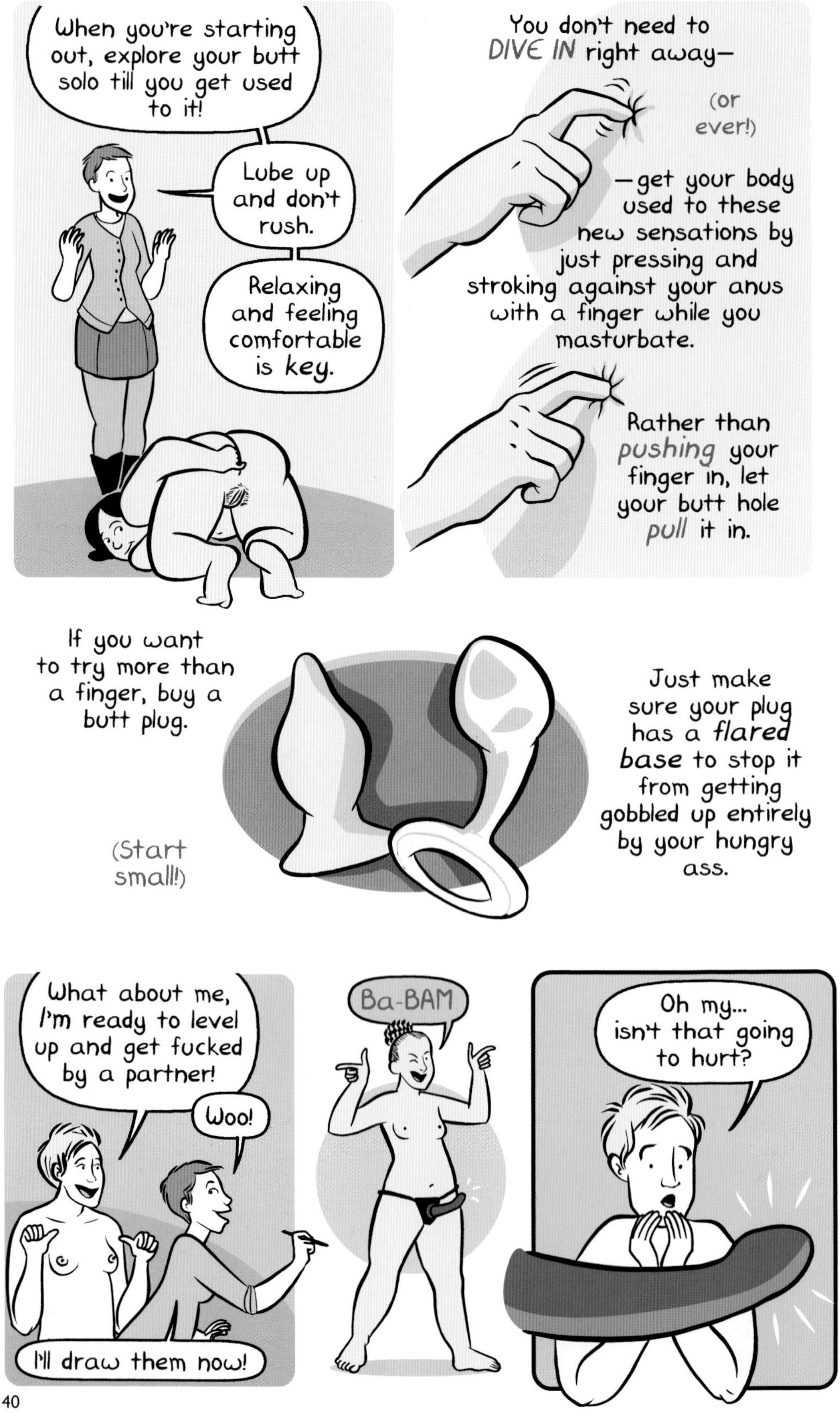

When you're starting out, explore your butt solo till you get used to it!
Lube up and don't rush.
Relaxing and feeling comfortable is key.
You don't need to DIVE IN right away—
(or ever!)
—get your body used to these new sensations by just pressing and stroking against your anus with a finger while you masturbate.
Rather than pushing your finger in, let your butt hole pull it in.
If you want to try more than a finger, buy a butt plug.
(Start small!)
Just make sure your plug has a flared base to stop it from getting gobbled up entirely by your hungry ass.
What about me, I'm ready to level up and get fucked by a partner!
Woo!
I'll draw them now!
Ba-BAM
Oh my... isn't that going to hurt?

Anal sex SHOULD NOT HURT.
Follow these three rules from the *Anal Safety Snails*:

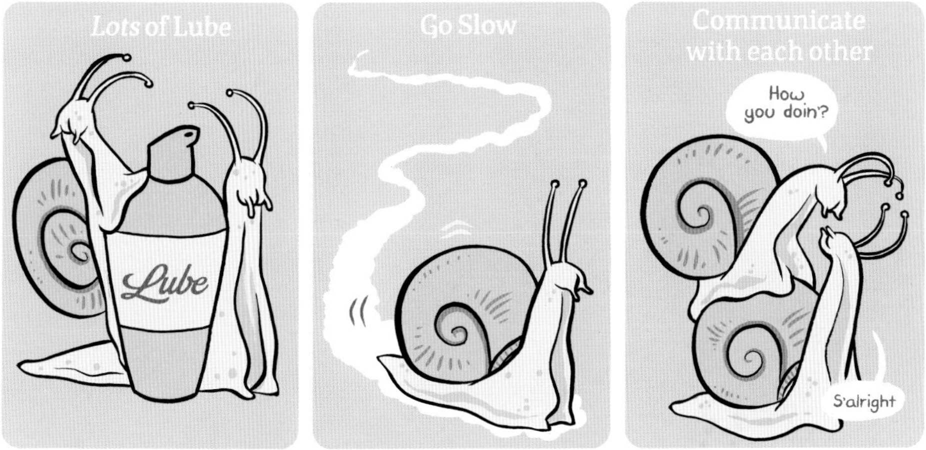
Lots of Lube
Lube
Go Slow
Communicate with each other
How you doin'?
S'alright

Mild, temporary discomfort while your body gets used to a foreign object being inside of it is normal...

...but if it *hurts*, STOP.

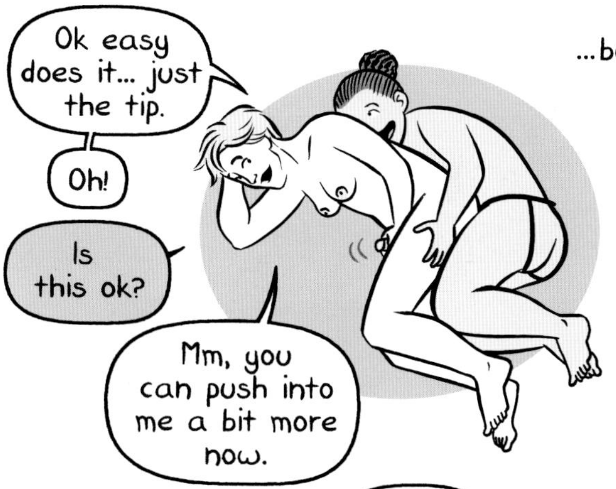
Ok easy does it... just the tip.
Oh!
Is this ok?
Mm, you can push into me a bit more now.

The spooning position is great for newbie anal sex, the receiver can back up onto the giver's cock in their own time, and still access their own genitalia.

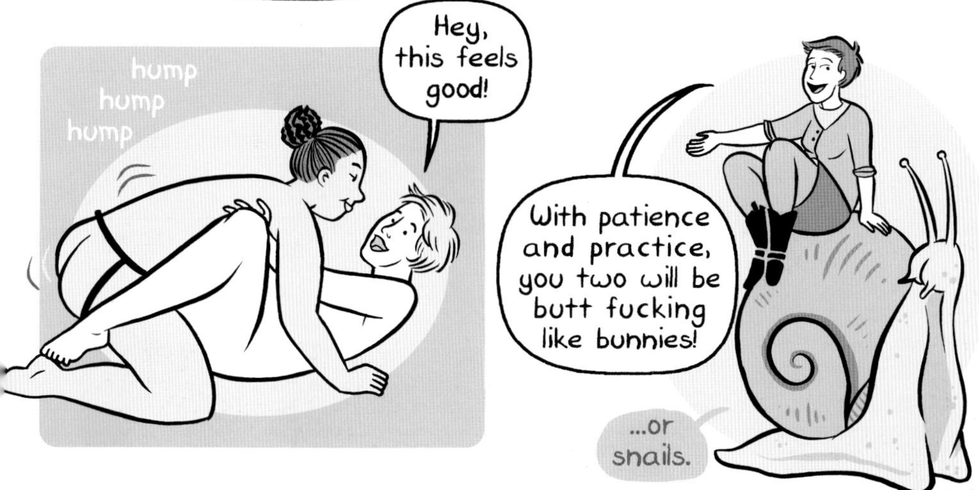
hump
hump
hump
Hey, this feels good!
With patience and practice, you two will be butt fucking like bunnies!
...or snails.

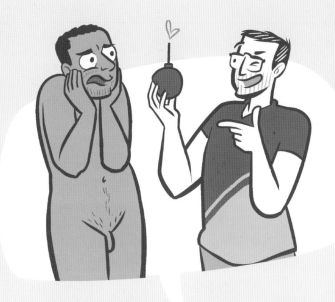

More Anal

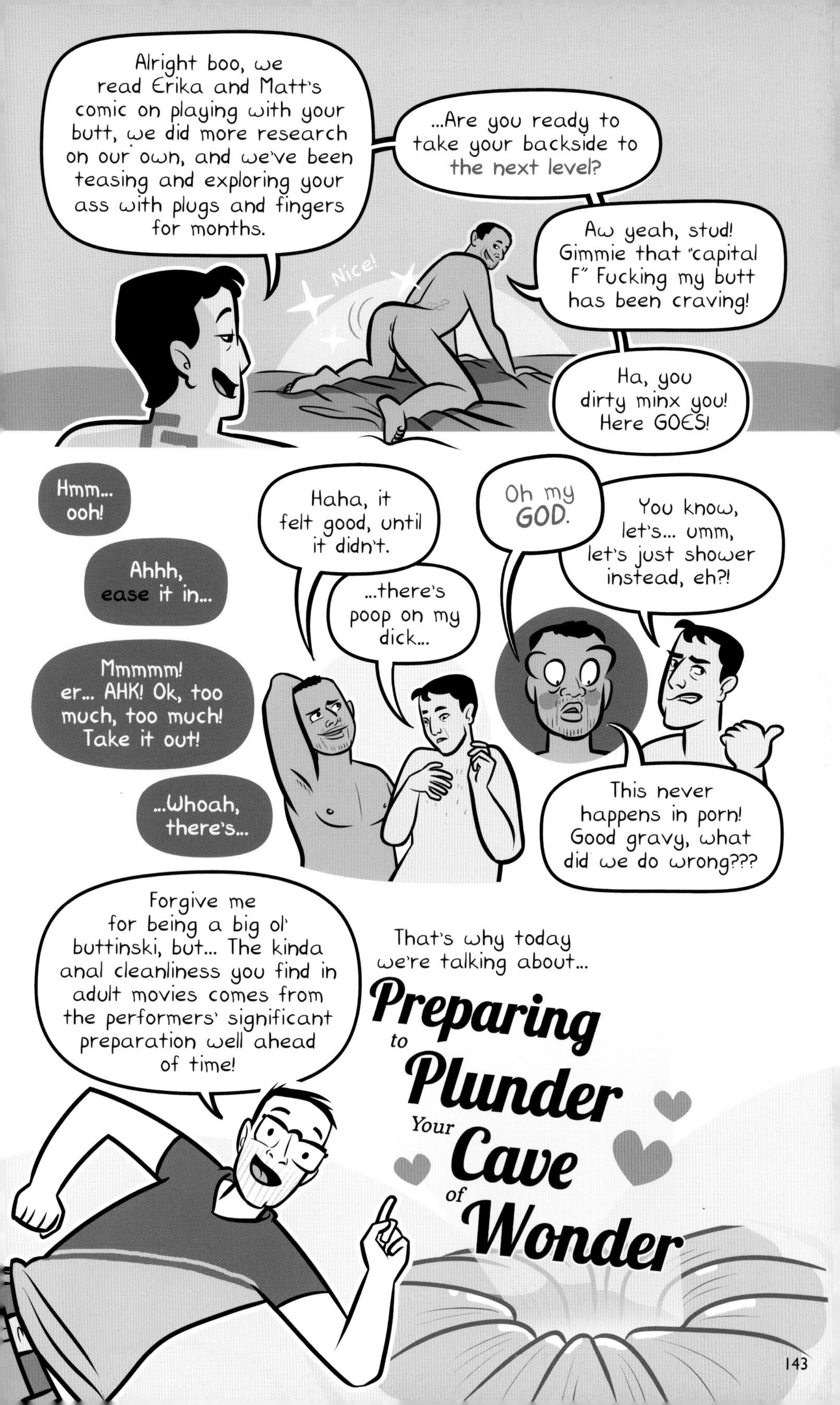

Alright boo, we read Erika and Matt's comic on playing with your butt, we did more research on our own, and we've been teasing and exploring your ass with plugs and fingers for months.
...Are you ready to take your backside to the next level?
Nice!
Aw yeah, stud! Gimmie that "capital F" Fucking my butt has been craving!
Ha, you dirty minx you! Here GOES!
Hmm... ooh!
Ahhh, ease it in...
Mmmmm! er... AHK! Ok, too much, too much! Take it out!
...Whoah, there's...
Haha, it felt good, until it didn't.
...there's poop on my dick...
Oh my GOD.
You know, let's... umm, let's just shower instead, eh?!
This never happens in porn! Good gravy, what did we do wrong???
Forgive me for being a big ol' buttinski, but... The kinda anal cleanliness you find in adult movies comes from the performers' significant preparation well ahead of time!
That's why today we're talking about...
Preparing to Plunder Your Cave of Wonder

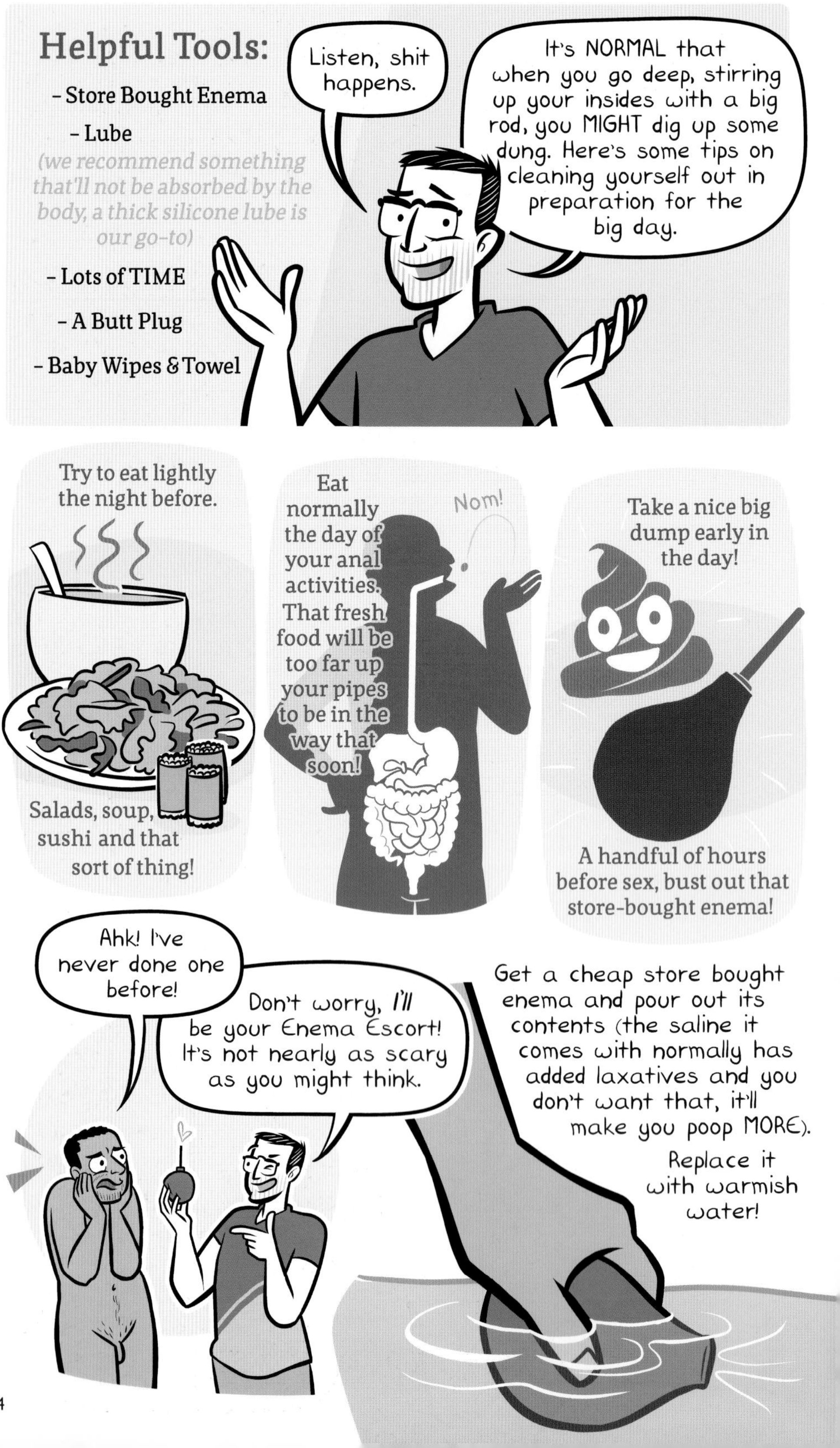

Helpful Tools:
- Store Bought Enema
- Lube
(we recommend something that'll not be absorbed by the body, a thick silicone lube is our go-to)
- Lots of TIME
- A Butt Plug
- Baby Wipes & Towel
Listen, shit happens.
It's NORMAL that when you go deep, stirring up your insides with a big rod, you MIGHT dig up some dung. Here's some tips on cleaning yourself out in preparation for the big day.
Try to eat lightly the night before.
Salads, soup, sushi and that sort of thing!
Eat normally the day of your anal activities. That fresh food will be too far up your pipes to be in the way that soon!
Nom!
Take a nice big dump early in the day!
A handful of hours before sex, bust out that store-bought enema!
Ahk! I've never done one before!
Don't worry, I'll be your Enema Escort! It's not nearly as scary as you might think.
Get a cheap store bought enema and pour out its contents (the saline it comes with normally has added laxatives and you don't want that, it'll make you poop MORE).
Replace it with warmish water!

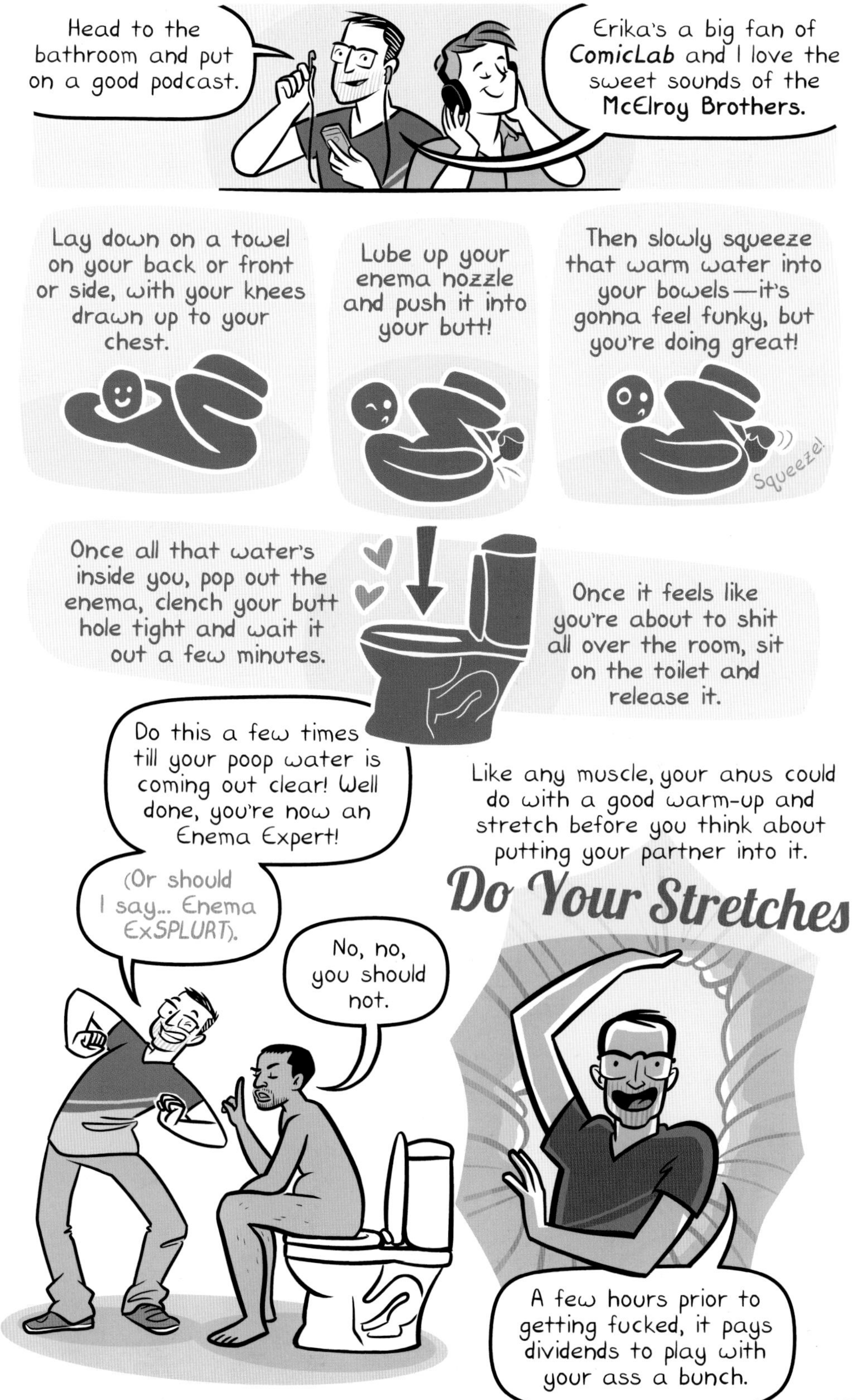

Head to the bathroom and put on a good podcast.
Erika's a big fan of **ComicLab** and I love the sweet sounds of the **McElroy Brothers.**
Lay down on a towel on your back or front or side, with your knees drawn up to your chest.
Lube up your enema nozzle and push it into your butt!
Then slowly squeeze that warm water into your bowels—it's gonna feel funky, but you're doing great!
Squeeze!
Once all that water's inside you, pop out the enema, clench your butt hole tight and wait it out a few minutes.
Once it feels like you're about to shit all over the room, sit on the toilet and release it.
Do this a few times till your poop water is coming out clear! Well done, you're now an Enema Expert!
(Or should I say... Enema ExSPLURT).
No, no, you should not.
Like any muscle, your anus could do with a good warm-up and stretch before you think about putting your partner into it.
Do Your Stretches
A few hours prior to getting fucked, it pays dividends to play with your ass a bunch.

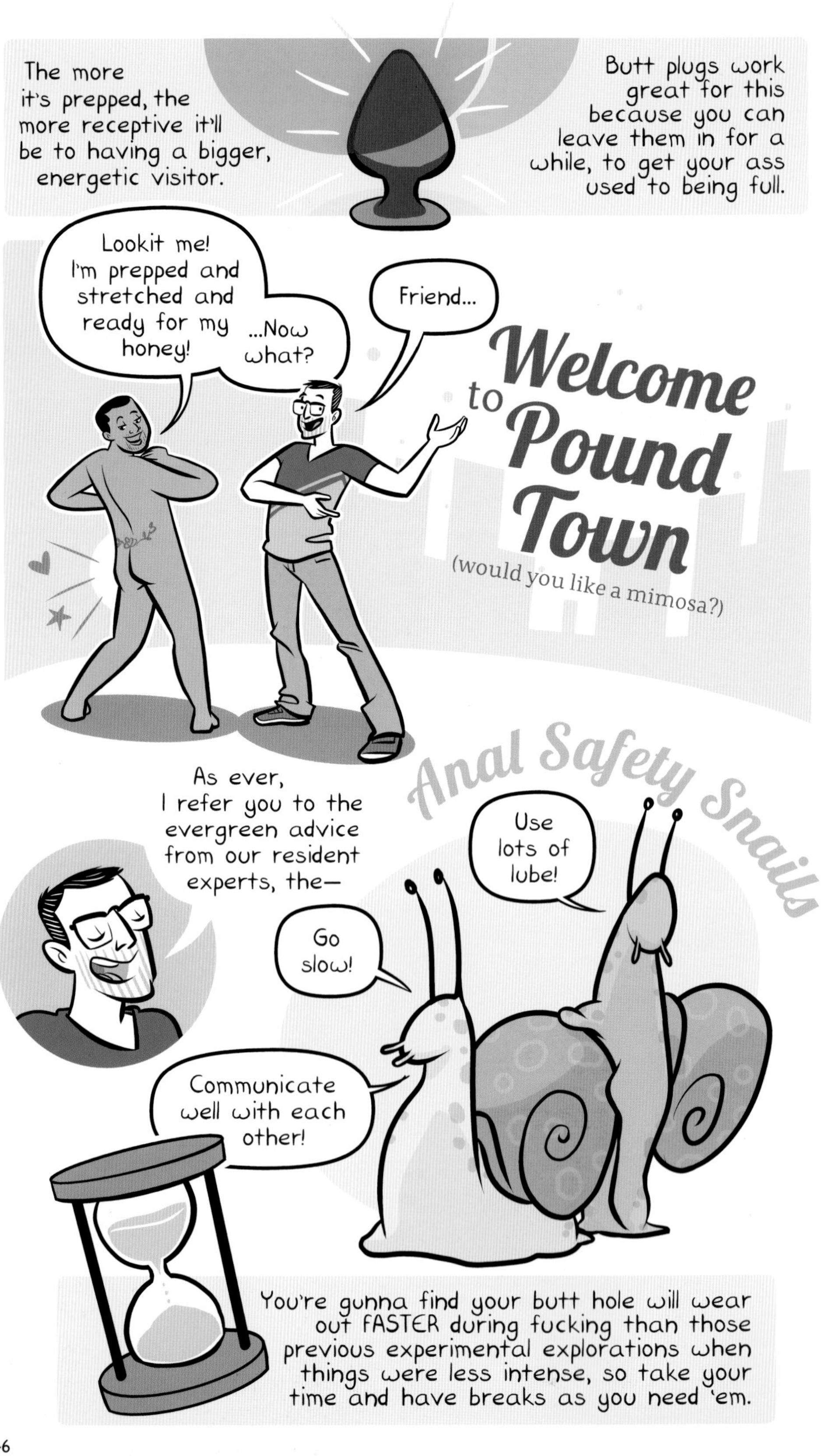
The more it's prepped, the more receptive it'll be to having a bigger, energetic visitor.
Butt plugs work great for this because you can leave them in for a while, to get your ass used to being full.
Lookit me! I'm prepped and stretched and ready for my honey!
...Now what?
Friend...
Welcome to Pound Town
(would you like a mimosa?)
As ever, I refer you to the evergreen advice from our resident experts, the—
Anal Safety Snails
Use lots of lube!
Go slow!
Communicate well with each other!
You're gunna find your butt hole will wear out FASTER during fucking than those previous experimental explorations when things were less intense, so take your time and have breaks as you need 'em.

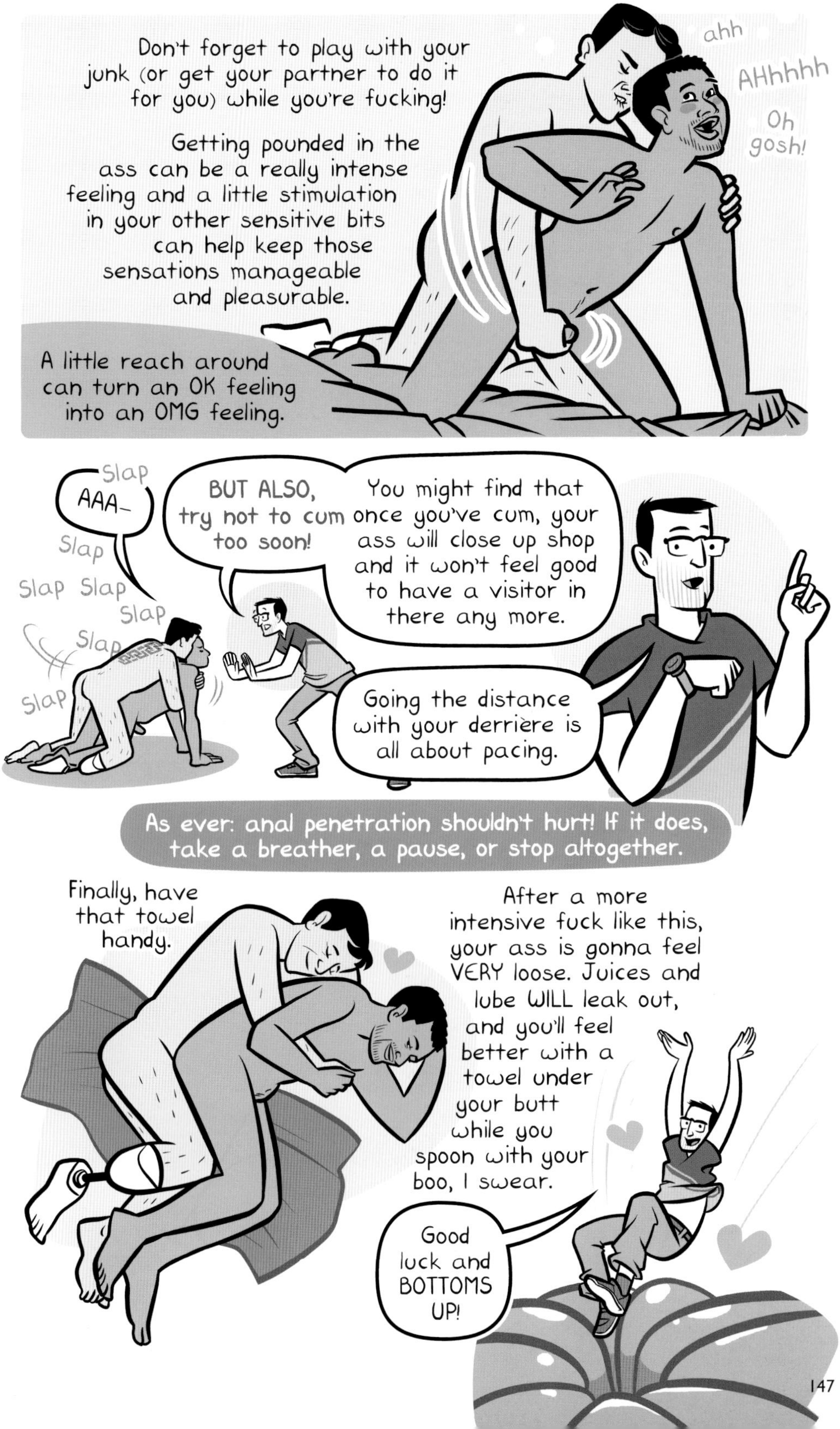
Don't forget to play with your junk (or get your partner to do it for you) while you're fucking!
Getting pounded in the ass can be a really intense feeling and a little stimulation in your other sensitive bits can help keep those sensations manageable and pleasurable.
ahh
AHhhhh
Oh gosh!
A little reach around can turn an OK feeling into an OMG feeling.
Slap
AAA–
Slap
Slap Slap
Slap
Slap
Slap
BUT ALSO, try not to cum too soon!
You might find that once you've cum, your ass will close up shop and it won't feel good to have a visitor in there any more.
Going the distance with your derrière is all about pacing.
As ever: anal penetration shouldn't hurt! If it does, take a breather, a pause, or stop altogether.
Finally, have that towel handy.
After a more intensive fuck like this, your ass is gonna feel VERY loose. Juices and lube WILL leak out, and you'll feel better with a towel under your butt while you spoon with your boo, I swear.
Good luck and BOTTOMS UP!

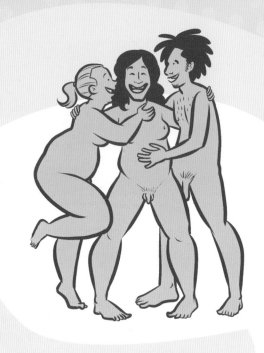

How to
Rock a Threeway

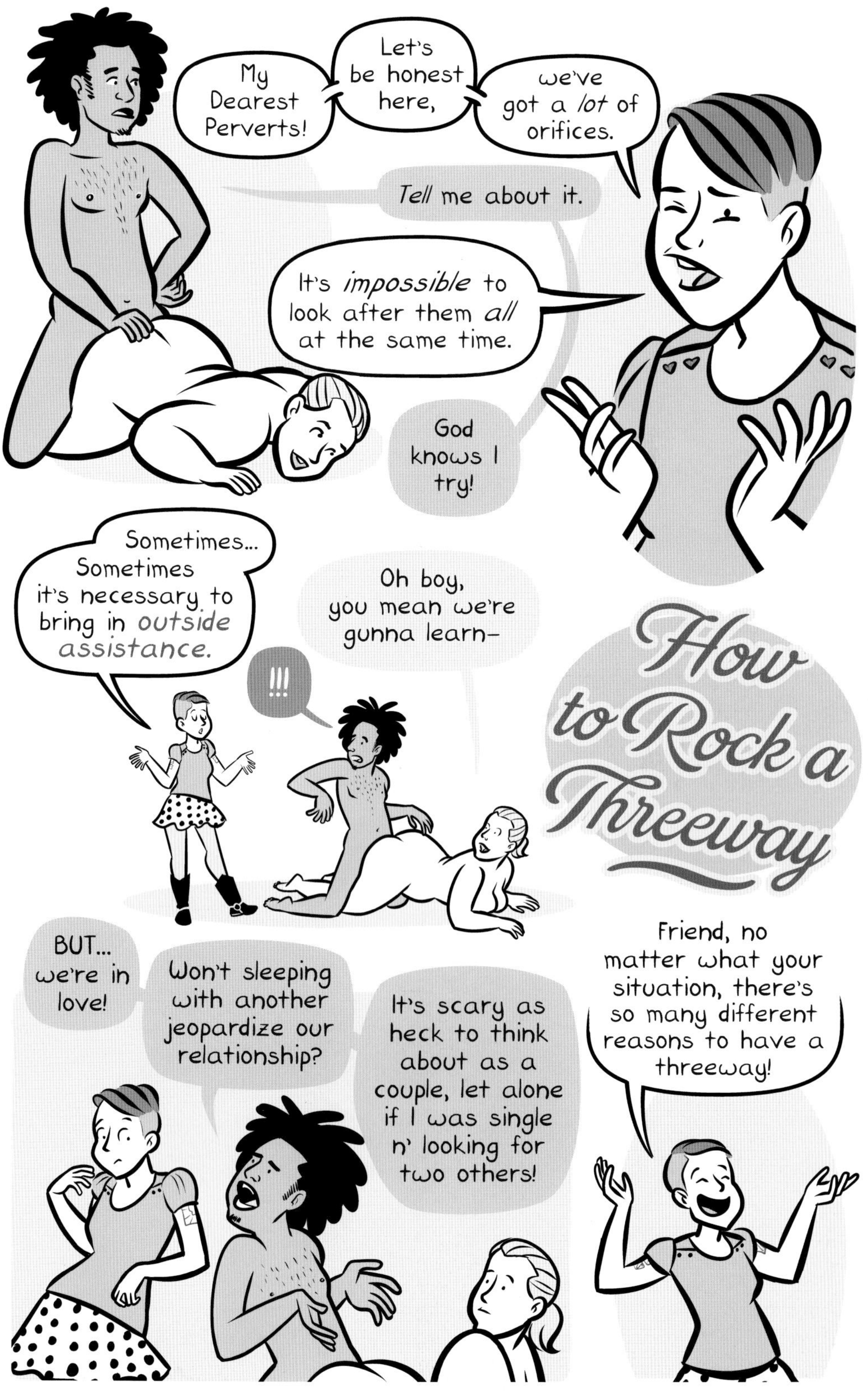

My Dearest Perverts!
Let's be honest here,
we've got a *lot* of orifices.
Tell me about it.
It's *impossible* to look after them *all* at the same time.
God knows I try!
Sometimes... Sometimes it's necessary to bring in outside assistance.
Oh boy, you mean we're gunna learn–
!!!
How to Rock a Threeway
BUT... we're in love!
Won't sleeping with another jeopardize our relationship?
It's scary as heck to think about as a couple, let alone if I was single n' looking for two others!
Friend, no matter what your situation, there's so many different reasons to have a threeway!

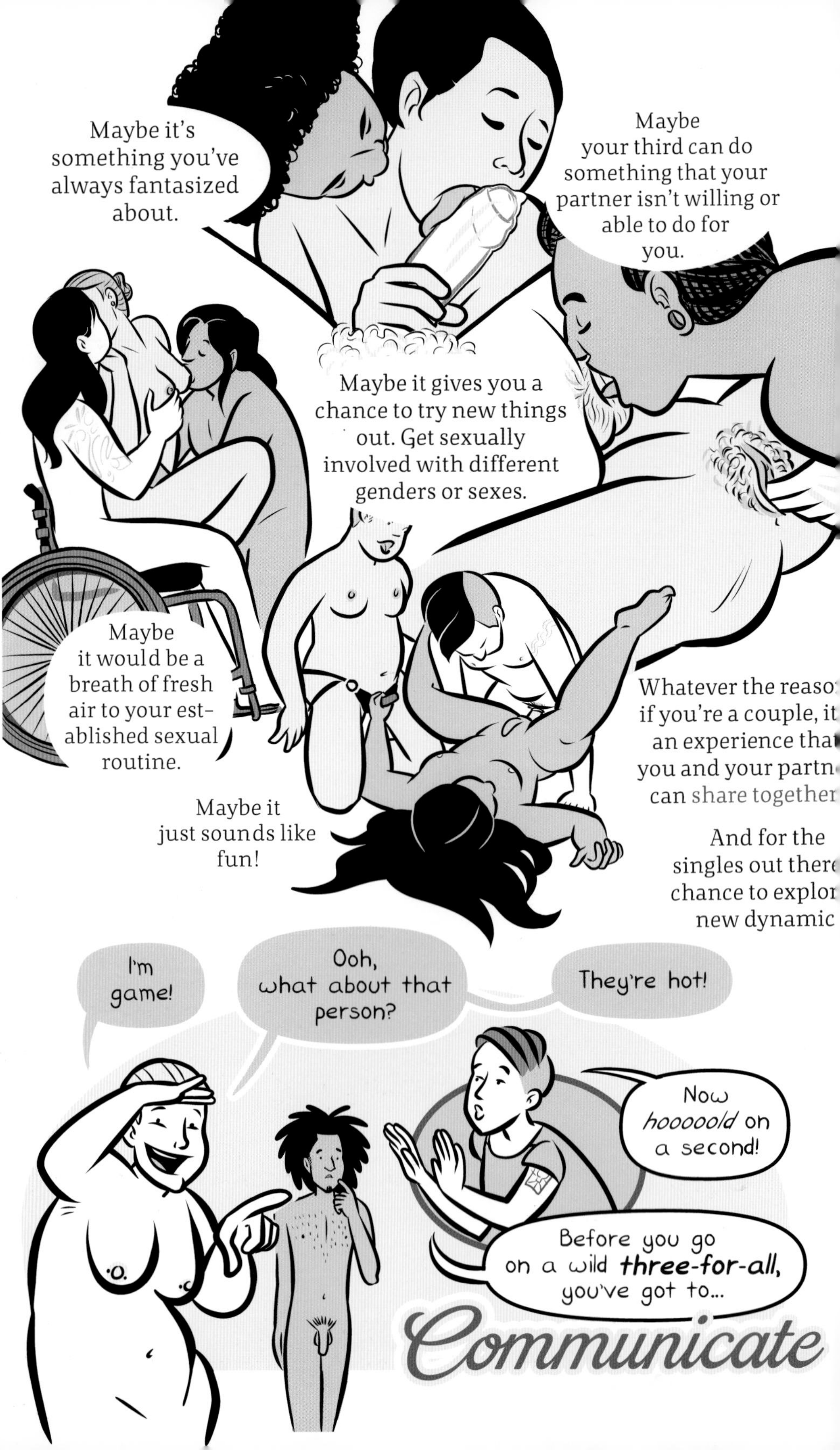
Maybe it's something you've always fantasized about.
Maybe your third can do something that your partner isn't willing or able to do for you.
Maybe it gives you a chance to try new things out. Get sexually involved with different genders or sexes.
Maybe it would be a breath of fresh air to your est-ablished sexual routine.
Maybe it just sounds like fun!
Whatever the reaso
if you're a couple, it
an experience tha
you and your partn
can share together
And for the
singles out there
chance to explor
new dynamic
I'm game!
Ooh, what about that person?
They're hot!
Now *hoooold* on a second!
Before you go on a wild **three-for-all**, you've got to...
Communicate

If you're a couple, it's time to talk honestly with each other about why you want this and what your fears are.

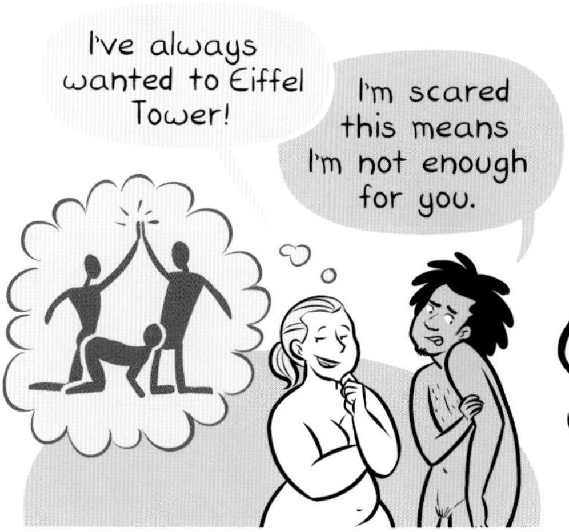

I've always wanted to Eiffel Tower!
I'm scared this means I'm not enough for you.

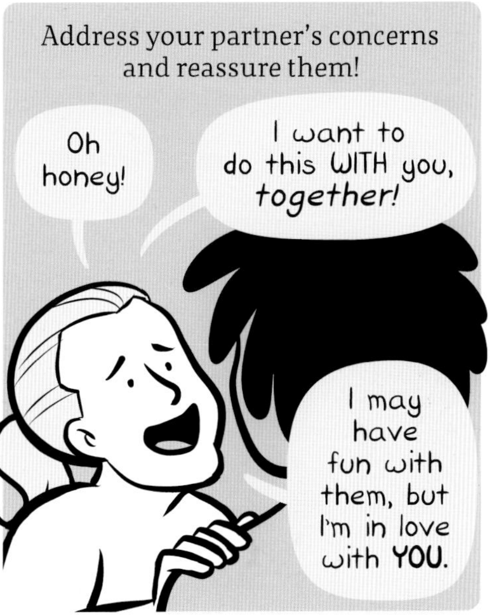

Address your partner's concerns and reassure them!
Oh honey!
I want to do this WITH you, together!
I may have fun with them, but I'm in love with YOU.

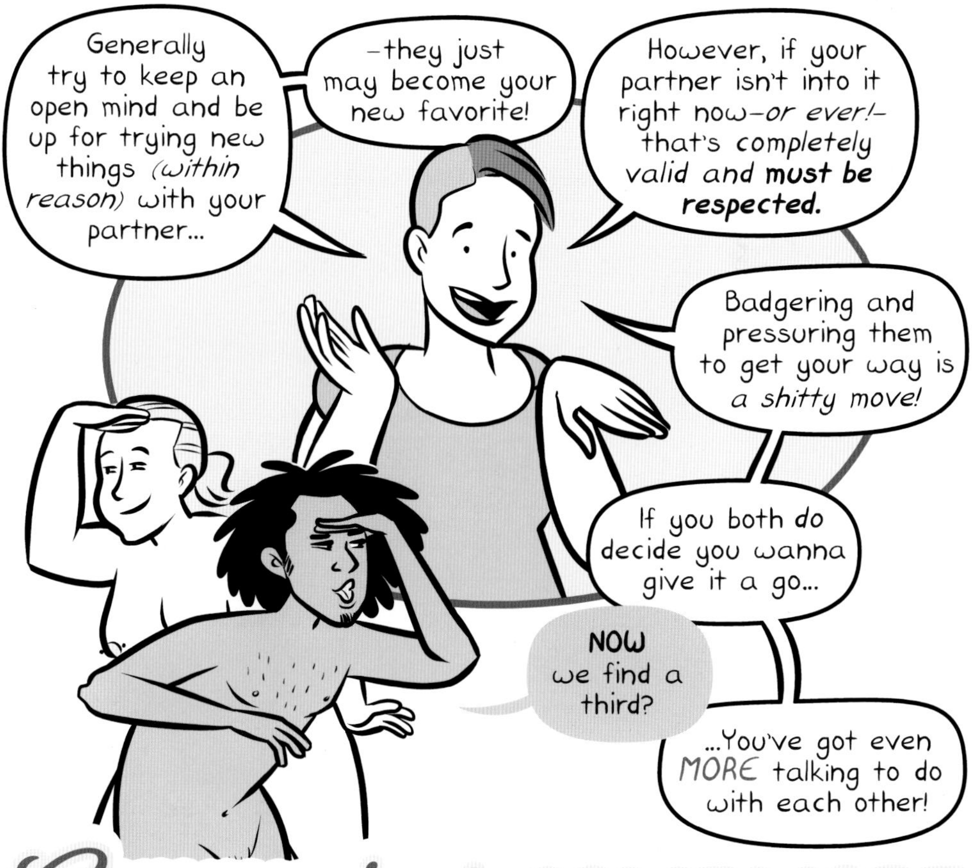

Generally try to keep an open mind and be up for trying new things (within reason) with your partner...
–they just may become your new favorite!
However, if your partner isn't into it right now—or ever!—that's completely valid and must be respected.
Badgering and pressuring them to get your way is a shitty move!
If you both do decide you wanna give it a go...
NOW we find a third?
...You've got even MORE talking to do with each other!

Communicate SOME MORE

For both couples and singles alike, it's important to sit down and invest some time into figuring out your expectations, desires and rules....

Figuring Out the Basics

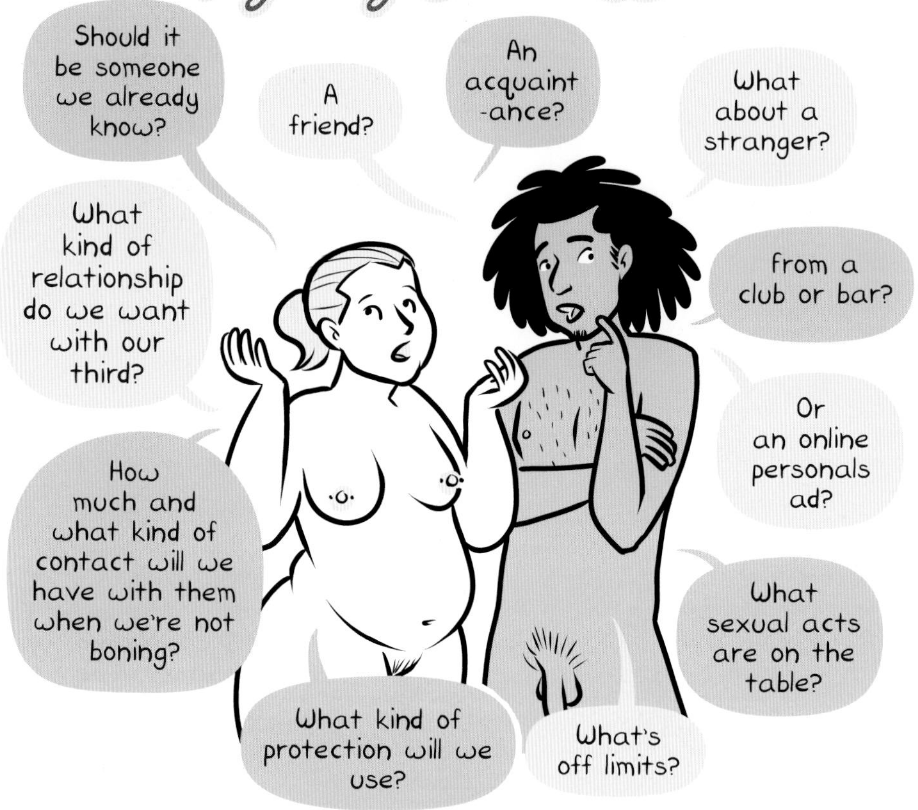

Should it be someone we already know?
A friend?
An acquaint-ance?
What about a stranger?
What kind of relationship do we want with our third?
from a club or bar?
Or an online personals ad?
How much and what kind of contact will we have with them when we're not boning?
What sexual acts are on the table?
What kind of protection will we use?
What's off limits?

It's pretty common to agree on some very restrictive rules in the beginning– –and then over time to relax a bit, as you both grow more comfortable and establish trust.

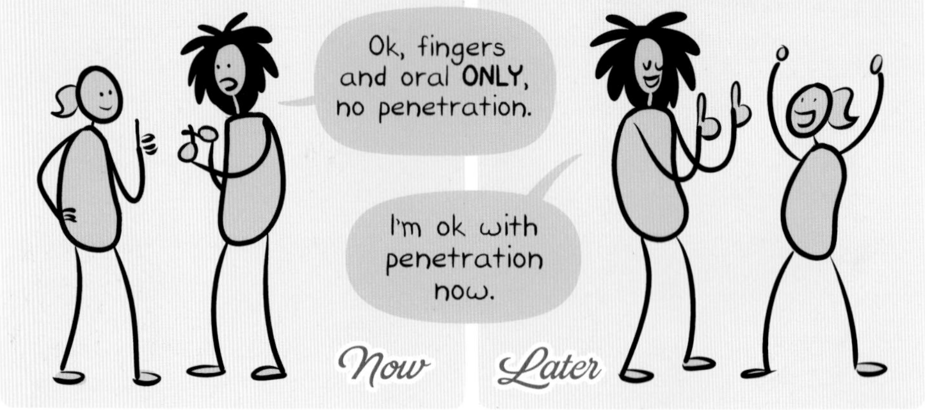

Ok, fingers and oral **ONLY**, no penetration.
I'm ok with penetration now.
Now
Later

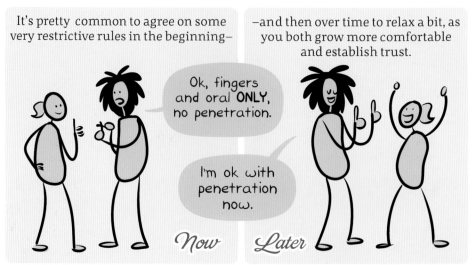

Talk about these agreement changes between everyone **in advance**, don't make sudden changes right in the middle of fucking!

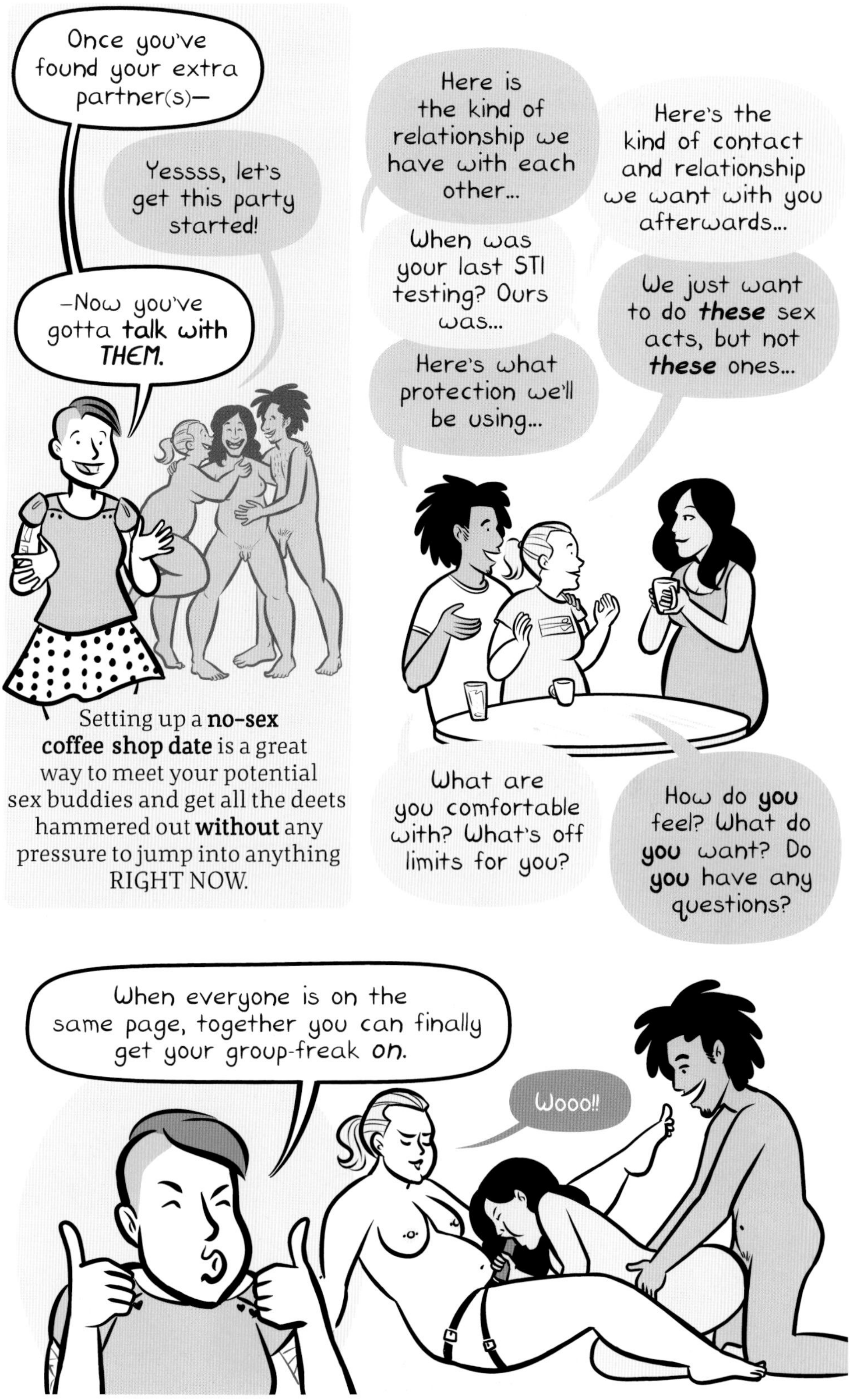

Once you've found your extra partner(s)—
Yessss, let's get this party started!
—Now you've gotta **talk with *THEM.***
Setting up a **no-sex coffee shop date** is a great way to meet your potential sex buddies and get all the deets hammered out **without** any pressure to jump into anything RIGHT NOW.
Here is the kind of relationship we have with each other...
Here's the kind of contact and relationship we want with you afterwards...
When was your last STI testing? Ours was...
We just want to do ***these*** sex acts, but not ***these*** ones...
Here's what protection we'll be using...
What are you comfortable with? What's off limits for you?
How do **you** feel? What do **you** want? Do **you** have any questions?
When everyone is on the same page, together you can finally get your group-freak ***on.***
Wooo!!

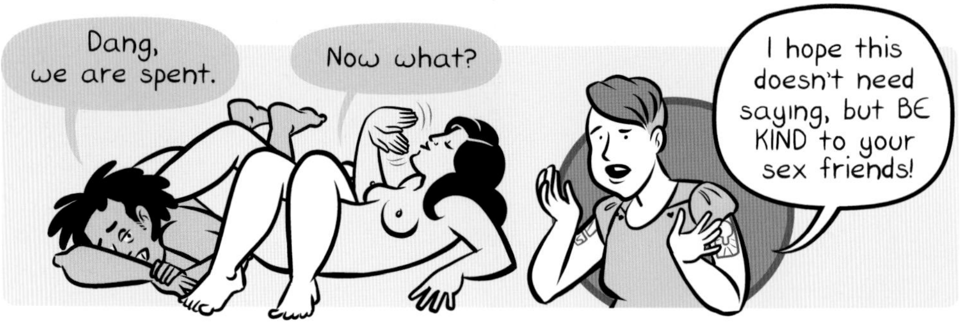
Dang, we are spent.
Now what?
I hope this doesn't need saying, but BE KIND to your sex friends!

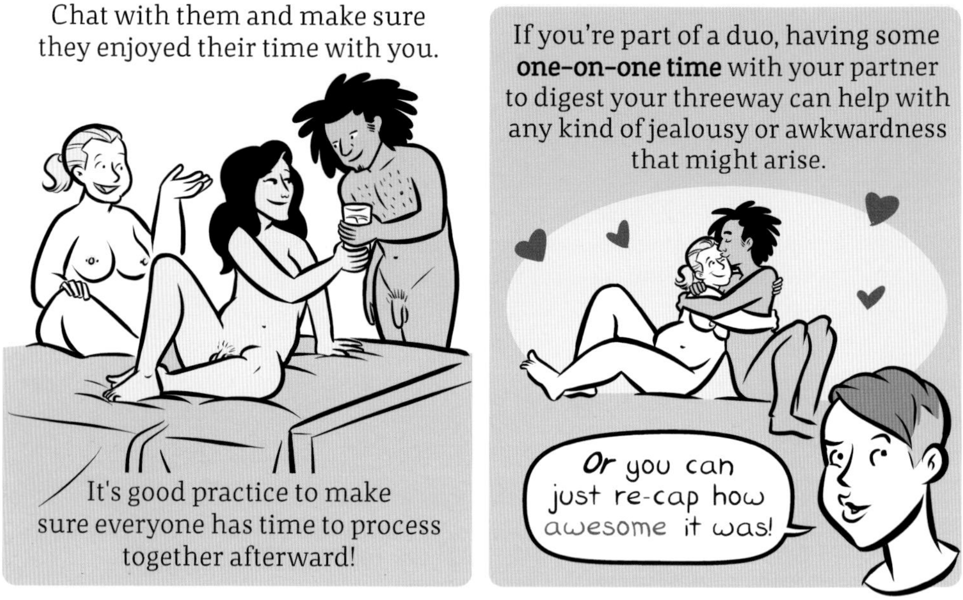
Chat with them and make sure they enjoyed their time with you.
It's good practice to make sure everyone has time to process together afterward!
If you're part of a duo, having some **one-on-one time** with your partner to digest your threeway can help with any kind of jealousy or awkwardness that might arise.
Or you can just re-cap how awesome it was!

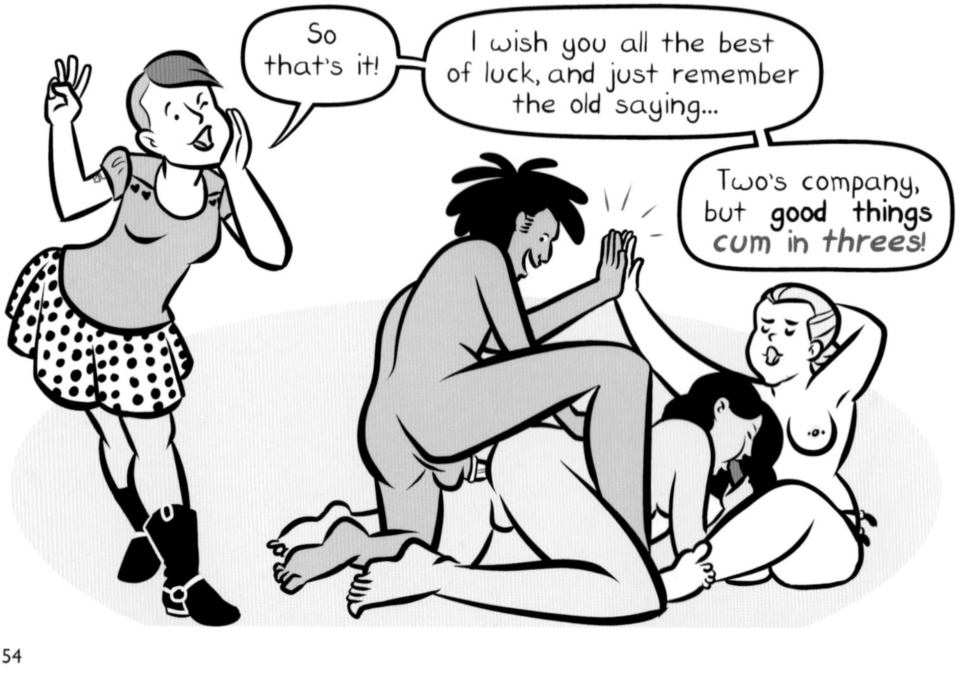
So that's it!
I wish you all the best of luck, and just remember the old saying...
Two's company, but **good things cum in threes**!

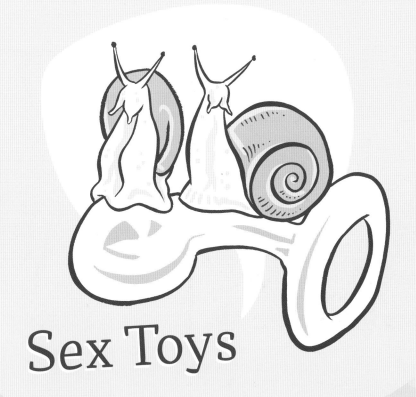

Sex Toys

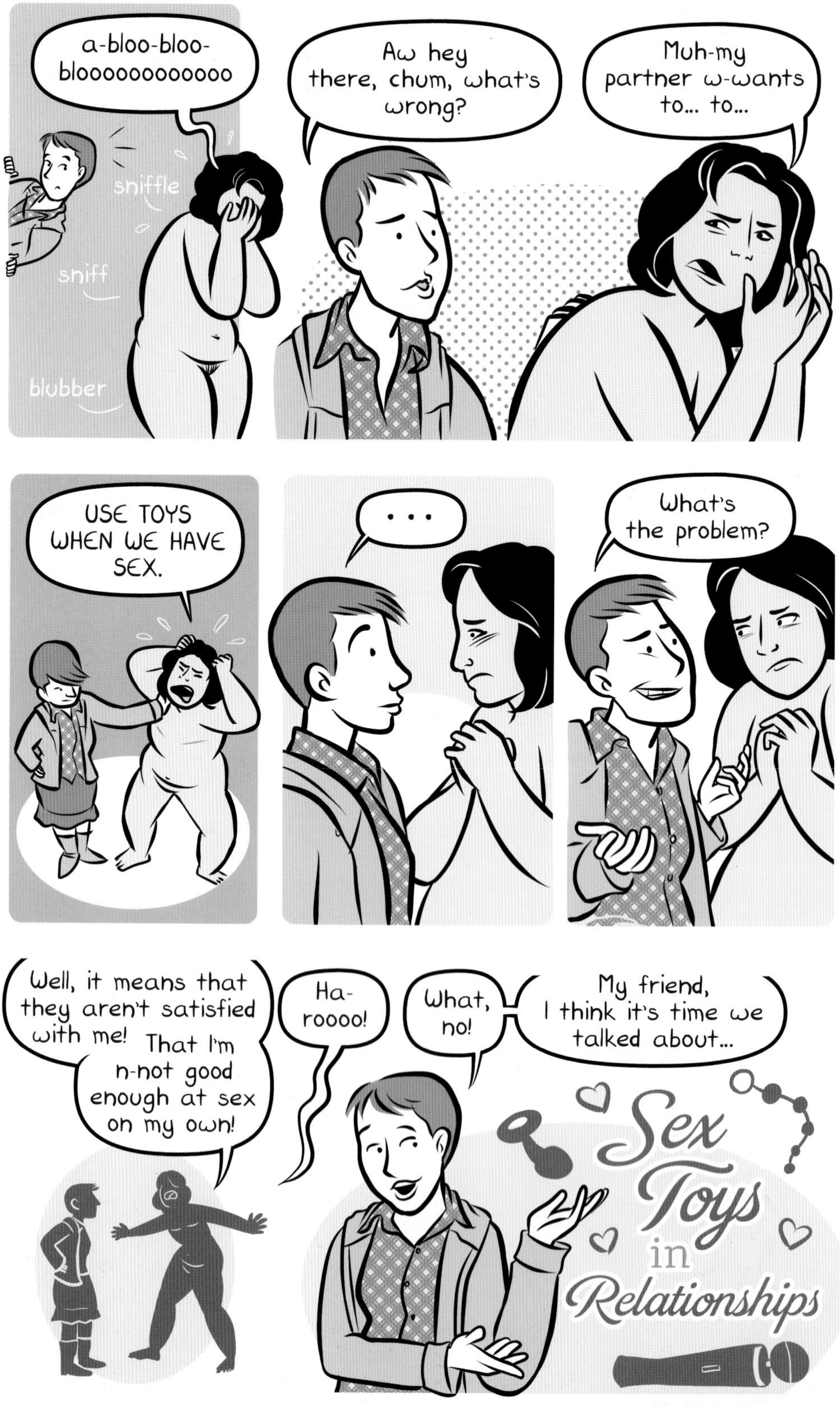

a-bloo-bloo-blooooooooooo
sniffle
sniff
blubber
Aw hey there, chum, what's wrong?
Muh-my partner w-wants to... to...
USE TOYS WHEN WE HAVE SEX.
. . .
What's the problem?
Well, it means that they aren't satisfied with me! That I'm n-not good enough at sex on my own!
Ha-roooo!
What, no!
My friend, I think it's time we talked about...
Sex Toys in Relationships

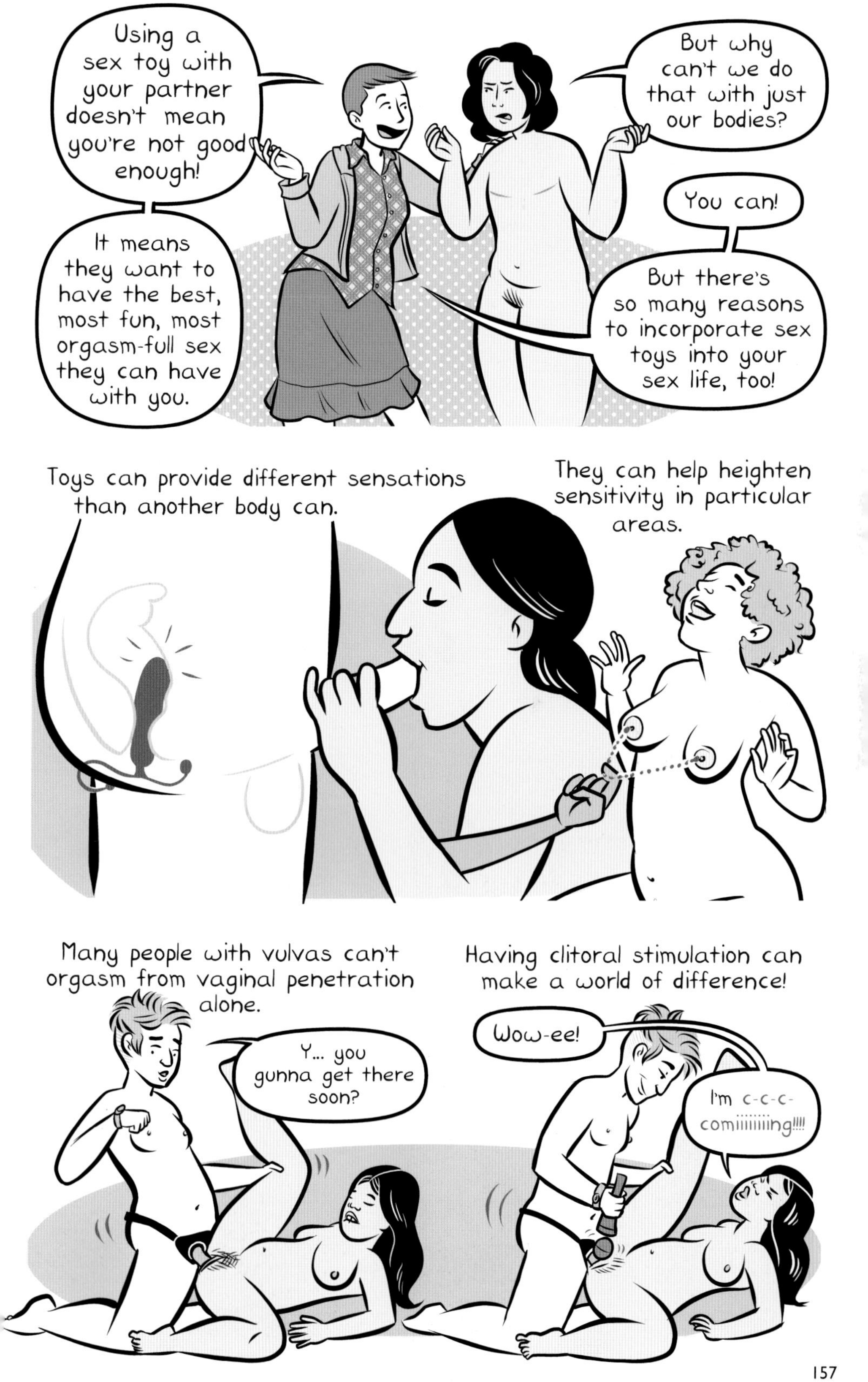
Using a sex toy with your partner doesn't mean you're not good enough!
It means they want to have the best, most fun, most orgasm-full sex they can have with you.
But why can't we do that with just our bodies?
You can!
But there's so many reasons to incorporate sex toys into your sex life, too!
Toys can provide different sensations than another body can.
They can help heighten sensitivity in particular areas.
Many people with vulvas can't orgasm from vaginal penetration alone.
Y... you gunna get there soon?
Having clitoral stimulation can make a world of difference!
Wow-ee!
I'm c-c-c-comiiiiiiing!!!!

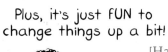
Plus, it's just FUN to change things up a bit!

It keeps sex exciting and new.

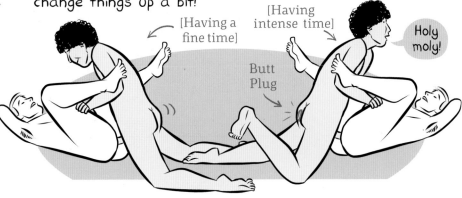

[Having a fine time]

[Having intense time]

Holy moly!

Butt Plug

A sex toy is a bonus to your fucking.

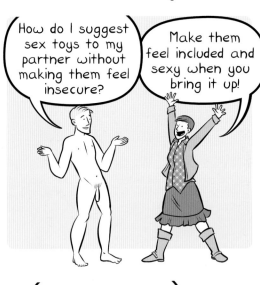

How do I suggest sex toys to my partner without making them feel insecure?

Make them feel included and sexy when you bring it up!

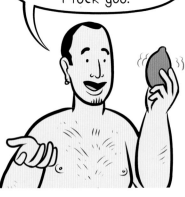

You know, I think it'd be really hot to watch you use a vibrator while I fuck you.

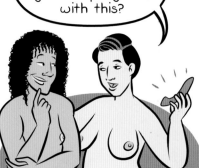

Baby don't you think it would be fun to lick my pussy while you fill up my cunt with this?

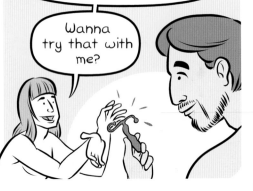

I've heard you can have amazing orgasms if your prostate is getting stimulated while you get head...

Wanna try that with me?

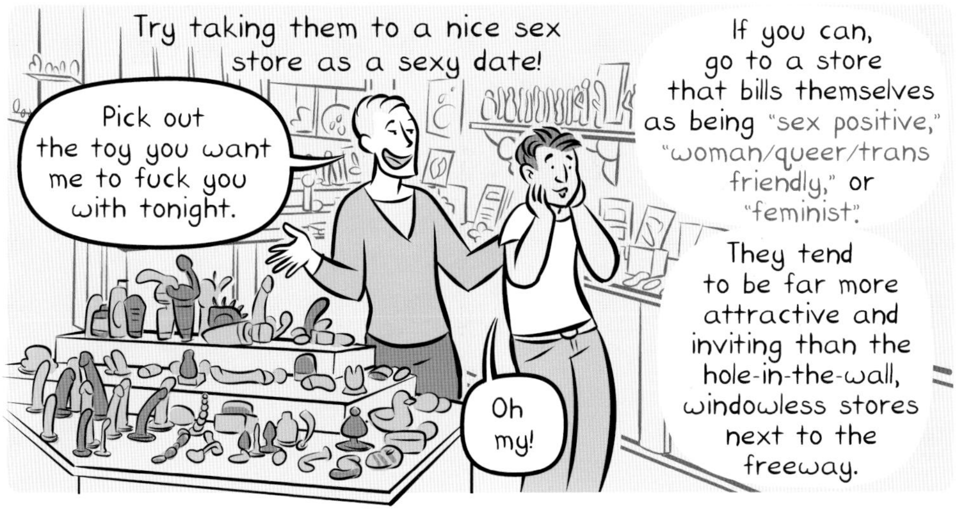
Try taking them to a nice sex store as a sexy date!
Pick out the toy you want me to fuck you with tonight.
Oh my!
If you can, go to a store that bills themselves as being "sex positive," "woman/queer/trans friendly," or "feminist".
They tend to be far more attractive and inviting than the hole-in-the-wall, windowless stores next to the freeway.

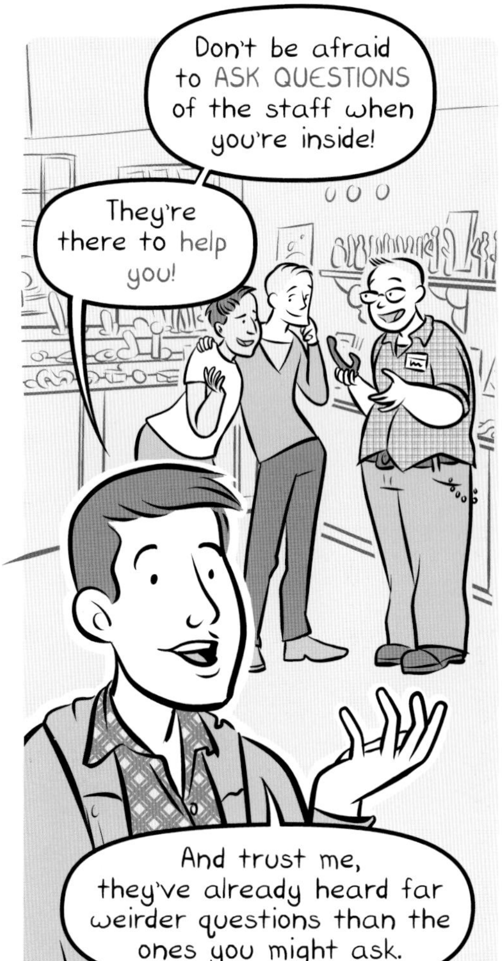
Don't be afraid to ASK QUESTIONS of the staff when you're inside!
They're there to help you!
And trust me, they've already heard far weirder questions than the ones you might ask.

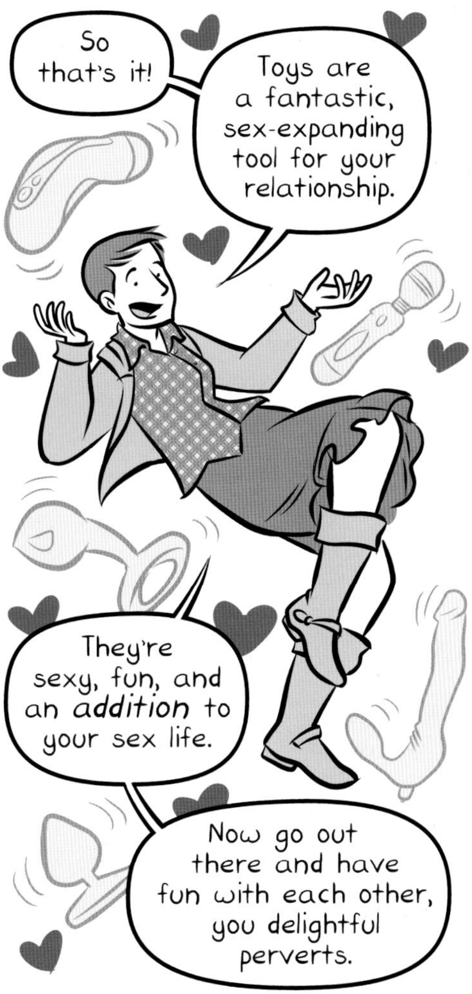
So that's it!
Toys are a fantastic, sex-expanding tool for your relationship.
They're sexy, fun, and an *addition* to your sex life.
Now go out there and have fun with each other, you delightful perverts.

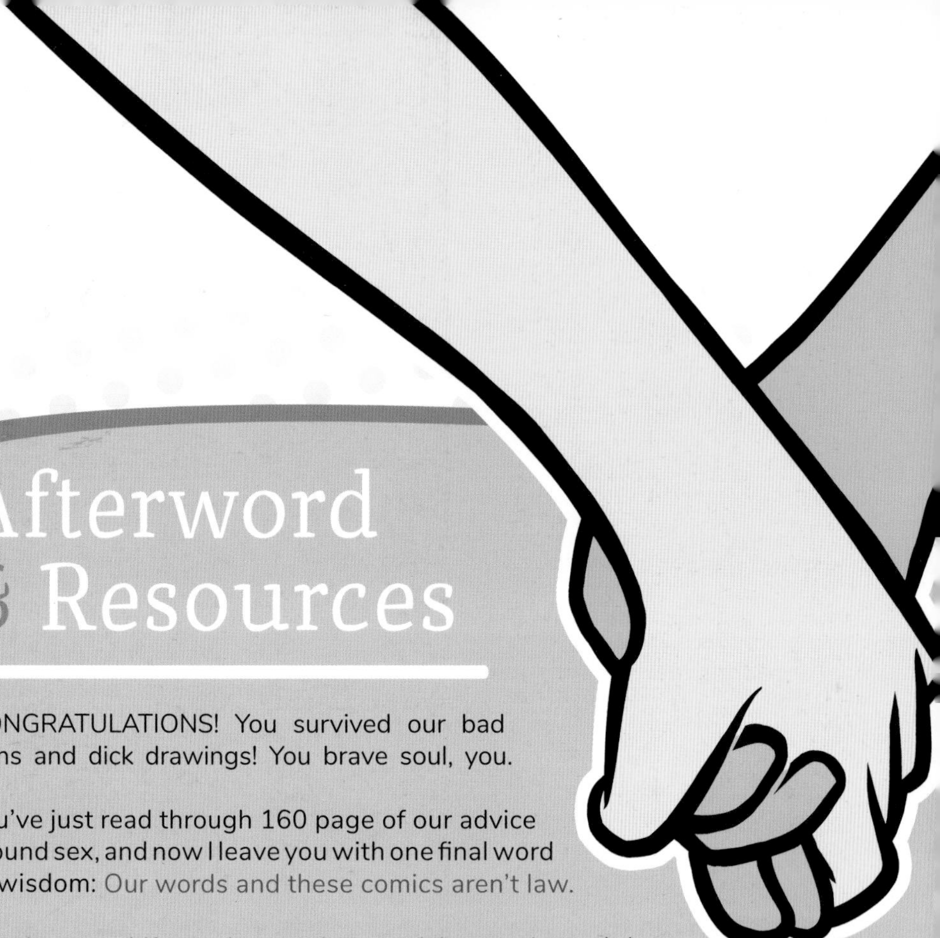

Afterword & Resources

CONGRATULATIONS! You survived our bad puns and dick drawings! You brave soul, you.

You've just read through 160 page of our advice around sex, and now I leave you with one final word of wisdom: Our words and these comics aren't law.

Sex is a multifaceted, complex, evolving topic and I don't think there will ever be a book that does the whole subject justice. Some advice and language in here may not age well! So embrace the information in here that you find helpful and discard what isn't. The fundamental goal of this book is to encourage you to pursue what feels right for you and whatever partners you engage with along the way.

I've always been the first to say I'm not a sex educator. I've never been professionally trained, I never went to doctor school, and everything I know I learned through my own research. But what I *am* is in love with the subject of sex. It's an incredibly vast topic that goes so much further than just the physical. Sex is a social, political, artistic, philosophical, cultural, technical, legislative, scientific, anthropological beast! It's this MASSIVE field that touches so many different aspects of our lives. I'm passionate about it and I not only want to share what I've learned with you, but encourage you to investigate and study up on your own too.

To expand on this book, visit PlannedParenthood.org and Scarleteen.com for indispensable, comprehensive, compassionate, accurate sex education. And then drop by OhJoySexToy.com for the abridged fart joke versions. Thank you for reading and I hope you pursue what's right for you!